PHYSIOLOGY AND HEALING
TREATMENT, THERAPY AND HYGIENE

Spiritual Science And Medicine

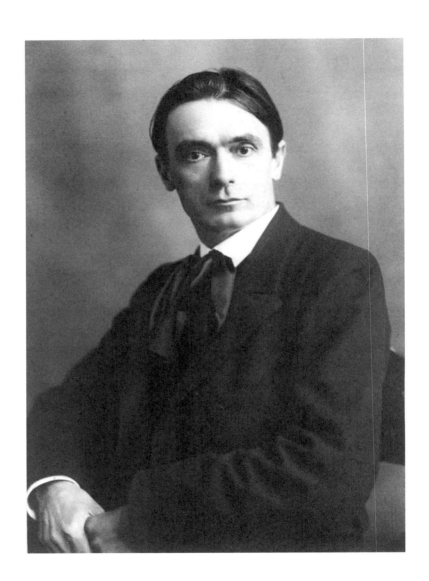

PHYSIOLOGY AND HEALING
TREATMENT, THERAPY AND HYGIENE

Spiritual Science And Medicine

Thirteen lectures, an address, two discussions and a question-and-answer session held in Dornach and Stuttgart between March 1920 and April 1924

ENGLISH BY ANNA R. MEUSS

INTRODUCTION BY ANDREW MAENDL, MD, AND
MATTHEW BARTON

RUDOLF STEINER

RUDOLF STEINER PRESS

CW 314

The publishers acknowledge the generous funding of this publication by Dr Eva Frommer MD (1927–2004) and the Anthroposophical Society in Great Britain

Rudolf Steiner Press
Hillside House, The Square
Forest Row, RH18 5ES

www.rudolfsteinerpress.com

Published by Rudolf Steiner Press 2013

Originally published in German under the title *Physiologisch-Therapeutisches auf Grundlage der Geisteswissenschaft, Zur Therapie und Hygiene* (volume 314 in the *Rudolf Steiner Gesamtausgabe* or Collected Works) by Rudolf Steiner Verlag, Dornach. Based on notes taken by members of the audiences not reviewed by the speaker, and edited by Hans W. Zbinden, MD. This authorized translation is based on the 4th German edition of 2011 which was reviewed and added to by Urs Dietler, working with Andreas Dollfuss and Eva-Gabriele Streit, MD

Published by permission of the Rudolf Steiner Nachlassverwaltung, Dornach

© Rudolf Steiner Nachlassverwaltung, Dornach 1965, Rudolf Steiner Verlag 2011

This translation © Rudolf Steiner Press 2013

I am indebted to my colleague Christian von Arnim, eurythmy therapist Ursula Browning, Dr Hans Broder von Laue and Prof. Peter Selg, all of whom have assisted me in fathoming the meaning of some of the more difficult passages (Anna R. Meuss)

A catalogue record for this book is available from the British Library

ISBN 978 1 85584 380 6

Cover by Mary Giddens
Typeset by DP Photosetting, Neath, West Glamorgan
Printed and bound in Great Britain by Gutenberg Press Ltd., Malta

CONTENTS

I PHYSIOLOGY AND THERAPY BASED ON THE SCIENCE OF THE SPIRIT

LECTURE 1

DORNACH, 7 OCTOBER 1920

The mission of spiritual science. Too little therapy in medicine, whilst experimental research is well developed. Unjustifiable hypotheses. The spiritual aspect is not taken into account. Abstractions in physiology and pathology. Development of cancer—from normal activity in the organism to the abnormal. Mania—from illusions that are organic in origin to hysteria. Schelling's way of making observations.

LECTURE 2

DORNACH, 8 OCTOBER 1920

Schelling. Inner powers of development up to second dentition. Creative activity arising from this—transforming powers of growth into powers of memory and power to develop thoughts. If transformation is inadequate—carcinoma. Troxler. Childhood diseases—excess of spirit and soul from life before birth. In old age—involution. Organizing power and principles of soul and spirit enter into the structural elements. Tumour development. Unconscious penetration with will activity from our organization—mania. Hypertrophic organizing power in liver and stomach—melancholia, hypochondria, hysteria. Griesinger (psychiatrist). Proletarians became materialists, aristocrats spiritualists.

LECTURE 3

DORNACH, 9 OCTOBER 1920

In spiritual science, the aim is to encourage not quackery but the art of medicine. Neoplasms and mental diseases. Threefold nature of the human organism with functions defined rather than spaces. See Steiner's *Riddles of the Soul*. Sensory perception and ideation bound up with degradation and elimination. Will processes with constructive processes in metabolism and limbs. Rhythmic system. Healthy balance—interaction between constructive and destructive processes. Poisoning and detoxification. Whole of nature—plant development process away from centre of earth. Goethe's metamorphosis of plants. Example of silver birch—development of root, bark, leaf. Potassium salt deposits in birch bark. Opposite direction—development of protein—albuminization. Development of rheumatic conditions and gout. Treatment—birch leaves. Development of inflamed skin eruptions—potassium salts from birch bark. Rational stage of science. Goethe. Study of medicine. For therapy—seeing natural functions together with functions of the inner organism to perceive the pathological aspect. With spiritual science the aim is to bring health to science.

pages 25–35

LECTURE 4

DORNACH, 9 OCTOBER 1920, EVENING

Trust between public and medical profession. Neurosensory system encroaching on metabolism and limbs and vice versa. Typhoid fever. Normal organization—full awareness of I nature or selfhood penetrates the etheric and physical in the sphere of soul and spirit. Awareness of I nature reduced. Mind and spirit go their own way. Look at purely spiritual I activity on the one hand, and the vehicle for it in the organism, the blood, on the other. Bridge from physiological and pathological to therapeutic—bringing about processes in the blood so that it withdraws from I activity but functions in a similar way. System of forces in human blood and alongside it I activity in mind and spirit. This system of forces may get independent if there is too much phosphorus. Hyperaemia in the skeleton as against calcification process. Phosphorus processes in brain and bone. Small doses for rickets—taking the physical I structure back to soul activity. Small doses of phosphorus cure rickets and other inflammatory conditions. Conversely, carbonates are effective if mind and spirit are bound up too much with the structure, and also for pulmonary tuberculosis. Life in head system conscious, in limbs unconscious. Massage improves connection between mind and soul on the one hand and physical on the other. Arms and hands constructive, legs and feet destructive. Diabetes—exaggerated I activity in organic sphere. Essential vegetable oils in bath are medicinal. Problem of heredity. Female organism develops more out of cosmic, male organism from earthly forces. Full meaning of Earth evolution through human I activity. Reproductive powers in male and female. Haemophilia. Future study of medicine. Progress in medicine only with spiritual research.

II   ANTHROPOSOPHICAL BASIS FOR THE PRACTICE OF MEDICINE

LECTURE 5
STUTTGART, 26 OCTOBER 1922

Basis of spiritual investigation for medicine and physiology other than mystical and gnostic approaches. No supersensible views in medicine since Galen. The four elements of Galen. Developing inner abilities—seeing the element of spirit and soul and the spiritual cosmos. In anthroposophy, full recognition of empiricism based on sensory perceptions. Guidelines for empirical research from science of the spirit. All factors taken into account. Liver, brain and blood cell compared to germ cell. Relationship of organic principle to universe not secondary. Stream of heredity. Structure of brain. Theodor Ziehen, Herbart. Brain—three-dimensional reflection of our life in ideas. Meynert. Image-based insight and structure of brain. Breathing process and inspired insight. Metabolic process and intuitive insight. Brain reflects mind and spirit; these enter wholly into metabolism. Act of will goes as far as metabolism. Recognizing the four structures of aggregation in human beings. Ascending and descending processes. Kidneys are organs of excretion to outside, liver to inside.

LECTURE 6
STUTTGART, 27 OCTOBER 1922

The different functions of human beings. The bodies or levels of existence. Living in the I point. Sexual maturity is peak of animal development. Human beings— physical body, laboratory investigations; etheric organization, structure of functions in enlivened fluid sphere. Solids are deposited in fluid element. Astral organization intervenes in airy element. Internal gas exchange in solid and fluid has laws. Fluctuating form given to airy organization. I organization intervenes directly in differentiated temperature levels. Route which foods take to lymph and blood streams. Ptyalinization means being taken into sphere of life. Then transmitted to vascular system, in cardiopulmonary tract, from the inorganic to sphere of life. Oxygen we breathe in takes the etheric into the physical. Carbon fixes the physical organization. Carbon—physical organization. Oxygen—etheric organization. Protein synthesis. Kidneys provide connection between the astral and the other organs—power of sentience, soul quality. Effects of cold and heat—excretion from kidneys. Significance of allantois and amnion for investigation of germ cell. Renal system and nitrogen—metamorphosis of uric acid and urea. I organization in warmth structure in hepato-biliary system. Animal sequence and hepato-biliary evolution. Lethal childhood diseases with secretion of bile. I organization—hydrogen. Annual plants, potatoes, cockchafer grub. Different structures of substances in flowers, leaves, roots, seed. Medicinal teas.

pages 72–87

LECTURE 7

STUTTGART, 27 OCTOBER 1922, EVENING

Threefold nature of human organism, important in pathology and therapy. Relationship of bodies to organ systems. Second dentition. Sexual maturity, voice breaking. Semi-radial emanations from kidneys and liver meet with sculptural forms coming from head system. Human growth. Modelling principle of neurosensory system is four times slower than metabolic organism. Variable incidence of morbidity in the seven-year periods. Activity of I organization in hepato-biliary system, of astral organization from the kidneys, blunted from head organization. Physical system acts from below upwards from the digestive system, the etheric organization from system of heart and lungs. Diseases in second seven-year period. Mercury to treat venereal diseases. Liver and kidneys working together and against one another, as do circulatory and breathing rhythm. I organization in warmth human being. Origin of childhood diseases. Vibrations of air and warmth going from above downwards, in the physical and etheric from below upwards. Fluid and gaseous principles, interpenetration in the middle. Intermediate states of aggregation between solid and fluid, also between fluid and gaseous and between gaseous and warmth quality. All working together = normal human being. Differing from this—pathological metamorphoses. Development of sense organ in case of cancer. Share of warmth and air organism in child. Neurosensory system giving metabolic organism three-dimensional form. Wrong proportions—tumour development. Creating mantle of warmth with Viscum.

pages 88–103

Treatment goals—to bring about metamorphosis. Food taken from inorganic to sphere of life, vehicle for sentience, I organization. Plant the other way round. Vital element in seed is sun's warmth from previous year. In root sphere, vital energy. Devitalization processes by petals rich in essential oils. Sulphur in essential oils. Digestion = beginning of poisoning, renal function = detoxification. Iron in human blood protects from diseases we bear in us. Pressure exerted by brain only 20 g, which makes I activity possible. Iron in blood important for relationship of ether body to astral body. Things taken in by human beings are taken towards vitalization by activity of heart and lungs. Renal function takes them on to astral organism. Iron levels regulate blood circulation and interaction between ether body and astral organism. Whole human organism is sense-perceptible reflection of something spiritual. Functional diseases are neural disorders. Rounding-out powers of neurosensory system. Function of vision is main part of the neurosensory system for configuration of form, rest of it is soul principle. Metabolic processes radiating from kidneys with rounding of forms. Rounding off through the nerves of sense organs. Adaptation of higher sensory function to individual organ tracts through soul principle. Astral organization too powerful—flatus, renal function too powerful. In upper human being, I organization held back. Spasms—astral lags behind. If spasms arise in stomach and genital organs—tea of flowers, contains sulphur. Physiology of the senses—eye as camera. Affinity of silica to inorganic in periphery. Silica drives out astral organization. Flowers containing silica are spiny. Supply of sugar for sense organs. Alkaline salts relieve nervous system of astral activity. After-effects of sugar in the nerves. Silica pushes towards periphery—medicament—alkaline salts, sugar, silica. Chamomile root—vitalizing at transition from intestine to blood, acting on neurosensory system via renal function, relieving of astral functions. Medicament corrects neurosensory system's modelling activity as if with a kind of phantom. Excessive renal activity leads to development of mucilage, weak renal activity to haemorrhoids, menorrhagia. Regulate relationships of ether body to astral body with iron levels, increase secretion of urea. Action of sulphur in digestive tract. SiO_2 and alkaline salts help in neurosensory system. Iron, gold and copper regulate the balance between gravity and buoyancy. Action of iron in relationship of lungs and heart to kidneys. Inadequate form function of nerves—organs deformed. Treatment—mercury, plus iron (rhythmic system), sulphur (metabolism), alkaline salts (neurosensory system). Metabolic diseases and sulphurous principle. Colchicum for goitre. Synthetic medicines.

pages 104–121

III   ASPECTS OF THERAPY

LECTURE 10

DORNACH, 31 DECEMBER 1923

Syphilis. Medicament—mercury. Action of ether body in system of metabolism and limbs. Ether body and physical body and I acting together in neurosensory system. Diagnosis is a whole case history. Syphilis—I organization predominates over ether body in pelvic region. Treatment with mercury ointment. Side effects. I organization lives in cosmic rounding-off powers. Problem of mercury dosage. For treating syphilis—find phantom of I organization with *Astragalus exscapus* (hart's milk vetch)—I organization going its own way. Also meditate abstract ideas—varying triangular form. Polarity of glaucoma and otitis, hypertrophy of vitreous body activity. Treatment for glaucoma—calcium carbonate and extract of aerial root. Astral body activity above diaphragm polar opposite to its activity below. Development of nerve substance. Essential oil of flowers for lower astral body. Substance from cosmic surroundings via respiration for neurosensory system.

LECTURE 11
DORNACH, 1 JANUARY 1924

Salvarsan. Bismuth. No antimony in case of syphilis. Schizophrenia due to Salvarsan possible. Hart's milk vetch preparation for acquired and hereditary syphilis. Glaucoma process and ear process. Development of eyes = inflammatory process, while ear development = tumour process—polar opposites. Levisticum and eurythmy therapy for otitis. Questions and answers—arthritis deformans—phosphorus and Stannum. Worry and shock, grouchy teacher. Measles. Arsenic, Stannum, sulphur baths, arnica, Equisetum. Adapting astral body to ether body. Astral body shift in sexual region in case of shock. Oxalic acid, Argentum. Treatment for enuresis.

LECTURE 12
DORNACH, 2 JANUARY 1924

Gonorrhoea. Toxic effect of male and female seed. Parasites. Treatment—alkali carbonate, oil of eucalyptus compresses. Asthma close to purely physical. Mental diseases may be purely physical. Cause of asthma in embryonic life—mother subject to shock and worries—action on mucosa of respiratory organs. Inner lack of appetite. Proper connection between ether and astral body interrupted—sage leaves, nut leaves, oak bark, willow bark, *Veronica officinalis*. Meditation on breathing. Nervous breakdown, sleeplessness, automatic thinking—eurythmy therapy, Equisetum baths, work with vowels. Proliferation of palatal mucosa—weakness of ether body—Apis, Vespa, honey, milk. Diseases of spinal marrow—difficult to treat—phantom of I and astral body due to silica action. Arnica, potassium salt, calcium salt, tannic acid. Latex-type protein in Arnica. Phosphorus, Quadrigeminal preparation for diseases of spinal marrow—tabes dorsalis, locomotor ataxia. Neural disease in digestive tract—Chamomilla injections. Tendency to myopia, hyperopia. Treatment. Glaucoma—start with Belledonna before third year of life.

IV HYGIENE AS A SOCIAL ISSUE

LECTURE 13

PUBLIC LECTURE, DORNACH, 7 APRIL 1920

Intellectualism a fundamental evil. People longing for democratic order in all affairs. In field of hygiene, undemocratic faith in authority today. Public health. Basic conviction in modern science—everything is a mechanical, physical or chemical process in the material world today. Explanation in terms of atoms and molecules. Anthroposophical science of the spirit helps clear confusion by distinguishing between diseases in body, soul and spirit. Spiritual philosophy of life—the physical body created by soul before birth. In the organs, soul principle differentiates into concrete processes—liver, respiratory, cardiac and cerebral actions. View of mind and spirit. Abstract ideas are objects of modern science. Handbook on nervous system says nothing about value, nature and dignity of human being. Spiritual science takes us to the whole human being. Deviations take us deep into the nature of the world. Deeper meaning of life. Understanding the other person. The healthy and the morbid aspects of another. Social effects of factual knowledge—social reform, health care take us to fellow human beings. Psychoanalysis is materialistic in thinking. Diseases of mind and soul are due to organ disorders. Impressions made on soul meet with faulty organs. Psychoanalysis = diagnosis but no treatment. Treatment of body needed. Bodily aspect of temperaments. With physical diseases, look for mind and spirit. Social institutions influence physical health care. Children should enunciate vowels and consonants loudly and clearly. Take specialized things to comprehensive view. Children should learn to use up the air when speaking. Sound of mind means sound in body. Educational issues are often medical issues. Help for mental illness only with healing of organs. Vision in images, Inspiration and Intuition are health-giving. Not just amass notes. Spiritual science spreads social hygiene. Salutogenic action of spiritual science thanks to sound common sense. Disposition for epidemic diseases due to too much sleep. Seven hours of sleep adequate. Independent, free life in mind and spirit also where hygiene is concerned—government standards should not inhibit individual endeavour, nor should economic forces. Hygiene from social insight. Threefold Social Order. Garden spider. Henbane. Sleeping with window open. Abnormal organ disposition of criminals. Emotions and feelings influence glandular functions. Defective organs with mental diseases and criminals. Theosophy and anthroposophy. Origin of epidemics. Parallel processes in mind and spirit and in organs. Atmosphere for micro-organisms. Typhoid fever. Bodily, organic disorder the case of problem in mind and spirit. Hypochondria, chronic pulmonary defects. Temperaments and organs. Iris diagnosis. Diseases as world history progresses—

spiritual stream behind them. Diseases must be cured. Wrong to let karma take its course and not help.

V   ASPECTS OF PSYCHIATRY

QUESTIONS AND ANSWERS
DORNACH, 26 MARCH 1920

Study of psychiatry today. Influence of spiritual science. Problems with transition from relatively well to relatively sick. Fundamental—consider whole social environment. Various conditions in robust country people and weak city people. Transitions from pathological to normal. Psychiatric medicine in need of reform. Raving madness, feeblemindedness, difficult boundary between mentally normal and abnormal.

VI   ADDRESS (FOLLOWED BY DISCUSSION) AT A MEETING WITH
MEDICAL PRACTITIONERS

ADDRESS
DORNACH, 21 APRIL 1924

Realities have lost value. Higher levels of human existence not known in modern medicine. Astral body and I organization predominantly active in human head. Physical body and ether body inducing more destructive processes in head, more constructive processes in system of metabolism and limbs. Liver comes to resemble head more when astral body and I withdraw. Reverse in the head. Too many vegetative processes in the head with diseases in system of metabolism and limbs. Identification of medicinal agents and cosmic activities. Lead, antimony. Telluric and cosmic processes. Soul at one on awakening. Levels of existence when walking and thinking. Liver disease and treatment. Loving study of morbid processes. Religious mood for healing processes. Insight processes for diagnosis and treatment. Treatment of excessively stimulated kidneys with silica. Statistics or full insight into single case. Stimulating astral body with arsenic to treat syphilis. Good medicines outside anthroposophy. Asthma treated with meditation. Courage to heal. Put aside thoughts of death. Medicaments as far as possible from plant world.

DISCUSSIONS WITH MEDICAL PRACTITIONERS (FRAGMENTARY NOTES) I
DORNACH, 22 APRIL 1924

Leukaemia—Various causes. Disorder in rhythmic human being—treat with resinous or latex-type saps and vegetable wax. This treatment ineffective if disorder is in metabolism. Ether body and astral body interact.

Smallpox—Weakness of I organization and affinity to spiritual world. Inwardly shaken when realizing influences of zodiacal configurations. Risk of infection great because it may be physical and psychic. Avoid infection by developing objective view and shutting oneself off.

Smallpox vaccination—No harm if anthroposophical work is done. Different if thoughts materialistic. Vaccination enhances ahrimanic power—no longer able to rise to things of the spirit. Statistics. Maintaining oneself in face of unwarranted spiritual elements also protects. If this education not possible, you have to vaccinate, do not oppose fanatically.

Restlessness and problems going to sleep—Possible reason years of problems with diet in the war. Astral body and ether body unable to interact in intestinal region. Transformation of foods in digestion. Ether body comes free, is born, in seventh year. Should be fully organized by coming from astral body = 'digestive disorder' there. Fight processes outside the human being rationally at physical level—calcium carbonate and phosphate. Dyspnoea and anxiety.

Local disease of thoracic vertebrae—Traumatic or lung shrinking or TB. Treatment— dilute tobacco injections, possibly phosphorus, and also stimulate vital energies.

Treatment for damage due to mercury—Hot baths followed by sweating. Possibly arsenic bath. To combat destructive tendency of mercury—follow up with geometry exercises, half hour daily.

pages 236–249

DISCUSSIONS WITH MEDICAL PRACTITIONERS (FRAGMENTARY NOTES) II
DORNACH, 23 APRIL 1924

Viscum as a specific. Carcinoma. Pre-publication passages from *Extending Practical Medicine*. Fundamental Principles based on the Science of the Spirit. Example: From diagnosis to treatment. Case 4—paralysis, atrophic sites in ether body, astral body not penetrating. Astral body intervening too powerfully in physical body. Rheumarthritis—astral body intervenes directly in physical body in the joints— spasm or inflammation. Teeth getting worse. Cause of frequent dreams—weakness in ether body. Urinalysis. Weakness relating to smells. Prefers sweet dishes— weakness in astral body. Occult finding—allantois not fully developed. State of allantois may be discovered from that of astral body. Allantois—physical correlate of astral body. Chorion—physical correlate of I organization. Often deep-seated damage there for generations. Influence I organization to harmonize astral body and ether body. Effects of pyrites ointment—astral body more lively. Action of golden agaric ointment. Solidago, Stellaria. Tea of willow bark, Stannum—highly effective for difficult child. Problems of history-taking. Case 5—Weakness of I organization means digestion of fats inadequate. Weakness of astral organization means carbohydrates not adequately digested. Ether organization too weak means protein not properly digested. Treatment with silica reduces sensitivity of astral body and I organization. Artificial sensitivity produced with mustard plaster—subtle stimulus. Guiding astral activity to ether body with copper and Carbo animalis. Pancreas preparation for ether weakness in digestive organs. Silver injections strengthen ether body in cases of pyrexia. Damage caused by metabolic deposits due to I organization. Insidious destructive damage due to astral body. Development of carcinoma corresponds to development of a sense organ, e.g. eye. Processes from outside the human being act like foreign bodies. Etheric deposits develop. Levels of existence relate in different ways. Very different in the ear. Breast cancer due to mechanical insults. Viscum injections for tendency to develop cancer. Heredity. Meditate on things it is possible to establish through spiritual science in disease processes according to the symptoms. Meditate on spiritual-scientific causes in relation to symptoms. Eurythmy—in the human organism things that are conscious are derived from the unconscious. Movements of limbs held back after birth (wrapping legs tightly) later helps speech development.

pages 250–266

EDITOR'S PREFACE

Before the beginning of the twentieth century, Rudolf Steiner devoted himself in his intensive studies of philosophy and Goethean science to a critical assessment, open to the future, of the basic methodological questions in natural science and medicine. When the new century began—Steiner had joined the theosophical movement and was beginning to bring his own approach to it—new subjects for research (Paracelsus, homoeopathy) came up and so did first contacts with physicians interested in theosophy who wanted to devote themselves to a medicine broadened through the science of the spirit. Rudolf Steiner made many suggestions and gave his support to the initiatives of individual people, also opening up areas for research. The breakthrough to establish anthroposophic medicine was not made until the spring of 1920 though, when he gave his first course of lectures for physicians (*Introducing Anthroposophical Medicine*, CW 312). During the next five years, until his death on 30 March 1925, it proved possible, in connection with intensive lecturing activity, to begin or realize some of the things which Rudolf Steiner wanted to achieve for a medicine broadened through spiritual science—to build bridges between empirical science, which he always supported—and a newly initiated science of the spirit; to combine the insights arising from this with clinical work and medical practice; to develop and produce new medicines, and to establish innovative research and training.

The lectures Rudolf Steiner gave and statements he made on medical subjects in this volume are certainly heterogeneous, covering the period from 1920 to 1924, apart from the major courses (the first and second medical courses, *Understanding Healing*, *Education for Special Needs* and *Broken Vessels*). They range from a question-and-answer session and the concluding lecture in a course of public lectures on the subject of anthroposophy and specific sciences, to lectures given in someone else's place at the first anthroposophical tertiary education course and discussions with small groups of medical practitioners. (For further details on things said on other occasions, see below.) In view of this heterogeneity it seems particularly important, if Rudolf Steiner's words are to be properly understood, to note the given context in every case.

As has been said, this volume contains the spoken words of Rudolf Steiner on medical subjects in all kinds of different ways (lectures, discussions, questions and answers), addressed to very different audiences (public, physicians, students):

Part I, Autumn 1920: Physiological and therapeutic studies based on spiritual science

From 26 September to 16 October 1920 the first of the 'anthroposophical university-level courses' was the first event to take place in the main auditorium of the Goetheanum in Dornach, with the building not yet quite finished. The aim of the organizers (Verein Goetheanismus and Bund fuer anthroposophische Hochschularbeit) was to have various speakers present the spiritual-scientific work in many different spheres of life to the public (see programme on pp. 268–75). A series of lectures by Ludwig Noll, MD, Kassel, was planned for the second week, the title being 'Physiological and therapeutic studies based on spiritual science'. At the last minute Dr Noll was unexpectedly unable to come to Dornach. Rudolf Steiner then spoke on the theme in four lectures in his place.

Part II, Autumn 1922: Anthroposophical foundations for the practice of medicine

These lectures were given to an audience of physicians and medical students as part of a 'medical week' at the Institute of Clinical medicine established in Stuttgart on 15 August 1921. The aim of this conference was to make medicine broadened on the basis of anthroposophy known in the general medical world and in the public domain. On the last day of the medical week Rudolf Steiner spoke to the physicians and medical students of eurythmy therapy. As the programme shows, practical demonstrations of it were made daily from 5 to 7 p.m.

Part III, Winter 1923–24: Therapy

During the 1923–24 Christmas Conference, at which the General Anthroposophical Society was established, three discussions were held with anthroposophical physicians in the 'Glass House' (at 8.30 a.m. on 31 December 1923

and 1 January 1924, and at 10 a.m. on 2 January 1924). Rudolf Steiner gave his views on individual issues raised by the physicians. Apart from Drs Friedrich Husemann, Ludwig Noll, Otto Palmer and Felix Peipers from Stuttgart, the meetings were also attended by physicians from the Arlesheim clinic—Ita Wegman, Hilma Walter, Margaret Bockholt, Julia Bort and Eberhard Schickler. Eugen Kolisko from the Stuttgart Waldorf School was present, as were eight anthroposophical physicians from a number of other European cities.

Part IV, Spring 1920: *The lecture on 'Hygiene as a Social Issue' was the concluding talk Rudolf Steiner gave at a fortnight's public event on 'Anthroposophy and Different Fields of Science' where a number of anthroposophical speakers had spoken on sciences, education, the arts, social and other issues. This conference may be considered to have been the precursor of the first anthroposophical university-level course in the autumn of 1920 (see above). The time when the lecture was given was between the 18th and 19th lectures in the first medical course* (Introducing Anthroposophical Medicine). *The written questions addressed to Rudolf Steiner after the lecture were probably put by people attending the medical course. This lecture is also published in* Fachwissenschaften und Anthroposophie *(not publ. in English) which documents the conference as a whole.*

Spring 1920: *At the beginning of the above conference Dr Friedrich Husemann gave a talk on 'Nervousness, Philosophy of Life and Anthroposophy' which was followed by discussion. The questions and answers on psychiatry were Rudolf Steiner's concluding words in the discussion. See also the above-mentioned Fachwissenschaften volume, which included this question-and-answer session.*

Spring 1924: *The discussions with medical practitioners on 21, 22 and 23 April 1924 took place at medical meetings during the Easter course for young doctors. Apart from older physicians who had been practising for some time, the meeting was also attended by younger physicians and medical students.*

The chronological table of medical lectures and discussions (over) may help to gain a clearer picture of Rudolf Steiner's lecturing activities in this field.

[GA = Collected works in German]

Date	Venue	Occasion
21 March–9 April 1920	Dornach	First medical course (*Introducing Anthroposophical Medicine*) GA 312
26 March 1920 7 April 1920	Dornach	Q&A on Psychiatry Hygiene as a social issue (both GA 314, *Physiology and Healing*)
7–9 October 1920	Dornach	Lectures on 'Physiological and therapeutic themes based on spiritual science' (GA 314)
11–18 April 1921	Dornach	Second medical course, GA 313 (*Illness and Therapy*)
12–18 April 1921	Dornach	Eurythmy therapy lectures for physicians and eurythmists, GA 315 (*Eurythmy Therapy*)
26–28 October 1922 28 October 1922	Stuttgart	Anthroposophical Basis for the Practice of Medicine (GA 314) Lecture on eurythmy therapy (GA 314)
31 December 1923/ 1 January/2 January 1924 28 August 1923–29 August 1924	Dornach (various cities)	Discussions with anthroposophical physicians on Therapy (GA 314) *The Healing Process* (GA 319)
2–9 January 1924	Dornach	GA 316 (*Understanding Healing*)
21–25 April 1924 21–23 April 1924	Dornach	Easter course, part of above (GA 316) Discussions with medical practitioners (GA 314)
25 June–7 July 1924	Dornach	GA 317 (*Education for Special Needs*)
8–18 September 1924	Dornach	GA 318 (*Broken Vessels*)

Summary of Medical Courses in English Translation (latest editions shown):

GA/CW 312   *Introducing Anthroposophical Medicine* (SteinerBooks 2010)

313   *Illness and Therapy* (Rudolf Steiner Press 2013)

314   *Physiology and Healing* (Rudolf Steiner Press 2013)

315   *Eurythmy Therapy* (Rudolf Steiner Press 2009)

316   *Understanding Healing* (Rudolf Steiner Press 2013)

317   *Education for Special Needs* (Rudolf Steiner Press 1998)

318   *Broken Vessels* (SteinerBooks 2003)

319   *The Healing Process* (SteinerBooks 2000)

INTRODUCTION

Medical science is of course concerned with the human body in all its complexities and wonders—but what skills or capacities do we need to fathom these? Steiner repeatedly suggests in this volume, and elsewhere, that scientists and physicians fail to understand the body precisely because they see it only as a physical organism. It is not just that the psyche is ignored or dismissed. Very often, in fact, this is not the case: the realities of both body and soul are acknowledged, and inclusion of complementary therapies in national health programmes has gone some way to addressing our sense that 'we are not just bodies', as has the whole realm of psychotherapy. Nevertheless, this acknowledgement of the reciprocal effect of body and psyche remains largely abstract, or vague at least. Meanwhile, Steiner's medical lectures are probably unique in, firstly, seeing the human body as inconceivable without the higher levels of soul and spirit which inform, and in diverse ways in different organs and systems, act within it; and secondly, in deriving from these highly varied interactions, medicines and measures that very specifically address different diseases and disorders by re-establishing the organ-specific degree of healthy engagement between spirit, soul and body.

Steiner's accounts of these extraordinarily complex interactions give one a sense of dynamic reality that continually changes in the ebb and flow of withdrawal and engagement between physical, etheric, astral and spiritual levels. He sees the human body as, literally, the embodiment of all these reciprocal realities. The capacities physicians need therefore—alongside thorough insight into physical processes—include well-grounded imagination and intuition, an artistic appreciation of the full spectrum of diverse and, if you like, almost musical interactions between different levels at work in us. How does the spirit (our core being) work in the body? Not just as some static constant or general principle. Nor are disease and health just distinct and easily distinguished sides of the human coin, one 'normal' the other 'abnormal', but both are intrinsic to an essential mutuality and flux. To take just one example: the 'I' and astral body (the human spirit and soul) are, in Steiner's account, most deeply engaged in us in metabolic and motor processes, whereas in the neurosensory system focused (but not confined to) the head—in our thinking therefore—these two levels are furthest withdrawn from physical involvement. As a surprising reversal, then, of our usual perception of the head as 'more spiritual' and our metabolic processes as 'more physical', we find our highest spiritual principle 'vacating the premises' of the head in healthy conditions, creating a free space for thoughts to be 'mirrored', whereas this same highest principle really 'gets down to work' in our metabolism and movements and is most fully engaged there. Very simply—and Steiner goes into far more complex, sometimes bewildering detail, which requires all our alert attention to follow—disorders of the metabolism can arise where, for whatever reason (including a range of traumas), the I and astral body withdraw, allowing lower principles to burgeon unchecked. Here therapy will involve interventions, medicinal, physical or psychological, or all at once, that induce the higher principles to engage again as they should. Such measures cannot really be carried out without yet another vital element emphasized by Steiner: the physician's loving attention as intrinsic to the healing process. Thus we find that 'physical' disorders cannot only be treated physically nor can 'mental' disorders be treated only psychologically. The latter are also invariably rooted in specific organs.

The range of Steiner's observations in these lectures is staggering. It is as if we are asked to look up from the small focus of the microscope and the narrow field of view of a particular medical specialism and encompass in inner vision a far broader panorama of human nature, though without for a moment relinquishing attention to the tiniest detail. This stance is, indeed, part of what Steiner calls the 'courage to heal': the capacity to observe the whole cosmos of the human being, all the varied and interacting laws at work in us, in order then to intervene with detailed understanding, with loving compassion and respect for each human biography. A daunting challenge, but surely the true task of medicine.

Andrew Maendl, MD, and Matthew Barton, September 2013

I
PHYSIOLOGY AND THERAPY BASED ON THE SCIENCE OF THE SPIRIT

Lecture 1

THE speaker has not yet arrived.[1] I hope he'll be here soon, but for now, I don't wish to have you sitting there waiting. It is self-evident that this series of lectures carries particular weight as part of the course. The intention is to take a practical subject and show how our spiritual science with anthroposophical orientation truly can play an effective role in everyday life. Now as everyone knows from personal experience, medicine, medical treatment, is a most important sphere of life, and for this reason if no other we must not fail to take anthroposophy into the field of medicine right from the beginning of our anthroposophical endeavours.

In this course we endeavoured to have the individual subject areas covered by people who are qualified specialists also in everyday terms. It is necessary to do so when we, representing spiritual science, present the different subjects to the world, for otherwise they are not taken the way they are meant to be taken. I will therefore try and say a few things about physiology and how it relates to medical treatment until the speaker arrives, doing so from the spiritual-scientific point of view. That was more or less the proposed subject matter. And I want to show you how much spiritual science is needed in the study of medicine and then also in medical practice, in the whole art of medicine.

As you know, at our universities the study of medicine is usually preceded by a study of the sciences. The actual study of medicine comes after this. Having got to know the phenomena more of biology and physiology, one then gives consideration to the pathological phenomena, until one finally comes to the subject of therapeutics. Many members of this audience will no doubt know that therapy really gets a poor deal in the process. It is indeed true that with the study of medicine given this scientific approach people concentrate on the natural processes relating to human beings. When the future physicians then come to the subject of pathological processes they do so with a mind concentrated on natural processes and are hardly able to see pathological processes in the right light. Now there is an opinion which I think has come up more or less of necessity in more recent times. We tend to gain a particular view of processes in nature, their inner connection and the underlying causes. In a healthy individual we must therefore under these conditions quite evidently look for certain natural processes in a necessary causal relationship. In a sick person, or let us say in a sick organism, what can we look for but basically also natural processes subject to causal necessity?

Yet we are compelled to say that compared to a healthy organism the natural processes in their very obviously causal development of a disease are abnormal, in a way dropping out of the system of causal relationships that exist in a healthy organism. In short, as soon as we enter into the field of medicine doubt and scepticism arise concerning our actual approach to the study of nature when it comes to considering natural events from the modern point of view. Many medical people therefore develop a real scepticism, downright nihilism, as I have said here on other occasions, when it comes to treatment. I have known famous professors at the faculty of medicine in Vienna—at a time when that faculty of medicine was at the height of its glory—who at heart really were nihilists when it came to treatment.[2] They said that one can really only let a disease take its course—and they took the particular disease where such a view does certainly apply, pneumonia, as an example. One can guide the course it is taking with external measures that will ameliorate or promote it, until the crisis comes and the whole then dies down again. Essentially we cannot speak of a cure in the true sense of the word, though people have done so for centuries if not millennia.

If such a view were to be consistently taken further, medicine would gradually develop into pure pathology. For in the study of diseases, albeit from the point of view of a natural science based on materialistic thinking, an extraordinary degree of perfection has been achieved in this age of therapeutic nihilism. At this point I'd also warn you against the potential misconception that in Dornach and in spiritual science with anthroposophical orientation we fail to recognize and tend to underestimate the full significance of modern science. That is not at all the case. Someone who has taken even just a brief look at the methods of investigation in pathology in the second half of the nineteenth century and how they have developed can only do so in amazement and admiration for the brilliant, tremendous progress made. Yet beyond this he must also make a very different admission. He has to say to himself: Yes, materialism has arrived. But it cannot meet certain needs in the human heart and mind; nor can it cast an adequate light on vast areas of human insight.

Materialism has however had its own kind of mission, I'd say. It has made us develop our ability to experiment and observe in an extraordinarily careful and thorough way. We are entirely indebted to this materialism for our modern pathology, even if it does have that materialistic bias. People will always complain if one is not biased in our present age. As editor of the journal *Magazin für Literatur*,[3] I was labelled a materialist when I had written an article after Buechner's[4] death that did not condemn him but did indeed express appreciation of his merits. This is what matters when we live with and practise the science of the spirit, that we are able to enter into everything, everywhere finding the thought form, the form of sentience, on which approaches and philosophies that may be complete opposites may draw, and we are also able to appreciate the merits of something which has its root in such a thing as materialism. At the present time—and this is simply the need of our time—we must, however, overcome materialism.

There is something else to which I'd like to draw your attention. You will have heard in the lectures given here that we seek to establish a phenomenology in science. You will also have heard, with full justification, that there is need to look for a chemistry free from hypothesis.[5] I am keen to discover if someone might not find that with regard to one thing or another which indeed has to be presented with reference to medicine and the practice of medicine, the discussions do not also cover elements that will seem to him to be hypothetical. But we must first clearly establish the concept 'hypothesis', especially when moving from the study of the inorganic to the organic.

What is a hypothesis? Well, let us take a perfectly ordinary thing from everyday life. When I have walked along a road and seen someone along this road and walked on and then did not see him any more I am unlikely to assume at first that this person has disappeared into the ground, something most unlikely to happen. No, I'll look around and perhaps see a house. I can limit my ideas and say to myself: Well, he's gone into that house. I don't see him now, but he's in there. It would be a justifiable hypothesis if I were to take the thoughts, as it were, that come to me as my senses perceive this, and then something occurs that needs further explanation, so that I have to presuppose something, take it as a hypothesis. This will arise from my train of thought but cannot be seen or observed directly, so that it is not a direct phenomenon for me. I would not be setting up a vague hypothesis in making such an assumption, just as I'd not be setting up a vague hypothesis when on using a thermometer I first perceive an increase in temperature, and then see this temperature disappear—due to freezing or something of the kind—and speak of the loss of latent heat.

If investigation is to be fruitful it is now and then necessary, therefore, to take the sequence of sensory concepts further. An unjustifiable hypothesis is one where we arrive at ideas where if we take them further, and consider them with insight, it becomes evident that the things on which it is based simply cannot ever be perceived. We must then provide the ideas we arrive at—ideas on atomism, molecularism—with ingredients that can never be perceived, otherwise we would be able to perceive them. For we could never, for instance, cherish the illusion—if there were some kind of process by which it would be possible to see even the smallest particles of bodies—that we could then still explain light as arising from motion. In that case we would actually be taking light into those smallest particles.

I would ask you to make occasion at this point to develop a clear idea of justifiably continuing in thought within an experience on the one hand and of establishing unjustifiable hypotheses on the other.

To come back once more to that earlier thought, we have to say: We see someone before us whom we consider to be 'normal'. And we see someone else who has fallen ill. We must of necessity acknowledge a process taking its natural course in either case. Yet how does the one process relate to the other? The fact that we keep physiology, pathology and medical treatment separate, as has become the custom in recent times, prevents us from gaining the relevant ideas as we move from one to the other. Apart from this, modern medical people really cannot include the spiritual in their considerations when working with physiology or also pathology, for the spiritual is really something unknown in the modern approach to science. And so it is not included in any of their considerations.

It is possible to contrast the two natural processes, one physiological, the other pathological, definitely and clearly, initially in abstract form, choosing certain final forms in pathology, I'd say, and the study of such final forms may perhaps allow us to arrive at fruitful ideas. You need not think of there being an absolute necessity, of it being demanded, when you are at the beginning of a science. This correctness, something we call inner necessity, can only develop in the course of our studies. And we may therefore start at any point, I'd say, if we want to study a particular thing in nature.

Let us take a truly extreme case within the sick human organism. One most extreme case which presents many problems in modern medicine is the development of cancer. With this we see—as may also be seen under the microscope—something organic, or at least looking organic, developing in such a way in the ordinary organism that it will gradually destroy life in the rest of that organism. At first all we can say is that within the body of the human organism we see something arise where we see how, rising from unknown depths, something enters into the usual natural course which interferes with the development of that natural course.

We may also turn to the other extreme of a pathological organism. We can perceive something arising, something where, in a sense, normal activity in the human organism proliferates, becoming 'unnormal'. We then consider the human organism to be abnormal. I don't particularly wish to operate with the terms 'normal' and 'abnormal', but they will serve our purpose for the moment. In due course of time it would then be evident, if this line of thought were to be taken further—which I hope it won't—that in transition the normal would also simply go over into the 'abnormal', as it is called. Just for the moment it will be reasonable to use the terms 'normal' and 'abnormal'. With reference to the 'normal' human organization we note that in the psyche, too, a specific form of will intent develops, a specific form of feeling and a specific form of thinking. In social life we have gradually let a kind of 'normal' image crystallize out of the ideas we gain from dealing with other people, an image which makes us consider a person as 'normal' who to a certain degree develops his will, feeling and thinking out of his own nature.

Concentrating that thought just a little, we will inevitably say to ourselves that if the organism functions too strongly, functioning like a body containing latent heat from which we remove that latent heat and which would then release too much free heat into the surrounding world so that we'd no longer know what to do with this heat— now if the human organism were to function in such a way, sending out too much in this direction, it would of necessity, if it were to present itself to us in reality, have to show the results which we've arrived at in our thinking, though the emotional element always comes into this through the element of feeling. In our thoughts such a human organism would seem to us to be affected by the abnormality we call mania. We see something appear in this human organism which results from powers of organization flooding it, powers that go very much in the direction of sensory qualities. Carcinoma-type developments are something where natural force appears in the organism, segregating itself, as it were, where this organizing power becomes embedded in the organism. On the other hand, the pathological phenomena of mania or the like are something which the organism is not able to hold on to, as it were, something which comes out of the organism. If I were to draw a diagram of this, I would do it by saying: If this is the normal development of the human organism, I'd draw in the occurrence of a carcinomatous growth like this [Fig. 1, over, red], putting something by way of powers of growth in some place or other, powers that now cling to the organism inwardly, so that it must there provide something which otherwise it would provide for the whole organism.

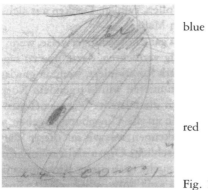

blue

red

Fig. 1

For a diagram of mania I would have to show something welling forth from the organism (blue), something pushing towards the sphere of mind and soul.

I have been referring to extreme situations, and you may consider them also in less acute forms. Imagine the problem does not go as far as developing into a carcinoma, but rather a carcinomatous change prevented from going all the way. In that case some organ or other—for these things do not happen in a vacuum, of course, nor in spaces between organs—is taken hold of, but the power which otherwise tends to go inwards and in there emancipate, growing quite independent, unites with the power normal to the organ. The organ is then affected by a disease which we may refer to in many different ways, as has come to be the custom in medicine.

Let us assume a tendency towards mania is stopped halfway. The abnormality of the individual's organization does not cause the element of mind and soul to be put outside completely, as is the case with full-blown mania, where it is completely beside itself, as it were, and the thought element emotionally goes its own way. The element which tends towards the other extreme goes only halfway, and we then have the different forms of 'mental illness' as it is called—as it is called, I say—which may take all kinds of different forms, from illusions, which are organic in origin, all the way to states of hysteria and so on where an organic origin is hardly demonstrable, though they do have their basis in the organism. As you can see, the aim has been to consider the phenomena that take us from the normal to the pathological in two different directions. We must consider these phenomena before we can form an opinion about them.

Let me now show you from another angle how it is possible to grasp, at least to a degree, what is behind it all, doing so not yet entirely out of the science of the spirit, the methods of which I have referred to as insight in images, inspiration and intuition, but by using a certain instinct, as we might call it, though unless there is a desire to progress to the spiritual-scientific way doing it from instinct will only take us halfway.

There is an extraordinarily interesting phenomenon in the evolution of German culture. Leaving aside one's personal view of Schelling[6] as a philosopher, he is an interesting phenomenon in the history of civilization. Perhaps everything he has developed as a philosophy may be wrong and askew, but there was a certain instinct alive in him for natural processes even in areas where people working in ordinary science are not at ease in following events in nature, relying more on a very crude empiricism. Schelling has indeed also tried to think in terms of medicine as occasion arose, and actually devoted quite some time especially to issues relating to healing processes. Little thought has been given in the more recent study of the history of philosophy to how Schelling actually came to leave more abstract and local philosophical deliberations aside and enter, quite instinctively, into a realistic study of nature and even the organic sphere. He actually published a journal[7] in which medical issues were extensively considered.

Where did this come from? We can come to understand it if we know, and learn to appreciate in the right way, the profound instincts for gaining insight on which Schelling drew for his truths and his errors. And so we find a remarkable statement made by Schelling, not based on clear insight, I'd say, but hewn from the instincts in his psyche. He said that to gain insight into nature was to create nature.[8] Now if these words were to be realized directly for human insight, we'd find it easy to enter into medicine. If we could have the creative powers entering into our search for insight, if we had powers of creation in our thinking, we would find it quite easy to enter into the field of physiological and pathological phenomena, for we would then be able to observe the steps taken by creative nature, as it were. From the empirical point of view one simply has to say that we are unable to do so. Someone who then takes this further would be able to say that the very fact that a demand like the one made by Schelling cannot be met, going beyond human capacities, is partly the reason why we are not able initially to see into a process of this kind, where new developments arise. Being unable to follow nature's creative work directly with our powers of insight, we are unable to see into the process where new forms, new developments arise. We are thus not immediately able to look into the facts of material processes such as the development of a carcinoma. However, if we rightly bring together this thing which is truly denied us, i.e. our inability to do with the things which do present themselves to us in the carcinomatous process, what a man of genius demands when he says that to gain insight into nature is to create nature—if we bring this together with the phenomena of the carcinomatous process it will become evident how one must tackle processes of this kind.

We have to admit that Schelling did not speak from instinct in other respects. Just consider how his utterances were polar opposites. On the one hand we have the words: To gain insight into nature is to create nature, something we are unable to do. On the other hand there are these words: To gain insight into the spirit is to destroy the spirit. So far only people involved in spiritual science have said these words, and even then only in a certain mysterious obscurity: To gain insight into the spirit is to destroy the spirit. Now if we are unable to achieve the creative work of nature, then—initially admitting this merely in analogous form, we may go further into this later—we are also unable, with our human capacities, to destroy the spirit. We cannot penetrate with our powers of insight to the point where the destruction of things spiritual begins. Yet you will have an inkling, I think, that here we have a certain relationship to manic or similar states where something destructive arises in mind and spirit. There is need to look for the connection between the normal human powers that cannot create nature by gaining insight into it, and those that cannot destroy the spirit by gaining insight into it. I have thus shown you the way initially, something which takes us from a normal, but instinctively more deeply stimulated conscious awareness to the relationship of the human being to nature. We shall see that along this road, which I have now indicated, there lies, as we go on, the element we must really look for as we move on from physiology to pathology.

Well, I hope that it won't be necessary for me to speak to you about this tomorrow as well, but I will try to take this line of thought further one evening during the next few days, at least in outline.

LECTURE 2

LET me pick up where I concluded yesterday. Reference had been made to an individual who was driven by his philosophical instincts, as it were, from insight in the sphere of mind and soul to a feeling that this sphere related to human existence in a physical body. This was Schelling, and I said that on the basis of these instincts Schelling became involved in practical terms not only in the theory of medicine but also with various forms of treatment. I do not know if this led to greater or less satisfaction, as is the case with physicians who are well prepared. For the question as to how much a treatment really contributes to a person's improvement is in most cases highly problematical unless, of course, one takes the inner view. Schelling did, however, gain a principle in the state of soul engendered out of that instinct, a principle of which we may indeed say that it would be good if it were to become a kind of inner principle for every physician, so that the physician would develop the whole of his practical view of the nature of the human being in sickness and health on the basis of it. I gave you the words Schelling spoke. He simply said that to gain insight into nature was to create nature.

I think you'll agree that the first thing to strike one when a man of genius says such a thing is that it is evidently absurd. No one would seriously believe that as an earthly human being in a physical body one would be able to create anything, whatever it may be, that exists in nature by gaining insight into nature. Yes, people are creating things all the time in industry, but there it is not a question of truly creating something in the sense Schelling meant it, but merely of putting together, combining, forces of nature that would give nature the opportunity to be creative herself in a particular way, in a specific arrangement. Essentially, therefore, we have here an absurdity on which a man of genius based really the whole of his thinking. And I quoted other words to you yesterday, words that may be seen as the opposite of 'To gain insight into nature is to create nature', which would be 'To gain insight into the spirit is to destroy the spirit.' Schelling probably did not utter these in such a fundamental way. But when one is again taking up the science of the spirit in a different age, developing one's own spiritual investigation, one realizes that essentially both statements take us back to most ancient inspired insights. Schelling was not an initiate in any way but simply a man of genius. He produced the one statement out of his own instincts. And when we do studies that were not done in Schelling's day this statement immediately brings to mind echoes of the most ancient maxims. This then takes one to the other statement, coming to us as the echo of ancient maxims in a similar way. Both cannot be grasped with our ordinary understanding today. Seen side by side or each on its own, they are really absurd. Yet they point to something of the greatest importance in the human organization in both sickness and health.

Looking at the natural world around us, the only thing we can say about finished processes in nature is that to gain insight into nature is at best to recreate nature in our thoughts. We thus really develop this principle which we call our thoughts and which can do no more than recreate nature since it lacks the inner creative power in our thinking, in an inner life filled through and through with thoughts and ideas. But it has already been said that this inner life filled with ideas essentially is merely something which emancipates from the physical and etheric organization as the second teeth develop, some-thing human beings have inside their physical and etheric organism up to that time. The powers at work in that part of us are truly creative in early childhood; they then become attenuated, toned down in the inner life as a world of images or of thoughts and ideas, in short, I'd say, as a cosmic power in our thoughts and ideas that is a dilution of the substantial creativity we had in our physical and etheric bodies. So the element which we come to know from our seventh year onwards simply sits in our organism and organizes things in childhood. There it is actively creative.

This creative activity is not such that we can see it creatively at work in the natural world outside; but we see it there being active in our own organism. If the child were to have wisdom already and were able to speak not only about the natural world outside but about the things happening inside him, and understand nature there, he would say what Schelling said: To gain insight into this nature is to create this nature. For the child would simply imbue himself with these creative powers, would be at one with them. And Schelling, with his medical instinct, his physiological instinct, did nothing else but take something which is an absurdity in the whole of later life, taking it from his childhood, and pushing it out, saying, as it were: All this gaining of insight in adulthood is nothing but a feeble tissue of images; if one were able to gain insight as a child, one would have to say: To gain insight is really to be active, to develop creative activity. We are, however, only able to see this creative activity in our own inner life.

So what is it really, this creative activity within us, something which a man of genius such as Schelling puts in words in the way I indicated? Now I think you'll agree that genius altogether arises when someone keeps some childlike quality later on in life. People who age absolutely, taking to ageing in a 'normal' way when the relevant age is reached, will never have genius. It is people who take something positively creative and childlike into later life who actually have genius. This childlike quality, positively creative, this creativity based on insight—to put it in what is perhaps a foolish way—does not have the time to turn the search for insight to the outside because it turns those powers of insight inwards and becomes creative. This is the legacy we bring with us when we go through birth to enter into physical existence. And someone like Schelling felt this instinctively.

Everyone who gains this kind of vision will know that these things are not, for instance, such that the powers of mind and soul that imbue the organism in childhood and organize it cease to be when the second teeth develop. They are merely going through a stage. They are, as it were, forced down to a smaller measure of activity. We do later on definitely continue to have organizing powers in us, but we have also gained powers to create memory. Those powers come to conscious awareness at second dentition and so free themselves from the organization. Memory has then left the latent state and been released, and our powers of growth, of movement, of balance have become powers of mental vision, which in early childhood had shown the higher degree of activity needed at that time. You can see from this that in normal human development this organizing power, this power of growth, must be transformed in a particular way, and taken down to a given level, to be powers of mind and soul, powers of memory, let us say, and the power to develop thought. If we assume on the other hand that due to some event or other too much of this organizing power active in childhood is held back, with development simply taking a course where not enough of the organizing powers are transformed into memory-creating powers, then they are held fast down below in the organism, are not taken properly into sleep every time the individual goes to sleep, but continue to be active in the organism, bumbling about in the organism from going to sleep to waking up.

Doing physiological and phenomenological medical research in the direction which I can only refer to briefly in the short time available for these lectures, one comes to see that in the human organism it is possible for powers that should really go into the sphere of spirit and soul at the right time of life to stay down below in the physical organization. This creates the situation of which I spoke yesterday. If the normal measure of organizing powers is transformed at second dentition, we have a measure of powers in the organism later on in life that can fully organize this organism in its normal configuration and normal structure. But if we do not have this, if we transform too little, then the untransformed powers remain down there, turn up in one place or another, and we get those neoplasms, those carcinomatous neoplasms of which I spoke yesterday. In this way we can follow the process of falling ill, or of being injured, as Troxler[9] put it in the first half of the nineteenth century, of injury in later life.

Comparison is then also possible with regard to the situation with childhood diseases, for these clearly cannot have the same kind of origin, seeing that they develop in childhood when nothing has as yet been transformed. Yet once we have come to know the causes of disease in later life we have also gained the ability to observe the situation with the causes of disease in childhood. In a way one sees the same thing, though in a different aspect. We find that there is also too much power of organization in mind and soul in the organism when childhood diseases develop. This shows itself particularly well to anyone who has developed the ability to see things in this direction when considering the phenomenon of scarlet fever, of measles, in childhood. They can then see how something which would otherwise function normally in the child's organism, the element of mind and spirit, begins to bumble about, is more active than it really should be. The whole course of these diseases can be understood the moment we are really able to see how this bumbling about in the organism is the underlying cause of the disease.

From there it is not far—please pay careful attention to this, for I never go a step further than the thoughts that have gone before do justify, even if I am only able to refer to things briefly, but I always make it clear how far it is possible to go—I am not saying that a conclusion is drawn here, but only that one is close to giving recognition to something which it is extraordinarily important to recognize for real knowledge. If we have reached the point where we are able to perceive that when disease develops later in life that goes in the direction of neoplasia—meaning that there is too much organizing power, resulting in a surplus, as it were, in an organizational island—we are close to saying to ourselves: If later life thus refers back to earliest childhood, then the principle apparent in childhood refers back to the time before birth, or let us say conception; it refers back to the individual's existence in spirit and soul which he had before being clothed in a physical body. Such an individual has simply brought too much of the spirit and soul element with him from life before being a human being, from life before earth, and this surplus comes into its own in the childhood diseases.

In future the only thing possible will be to allow oneself to drift from the fruitless materialistic thinking in which we are caught up today, especially in physiology and therapy, and consider things from the point of view of mind and soul. And it will be found that the things which arise in spiritual science do not do so because the spiritual investigator is not properly based in physical research, being an amateur, as it were, in physical research. In parenthesis I'd definitely say that many who call themselves spiritual investigators are indeed such amateurs, but that is not how it should be. A spiritual scientist does not have to be too limited in his knowledge of physical research to be a spiritual scientist; he will be a spiritual scientist when he is more knowledgeable in that field than scientists usually are. If he understands the phenomena more clearly the phenomena themselves will drive him into the sphere of mind and soul, especially where we have to speak of sickness.

Then there are the words 'To gain insight into the spirit is to destroy the spirit'. Well, it really is equally absurd. But these words, too, point to something that has to be perceived and understood. For just as the words 'To gain insight into nature is to create nature' refer us to early childhood, and in fact to the time before birth, if we broaden them in the right way, so the words 'To gain insight into the spirit is to destroy the spirit' refer to the end of an individual's life, to the principle in us that brings death. You only have to subscribe to those words—para-doxically, I'd say—that to gain insight into the spirit is to destroy the spirit, and you'll find that we must not go along with them, and yet they are there in life as something we are always asymptotically coming close to. For someone who does not simply rush into insight-gaining, as we might put it, but develops the right way of knowing himself, to gain insight into the spirit, it means to see, to gain vision of, constant pro-cesses of degradation, constant processes of destruction in the human organism. Looking into the creative age of childhood, we see continuous building-up processes which, however, have the peculiarity that they dim the conscious mind. This is why we are half dreaming, half asleep, in childhood, with the conscious mind not fully awake yet. Our own earthly spirituality—growth activity suppressing conscious mental powers—is something which really organizes us thoroughly. At the moment when this power enters into our conscious mind it ceases to organize us to the degree to which it has done until then. And just as we are looking at the up-building powers when we look into the age of childhood, powers which do however dim consciousness, we look at destructive processes when we direct our vision to the fully developed thinking processes—but these have the capacity to make our conscious mind bright and clear.

Modern physiology does not take this sufficiently into account, although the phenomena are as much in evidence as they can be. Take a look at the real phenomena of modern physiology and you'll see that nothing can be more clearly shown on the basis of everything known about the physiology of the brain and the like than that with conscious processes in mind and soul one is not dealing with some kind of powers of growth, some kind of powers to take in food, but with eliminatory processes, degradation, a slow, continuous dying process. Death is at work in us when we give ourselves up to the principle which is actually involved in our conscious awareness. And just as in looking at unconscious creative powers we look to the beginning of life, so in looking at the powers of conscious ideation, which prove to be powers of destruction, we see the principle emerging which begins to take hold of us more and more as we grow into life on earth, break down the physical body and finally take us towards earthly death. We are with those powers looking to the other end of life, to death. And we will not be able to understand birth and death, or let us say conception, birth and death, unless we also consider the non-physical.

The statement that to gain insight into the spirit is to destroy the spirit really is a way of saying: if we were to consider only the spirit, no longer looking at it more or less naively, but were to look at it the way we look at the natural world outside us, we would have to stem back the principle which lies in this conscious thinking, ideation and sentient, feeling activity, would have to prevent the breaking-down process. This means we would at that moment have to tone down the power over the mental aspect, take inner conscious awareness down to unconsciousness, with the mental principle active unconsciously. We would reach a point where we created something spiritual out of ourselves, pushing it out to the outside, as it were. But we would not be able to follow this with the conscious mind, for we cannot take the organization into this breaking-down process, this process in mind and spirit. We are therefore able to say that organizing processes are such that in a way we have the structural framework of the human organism [Plate 1, top]—though this is now an abstract way of looking at it—with the organizing power [Plate 1, below, red] entering into it as a principle in mind and soul. In the other case—the second case I spoke of—we have here the framework of the human organism, but do not allow the organizing power which to a degree dims down conscious awareness to enter into it but seek to drive out that organizing power into which we now seek to gain insight as spirit [Plate 2]. Yet our I or self cannot follow this, being bound to the organism. We have the other side, the side where human beings do begin to develop spiritual principles, above all will activity. Due to being filled with will activity, which remains unconscious and in a way is asleep, dreaming, we bring forth a spiritual and soul principle from our organization without conscious awareness. We have the other side, the manic, raging side, where the human being goes mad, and the various forms of mental diseases, as they are called, though these are nothing more than that here, with physical diseases, we have an element of mind and soul that does not belong in the physical organism [see Plate 1, below], and with the 'mental' diseases we drive forth from the physical and etheric something which should really be inside, but we drive it forth from the organism [Plate 2]. Today we see light cast on something which we discovered yesterday, but from another side. And the situation is that this point of view provides more guidance for us. Tomorrow we'll see the fruitful consequences we get exactly from these points of view, consequences that will definitely find confirmation in life, proving to be the most practical application in life, in medicine— therapeutic practice.

When we enquire into the causes of a physical illness, we must ultimately really look for them in a spiritual principle having lost its way in the organism. One should certainly not take an abstract view. People who know nothing of the way in which the principle of soul and spirit is connected with the physical organism really should not bring in their opinion here. For we can only identify the specific situation where there is too much organizing power somewhere in an organ, a hypertrophic organizing power I'd say, if we know the principle of spirit and soul, which in itself is just as real as the physical body has liver, stomach and so on as tangible organs (people have no idea of this in psychology), if we know it and its parts, its elements, just as we know elements that are physical and material. Knowing the relationships between the two we can consider the condition which develops in a person, often even in mind or spirit and soul, so that there is a kind of hyper-organization in some organ or other.

With everything but external injuries we would be able to refer to some such cause and origin.

If on the other hand we concern ourselves with mental diseases, as they are called, we will remain abstract if we think we can gain anything from half a phenomenology, if we think that we can gain anything by simply describing the abnormalities in mind and soul—though it is, of course, very useful to describe them. Such descriptions are very good for causing a sensation among lay people, for it is always interesting how someone who is foolish deviates from the normal in life. Rare things are always interesting, and in our day the situation is that something which deviates from normal life in this way is at least still a rarity. But there can never be a question of stopping at this point. Above all there can be no question of letting something move in the direction of the amateurish lay opinion that mind and soul are sick and it is possible to cure mind and soul somehow with measures in mind and soul. That is what abstract thinkers dream of. But it is especially with the 'mental' diseases that the most important thing to do is to point in every case to where the under-organization of some organ or other is to be found. Wanting truly to gain insight into a melancholy or hypochondria which has become a mental illness we should not paddle around in the sphere of the psyche but rather endeavour to consider the condition of the individual's abdominal region, how under-organization takes effect in the abdominal organization, how organizing power that is functioning below normal is in a way making something precipitate, to use the chemical term. A chemist precipitates something from a solution and the like, causing a sediment to form. We must endeavour to see how reduced organizing power causes something physical, material, to drop out, precipitate, that would otherwise be fully penetrated by the organizing power, how this then exists in the organism as physical matter, is deposited, and what is going on in the liver, bile, stomach, heart or lung. These processes are not as easy to investigate as we would like in an age when people turn to cruder methods—for histology, the study of tissues under the microscope, is also a crude method. Psychologies will be needed for such an investigation, but it is always necessary to trace 'mental' diseases back to physical conditions.

This does, however, make them less interesting. But that is how it is.

It is, of course, more interesting when a hypochondriac is able to say that his psyche is in some way or other involved in the cosmos of spirit and soul than if we are able to demonstrate that there is an under-organizing power in his liver. Or it is more interesting to look for the cause of hysteria in mind and soul, let us say, than having to point merely to metabolic processes in the sexual organs when speaking of hysterical phenomena or whatever other metabolic irregularities spread in the organism. But we won't gain insight into these things unless we study them in this way.

The aim in the science of the spirit is certainly not always just to look for the spirit. We may leave this to spiritualists and other interesting, because rare, people—sadly only too rarely rare! We do not speak of spirit, spirit, spirit all the time in the science of the spirit but seek to trace the spirit's influences, and it is exactly this which will get us to grasp the material aspect in the right place. Far from being proud to explain mental diseases in an abstract way, referring to mind and spirit, the way is to come to a material view especially for mental diseases.

We are thus able to say that the science of the spirit points to and explains the interesting phenomenon which existed in psychiatry just a short time ago—perhaps with Griesinger[10] or in the time before Griesinger. A relatively short time ago psychiatrists would at least still consider the physical condition as well when making a diagnosis. What has become more and more common today? That psychiatrists crowd their literature with syndromes that are merely descriptions of abnormalities in mind and soul. Materialism has actually taken people directly into an abstract sphere of mind and soul in this field. This is a tragedy for materialism, for it has in fact taken people out of the material sphere. This is what is so strange about materialism that at certain points it actually leads to lack of understanding, an inability to grasp, the material. Someone who follows the spirit as a genuine fact will also follow it where it influences the material sphere and then withdraws from it so that matter is deposited, as is the case with 'mental' diseases.

I had to present these things to create a basis so that tomorrow I may also suggest some guiding principles for therapeutic work. The things we find if we thus fructify the sphere of physiology and therapy with the science of the spirit also have a social aspect. It is a peculiarity of life that wherever in looking for knowledge today we do not withdraw, being abstract, into scholarly existence inimical to life but look for it in taking a view of human existence, human togetherness, that is full of life, such a living search for knowledge will actually take us into a social sphere. An extraordinarily interesting social phenomenon shows itself in current developments. We see humanity divided up into middle-class and aristocratic people above on the one hand and into proletarian life below on the other. The one-sidedly aristocratic style of life leads to people being caught up in a false seeking for the spirit, materialism in the spiritual sphere, whilst proletarian life is caught up in a a certain spiritualism in the material sphere. What does it mean to say 'spiritualism in the material sphere'? It means to stop in one's search for the origins of existence. Proletarians have developed scientific materialism as a philosophy of life at the same time as the aristocratic element developed materialistic views of the spirit. The proletarians have become materialists, the aristocrats spiritualists. For if you find spiritualists among proletarians this is not something grown in their own proletarian soil but 'mimicry'; it is copied, merely something which has come across from the aristocratic and middle-class element like an infection—I'll be talking about infection tomorrow.

If on the other hand you see materialism developed among aristocrats so that spirits let themselves be seen materially, as if looking at flames, so that materialism is taken into the most spiritual elements and the intention is to see the spiritual in material terms, this arises from the original decadent one-sidedness where people step outside their humanity as a whole, out of the totality, and turn one-sidedly to the aristocratic and the middle-class element, the latter having caught some of the aristocratic disease. If proletarians, feeling compelled to stop in matter when they want to use their minds, their spirit, because they are not lifted out of it through the appropriate education and the like, when they are forced to stay in the material sphere in their search for the spirit, their philosophy of life will be materialism. This has been developed by proletarians as a philosophy for instance in the materialistic view taken of history. Materialism was developed as spiritualism by more aristocratic people, for spiritualism is materialism, a masked materialism where one will not even honestly admit to it being such but lies and maintains that those who subscribe to it are spiritual individuals.

Following this reminiscence, let us continue tomorrow.

LECTURE 3

IT will, of course, only be possible to speak in general terms about specific methods of treatment, particularly as the time available for this therapeutic part of our conference is short. On the other hand it is also a somewhat doubtful thing to have to give details on specific subjects, particularly in medicine unless one has an audience wholly of professionals in this field, as was the case in the spring.[11] On the one hand it will be necessary in future human evolution for as many people as possible to come to understand the general principles of healing, the consequences of medicine, as it were, so that there can be a relationship of trust between physician and patient, based however on proper knowledge of the subject. Yet although there is need to have such understanding on the broadest possible basis in order to have social hygiene, it is on the other hand not desirable that too many amateurish lay opinions are given room in medicine, though this has been very much the case in more recent times, the system of medicine being what it is. It really must be stressed that it cannot in the least be my intention to encourage any form of quackery, and that in our spiritual science with anthroposophical orientation there certainly must be the endeavour to support genuine medical knowledge based on exact methodical study, the art of medicine, and to bring spiritual-scientific insights into this genuine art of medicine. So we do not wish to be in the ranks of people who out of an infinite ignorance concerning the subject they are talking about declare themselves up in arms against all kinds of things they label 'conventional medicine' and the like. No, we certainly do not wish to be counted among them.

Something else must also be taken into account when we discuss things of this kind. Something has entered into medicine in more recent times. In a sense it has been there for a long time, but it has made itself felt more recently with all the vehemence generally found in a social order seemingly as chaotic as ours. It is the tendency to form factions even within the medical community. And these factions are as aggressive towards one another as are political parties, I'd say. This cannot be helpful for medicine, as is only too evident, quite generally. The fight of allopaths with homoeopaths, 'conventional' medical professionals with those versed in natural medicine, and so forth, has brought much confusion into the understanding of medicine, which we need to have among wider sections of the community. This had to be said first, so that the things I will be saying today may not be given the wrong basis.

I spoke to you of how on the one hand we have the element of spirit and soul in the human organizing process and how it hypertrophies, as it were, when physical diseases develop, so that this element of mind or spirit and soul does not stand apart from the physical organ in the right way and therefore proliferates within it. Here we are dealing with all the diseases that go in the direction of neoplasms in the organism. On the other hand we have diseases where the element of mind and soul develops in such a way that it does not adequately intervene in the physical organism, and therefore leaves certain parts of the physical organism to processes that have not been taken up by the human organization but left to the subordinate processes of natural existence, I'd say, so that organs become physicalized, if I may use the word, to an overwhelming degree instead of filling themselves with qualities of soul and spirit. The element of soul and spirit then flows out and cannot be properly spanned by self-awareness, the conscious I, with the result that conditions rather incorrectly called mental diseases develop.

This view has to be modified, however; it has to be given a more precise form, I'd say, as soon as we move from sound physiology to sound pathology and therapy. It needs to come together with the view of the essential human being which has been presented here on repeated occasions, though in a very different context than the one we need today. It is the view of the human organism in its threefold nature. On the one hand human beings are threefold in their soul in forming ideas, in feeling and in their will impulses. But this threefold nature of the soul exactly corresponds with a threefold physical body, with a kind of head or neurosensory system, a rhythmic system and a system of metabolism and limbs. Let me stress that this differentiation of the human organism must not be considered with the intellect but as a particular view. Someone who would consider the head system to be the part that extends down to the neck, and then the circulatory or rhythmic system as the part that comprises the trunk, and then the system of digestion and limbs, also including the sexual system, making such an external differentiation, would not have the right idea. The point is that the neurosensory system is located mainly in the head but also extends through all the rest of the organism. In a sense, therefore, we have to say when referring to the neurosensory system in anthroposophical terms that it is the system of functions in the human organism—for we are dealing not with boundaries in space but boundaries between functions—which is mainly located in the head but extends head activity through the whole human being, so that in a way the whole human being would also be 'head'. It is the same for the other systems. And it was plain mischief when an irresponsible professor of medicine who had no intention to consider things properly but did want to cast aspersions on these things in the eyes of the world spoke of the 'belly system' to discredit what is really meant by 'metabolic system'. He showed that he failed to realize that with such a differentiation it is the functional aspect which counts and not boundaries that might be set in space.

Once you have grasped this differentiation, and one could give many lectures to describe every detail, you clearly understand the differences between the head system, that is, the neurosensory system on the one hand, the system of metabolism and limbs on the other, and the middle system, the rhythmic system, which essentially serves to maintain the balance between the other two systems. If we then want to encompass the whole of essential human nature we have the following. The actual idea-forming and sensory activity has everything which physically happens in the neurosensory system for its basis; we can't actually say instrument, but its basis.

The view held in more recent psychology and physiology that the processes which are primarily connected with the system of feeling and of will take place in the neurosensory system is not correct. It will not stand up to a more detailed study of the subject. You will find an indication of this more detailed study, or at least its guiding principles, in my book *Von Seelenrätseln* (extracts in *The Case for Anthroposophy*).[12] Much detailed work still needs to be done in this direction. Then the things which can today be said with certainty on the basis of spiritual science will also be evident from the other point of view, the physical and empirical point of view. It will be evident that human feeling is not primarily connected with the neurosensory system but with the rhythmic system. Where the neurosensory system relates to sensory perception and the forming of ideas, the rhythmic system relates to feeling. It is only because the rhythmic system interacts with the neurosensory system via the rhythm of our cerebrospinal fluid, a rhythm that comes up against the neurosensory system, that this system is made the vehicle for our life in ideas when we raise our feelings to ideas. Our dim, dreamlike life in feelings is then perceived by us and becomes inner idea. Just as life in feeling is directly connected with the rhythmic system and is indirectly mediated by it, so does the life in will connect directly with the metabolic system. This connection is then such that secondarily, for there is metabolism also in the brain, the functions of the metabolic system come up against the neurosensory system and we thus inwardly manage to produce ideas of our will impulses, impulses which otherwise would play in a dim life of sleep in our organism.

You see that we have three different systems in the human organism and each sustains the life of the psyche in a different way. These systems not only differ from one another but they are also opposites—as I said, I can only refer to these things briefly today. We thus have the neurosensory system on the one hand, and on the other everything that makes up the functions of the metabolic system, the system of metabolism and limbs [Plate 3]. You can, of course, develop ideas about the connection between metabolism and limbs by simply considering the influence which limbs in motion have on metabolism. This influence is much greater than people tend to think. But I'd say that these two systems— neurosensory system and system of metabolism and limbs—are in a way also polar opposites. This opposition must be thoroughly considered in order to develop a sound pathology and therapy, especially a pathology that develops in a wholly organic way into therapy, thoroughly studying every single detail—and the details are of course countless. The following emerges when we consider the detailed influences. Something to which I referred briefly yesterday then becomes evident. It is that this thing I referred to yesterday is present to a high degree. Processes of degradation exist within everything connected with the head system, the neurosensory system. When we form ideas in our waking state, making sensory perceptions and forming ideas, this is not bound up with processes of growth and development but with processes of degradation, of elimination. You will in fact arrive at this by looking in a sound way at the things which empirical physiological science has to offer today. Empirical proof is available today, or I might put it better by saying empirical proof of knowledge gained by contemplation in spiritual science. Study the things certain inspired physiologists are able to say about physical processes in the nervous system that run parallel to the forming of ideas and to sensory perception. You will see that the statement that we are dealing with processes of elimination and degradation, catabolism, and not of anabolism when we are awake and thinking, perceiving things, is very well substantiated today. We have anabolic processes, however, where processes of will come to realization in the system of metabolism and limbs.

All the individual functions of the human being are of course interactive. Looking at this in the right way we have to say that the anabolic processes act from below upwards into the catabolic processes, and the catabolic process down from above into the anabolic processes. Study the matter in these terms and you'll then have the rhythmic process maintaining the balance between catabolic and anabolic processes. Its functions drive catabolism into anabolism and anabolism into catabolism. If we study this in the right way, not just outwardly, to see what is going on in the 'circulation of the blood', as it is called, of the heart, as the human body is breathed through, you have everywhere in there special processes that are interrupted in some way, as I might put it. I can't go into this interruption, for good reason; but the curve of this rhythm which I have drawn here {Plate 3, right} is everywhere specialized. The breathing process is a special case of this curve, and if you draw the movement of blood from the heart upwards, to the head, or else to the lung and down into the body, these are special cases of this process. In short, if you bring life into the things which I am just touching on here you enter into the tissue of functions in the human organism not in the usual, rather dead way, but in a living way. You must, however, make your ideas themselves come to life. You'll need to visualize a three-dimensional image of the human organism, in a way. You cannot encompass the human organism with the static, abstract ideas people want to have in modern physiology and pathology. We have to grasp it in ideas that move, ideas that truly enter into the action of something that is inwardly mobile and certainly not mere mechanical interactions among organs that are at rest. We thus begin to see that essentially there is constant interaction in the human organism between catabolic processes, killing processes, and the anabolic processes of growth, processes of proliferation, and so on. We cannot comprehend the human organism unless we proceed in this way.

But what do we really have there? Take a closer look. When the destructive catabolic process of the neurosensory organization acts through rhythm into the system of metabolism and limbs, we have something which acts against the system of metabolism and limbs, is poison to it. Conversely, when the principle in the constructive anabolic system acts through rhythm into the head system, it is poison to the head system. As I said, the systems spread through all the rest of the organism, and so we have constant poisoning and detoxification everywhere in the human organism, with the rhythmic process balancing them out. We are not looking into a natural process of the kind one would generally like to have, a process going in a particular direction—easily understood direction, I'd like to say, so that we may simply refer to the healthy processes as normal. No, we are looking into two processes acting in opposite directions, with the one definitely harmful to the other, and we actually cannot live in our physical organism without our system of limbs and metabolism continually exposed to the causes of sickness from the head system, and the head system to the causes of sickness from the metabolic system. Just as scales that are not balanced go to one side, wholly according to natural laws, with the beam not in the horizontal, the state of balance that exists in life is unstable, not static, and may go in the one direction or the other, leading to irregularity.

To cure is simply that when the actions of a head system are too toxic for the metabolic system you relieve the head of its toxic action, taking it away. Or conversely, if the actions of the system of limbs and metabolism are too toxic for the head system, causing proliferation, the former must be relieved of its toxic action.

Our view of this area will only be complete, however, when we are in a position to extend anything observed in the human being to the whole of nature and are able to see that nature from the spiritual-scientific point of view. Looking at the way a plant develops, for instance, you very clearly see, in the most macroscopic way, a plant development process that strives upwards, seeks to move away from the earth's centre. It is most interesting to study these metamorphosing endeavours to develop in Goethe's *Metamorphosis of Plants*,[13] at least for the first, basic principles.

Goethe's *Metamorphosis of Plants* outlines the very first classification, the very first elements of plant nature to be studied in this way. The method needs to be further developed. The basic principles must be followed, and this will give us a living way of seeing everything that happens when plants grow. The plant roots in the soil, developing the negative of upward-striving, as it were, in the root. It then grows upwards, overcoming earth's powers of attraction that are still highly active in the root. It battles its way through other forces and finally comes into flower, developing fruit and seed.

Many things happen along that road. One is that an opposing force comes in again. You can observe this opposing force—taking some example, for instance. Take common birch, let us say silver birch, *Betula alba*,[14] and look more closely at the process that goes from development of the root to the trunk and there especially the bark, and then on the basis of everything that is involved in trunk and bark development we get leaf development. We can study this particularly well in the spiritual-scientific way by studying the young birch leaves when they are still brownish in spring. Studying all this we gain a view of how the forces involved metamorphose, forces that are active in the inner plant, and we see how on the one hand the direction of forces in plant development is from below upwards. And we also have the element which still causes retardation, which in the root, I'd say, still acted strongly as gravity; but then, as the plant struggles free of earth's substance, forces act from the air, working together with the upward-striving force in a different way. Then comes an interesting stage, though again wholly factual, to realize how in this upward-striving process in birch bark certain salts are deposited in the bark as the plant develops—potassium salts. These are simply the outcome of the downward-acting forces in their interaction with the upward-acting forces and tend towards protein production—I'd say to something I would like to call the development of albuminizing powers. And so one penetrates the plant development process, for instance. I can only refer to it briefly here. You see we penetrate into it by looking, as it were, how potassium salts are deposited in birch bark, how something then struggles free from this power that draws things down—I'd say a kind of process roughly comparable to a salt precipitating from a solution—and we come to the process which consists in the solution coming free of the salt. If we grasp this in a living way we come to the protein producing process, into something I'd like to call the albuminizing process. This is a way of studying, with vision, the outside world around the human being.

We then return to the human being and consider the catabolic process which acts from above downwards. We see that basically, let us say, human beings have the kind of forces in them which in plants act from below upwards. Looking at the forces that act down from the head system towards the system of limbs and metabolism, we are, as it were, seeing the forces acting downwards which in plant development were being sent up from below. If someone blocks this plant development active in him, doing so in the wrong way, so that the process is not coming from the sphere of head activity—the astral, I nature—to penetrate bodily nature in the right way, and the penetration comes to expression within the living body, we have something which is blocked, though it should take its course in the human organism. This is a pathological phenomenon which we see, for instance, when rheumatic disease or gout develops.

Looking from the inner organism, let us say, to a process in plant development like the one we found in silver birch, we learn the following. On the one hand we are considering what happens when salts form, and on the other when protein forms. If we understand the process of protein synthesis properly we find in there a process which is the opposite to the situation where something is blocked. The process is held up in the organism which should run in a way similar to the process which runs properly as albuminization in birch leaves. We thus see a connection between the processes found in birch leaves, for instance, and the processes in the organism. If we use the principle found in birch leaves to produce medicines which we give to people these will be therapeutic because they are correctly counteracting this blocking process which leads to rheumatic disease and gout.

We are seeing both what is happening outside, in the natural world, and what is happening in the inner organism. This gives us an idea as to how we should direct the healing powers. On the other hand, when catabolic processes proceed in a way where the organism is, as it were, unable to stop them, they broaden out in a downward direction, the rhythmic system is not sending them back in the right way, and they go to the periphery of the body, forcing their way outwards to the skin, as it were. This results in inflammatory changes in the outside part of the human being, skin eruptions and the like. Looking at our plant, *Betula alba*, again we find the opposite process, with potassium salts deposited in the bark, and are able to see how to combat this skin eruption process, which in human beings leads to hyper-exudation,[15] by making a birch bark medicine.

We are thus able to study the actions of vegetable and mineral processes, and see a connection between activities in outside nature and in the human being. In other words we see medical empiricism, therapeutic empiricism, raised to the level which Goethe in his terms, now not intellectual, called the rational stage of science. We gain a science for therapy where the connections are truly understood. Things are not too easy, for we really have to study things in detail, at least according to certain types, in the first place the hidden types of individual human nature and the secrets of existence in the natural world. Nor should you think that once you have studied the process in an example such as *Betula alba* you have fully grasped all that matters. These developmental processes are of a very different kind with some other plant development processes, in horse chestnut or the like. The things I have touched on here must not lead to general drivel and twaddle, but to very serious and extensive study.

But—and here I would particularly address the ladies and gentlemen who are students—done in a rational way this kind of study should not, if done rightly, make you afraid of its vast extent. I can assure you that when all the ballast of examinations—examination Tartarus to use Paracelsian terms—is eliminated, and instead you do everything which in this way leads to a rational view of therapeutic pathology and pathological therapy, medical students will not need to study more but indeed less. And being full of life this study will evoke greater enthusiasm in you than the things taught today concerning the human being, which essentially give you nothing but organs which are definitely not at rest and can only be understood if you grasp their living function and their interaction with other organs as you study this organization, if you grasp the way this goes wholly into the functional sphere, and you will also have a science of the natural world outside which likewise takes you to the functional aspects. It will always be necessary again and again to study the inner process in the human being, the particular processes of poisoning and toxic effects that are no longer in balance side by side with processes which do not follow the natural order and, the external being the polar opposite to the internal, must in a way also be used in polar opposite ways, and thus may certainly lead to pathology or, to use a better term, to therapeutic pathology and pathological therapy.

I have only been able to touch briefly on the road to be taken to make the study of medicine sound. And I was only able to hint at the way in which the science of the spirit needs to be brought into this study of medicine. This evening, when I'll again speak for half an hour after the eurythmy performance, I'll give you some further examples which will show how such intuitive vision of activities both in the natural world outside and in the inner organism can lead to the therapeutic aspect and to insight into the pathological element. I'd wish to go into individual substances then.

In the short time available to me I have only been able to demonstrate the principle on the example of *Betula alba*. Tonight I will go further, but will always make sure to speak of things meant for general human understanding. Medical professionals will have to build on this basis. They need to consider the specific, for to treat the specific in this way always also calls for individual assessment, and it will be necessary for all lay people to understand the medical principles so that understanding, a sympathy, develops for the things which the medical profession have to undertake in the world outside.

If you consider the line which we want to follow in spiritual science with anthroposophical orientation for the field of medicine—I'll have more to say on this tonight—you are bound to say to yourselves: Truly, in this spiritual science with anthroposophical orientation the aim is not to go for charlatanism, lay approaches and amateurism. The aim is above all to help science, genuine, serious science, to grow sound, and this will in itself no doubt have social consequences.

LECTURE 4

TONIGHT I'd like to add something to the lectures I was compelled to give here these last days. I'd like to point out some things, aphoristically, which may help to shed light on the principles according to which the science of the spirit can make the study of medicine and therapy more fruitful. It will, of course, not be possible to go into much detail—I gave the reasons for this earlier today. Time is short, and above all detailed insight must be reserved for consideration among professionals, again for reasons which I gave this morning. I nevertheless want to say a few things relating to this field that may contribute to a general understanding of it, so that a kind of social effect may result from this part of our spiritual-scientific consideration of medical matters, establishing a degree of trust between the public and the medical profession. The greater the understanding you will have for medical matters the better will the medical world be able to work.

This morning I spoke of how life in the human organism really consists in the neurosensory system, or head system in short, really working in opposition to the system of limbs and metabolism, with the rhythmic system keeping them in balance. All the most necessary breaking-down processes, catabolic processes in the neurosensory system, are continually brought into harmony and exchange with the anabolic, developmental processes in the system of limbs and metabolism. You can imagine, and it is possible to substantiate this in detail, that the two systems in the human organism are indeed working in opposite directions, and in a way also affect each other in such a way that anything going on in one of them, let us say the system of limbs and metabolism, must not be affected too much if, say, an activity suitable only for, say, the head system influences the system of limbs and metabolism without being corrected by the rhythmic system.

When one has gained sufficient insight into this one will also be able to understand how in other words the head system, the neurosensory system—where metabolic processes must also be active, as I have said—may on occasion also be overwhelmed by such metabolic processes, with these metabolic processes in a way inwardly, functionally, making the head system similar to the system of limbs and metabolism. And the opposite may also be the case. The functional system belonging to the head is certainly also active in the system of limbs and metabolism, though only in a subordinate way in normal life. It may however grow overweening, developing excessive intensity in the system of metabolism and limbs where it should function only to a limited degree, its real, full role being in the head.

In other words, neurosensory activity which is also present in the system of limbs and metabolism and bears the powerful imprint of head activity may grow overweening or too intense in the lower abdomen. The destructive, catabolic processes which normally should only occur in the neurosensory system will then affect the organs in the lower abdomen. Developments that should normally only be catabolic processes in the neurosensory system will then occur in the organs of the lower abdomen. They will, of course, have a different configuration in the lower abdominal system, but perform its nefarious activity there. Looking into the human organization like this, we can indeed see the development of a serious disease there, of typhoid fever. It is of course possible to observe typhoid empirically in its outward manifestations, but it can only be understood and placed within the whole human organization by studying the human being in this way, from the point of view of a rational medicine—to use Goethe's words. I also showed you this morning how it is possible to progress from physiology and pathology to therapy by seeking to gain insight into not only the things that happen within the human being but also those in the natural world outside. Processes in the natural world can, if rightly understood, be introduced into the human organism in the form of appropriate substances. That is because the natural world outside, plant nature for instance, in rising upwards acts in the opposite sense in the human being, like the element in it that seeks to go downward, and can stop certain processes that are proceeding in the wrong way between the three systems in the human organism.

It is interesting to observe that the principle which I showed to you this morning for the plant world and its connection with the human being can also be studied and understood for the mineral world. However, if we want to understand the matter with reference to the mineral world we must draw on certain anthroposophical insights relating to the human being.

The element of mind and soul, the etheric and the physical principles are active in human beings. This element of mind and soul acts in such a way—you were able to perceive this during this morning's lecture—that full awareness of I can be present in it. There we have the human being in his normal organization, as it were. But it may also be that awareness of I is reduced in some way and recedes. If the element of mind and soul is in some way roaming, going its own way, and not properly imbued with the I, the different kinds of mental illness develop. But everything that is mind and soul in the human being—the astral as we see it in anthroposophy, being the more subconscious, dreamlike or also wholly unconscious inner life, and I activity, meaning fully conscious inner life—all this has physical vehicles, in a way, that allow it to take effect in physical life. We are therefore able to say that when we look at the human being we must turn our attention not only to I activity, which is purely spiritual, but also to the actual vehicle for this I activity in the organism. And we find that the actual vehicle for this I activity is essentially anchored in the blood.

It would go too far for me to show in every detail—which would certainly be possible—how the specific activity of the blood, metabolic activity combining with rhythmic activity in the blood, actually enables the I to work together with the rest of inner or soul life. Something which should be of particular interest to us at this point, however, is the bridge between physiology and pathology on the one hand and therapeutic aspects on the other. There we find something that is extraordinarily important. We can, as it were, influence the physical scaffolding, the physical vehicle of something that exists in mind or spirit and soul, let us call it the fully conscious I, to such effect, through processes of one kind or another which we cause in it that it withdraws from I activity, as it were, but performs a function similar to that which otherwise occurs only under the influence of I activity.

Let me recall a particular instance of this kind. Please think of—I'll draw this in diagrammatic form—I activity built up in a kind of scaffolding, taking the form of scaffolding, as it were, through the human blood system. I would like to show the I activity itself by drawing strips of colour along the lines of this scaffolding, those strips to be the mind and soul element in the I activity [Plate 4, red]. If we are then able to influence the organization of forces underlying I activity, it can happen that this organization of forces makes itself independent, as it were, tears itself away and separates out as physical activity, a scaffolding of physical forces separate from the mind and soul element, but still a kind of image of that activity in mind and soul, though its actions are wholly physical. One is creating a kind of inner double in this way which is at work down in deep subconsciousness. But its actions are similar, though only spatial, that is, only physical, to when it merely devotes itself to be the instrument for I activity.

We can evoke this—no need to do it, as in elementary cases one can, by merely following the right route, always find the point which Goethe called the point behind which nature reveals her open secret. We can evoke this condition when a person gets too much phosphorus into him, or is treated with a powerful dose of phosphorus. It is possible, as it were, to separate the vehicle of I activity in the body out of that I activity, with the result that this I activity would be performed separately in the body, as in an image. What would be the consequence of this? It would be that especially under the influence of phosphorus powers, blood activity would go beyond its usual measure, especially in the skeletal system, and a kind of hyperaemia would develop in that system. Due to the hyperaemia, the principle which comes right next to such excessive blood vessel activity in cartilage would then proliferate and calcification of bone would be counteracted.

I have told you what might happen when someone is given too much phosphorus, treatment where the function which phosphorus is able to perform in the human organism is made too powerful. But the forces which exist in the world outside, forces anchored in the individual minerals, also exist in human beings though in another form, let us say a supersensible form, and may indeed be active in the human being. The human being is in a way a microcosm. When the forces which otherwise are anchored in the natural world outside are active in the human being, which may be the case particularly at an early age, rickets will develop. Understanding the way the human being is connected with the surrounding world we come to see that the development of rickets in the human organism is a process similar to the one which occurs when phosphorus comes into existence in the outside world. Aphoristically and in a way of course where it is not possible to refer to every link in a chain of evidence, but in a particular instance, I am indicating the direction and method one uses to look for this connection of the human being with the rest of the world in the science of the spirit.

We can take things further. This morning I showed you how the system of limbs and metabolism on the one side and the neurosensory system on the other work together in the way I indicated by referring to the two systems and to the rhythmic system maintaining the balance between them [Plate 5]. Now you see the situation is that something which is irregular, causing sickness in the system of limbs and metabolism, actually brings health to the head system. This is why we always have certain functions in the human head system that are due to phosphorus, but an extremely small amount of phosphorus, which is in the human brain. As I have shown, in the system of metabolism and limbs this phosphorus activity inhibits the proper degradation or catabolism that goes into calcification processes. They must, however, be present in the brain, these phosphorus processes, where degradation has its place and above all must be continually in progress. In other words, having the phosphorus process present in the brain we have a continuous nascent state, I'd say, a kind of rickets development in the brain. Cerebral activity depends on it that bone wants to form all the time but is continually prevented from doing so once the cranium has properly developed around the human brain. In the human brain—as is evident on consideration—there is a constant tendency to develop bone. But this bone development comes to its conclusion at a certain age.

After this the bone-development activity is blocked. So here we really have a process that causes disease but is balanced out from the other side, the other pole of the organism. We see a constant tendency to develop rickets.

The remarkable thing is that a rhythm like this, the rhythm we observe in the human being, also exists in all the rest of the natural world, only that in some respect it goes in the opposite direction. Considering the remarkable significance of phosphorus for the human brain we have to say to ourselves: The phosphorus that is taken in is processed all the way up to the head. It goes through changes itself within the human organism. It follows the direction which is the direction of growth in human beings. It makes itself part of this direction. This reduces its activity to a minimum, dilutes the phosphorus, and in this attenuation its action is such that the rickets prevented from developing in the head can be the vehicle for exactly the processes in soul and spirit that have to be mediated by the human head.

The peculiar thing is that if people are given extremely small doses of phosphorus rather than somewhat larger doses, appreciable in the ordinary way, something else will be achieved also with regard to the functions of phosphorus. Introduced into the human organism these small doses act in that organism in the way in which phosphorus acts in the human brain. Their action in the rest of the organism will be to stop the rickets process when it has started in children. In this case, small amounts of phosphorus, minimal doses, are a medicine for rickets. In a wider sense phosphorus is altogether a medicine which restores everything in the I scaffolding—drawn here {see Plate 4, white} underneath the red—which due to sickness has emancipated itself from its real function in the soul, restoring its function in the soul, that is, changes it back to normal.

I had to speak in a highly complicated way about human nature so that you may see what is really behind the dispute between allopaths and homoeopaths. In certain areas, we may say, the principle behind homoeopathy is very evident, as in the case to which I have been referring. Rickets and also some other inflammatory conditions can certainly be cured with certain small doses of phosphorus or also sulphur, in short something combustible—I'll come back to this later—if they are due to blood activity having become emancipated from the I nature.

So you see that the connection between human beings and inorganic nature outside grows transparent if we are prepared to consider the human being in the way shown in the science of the spirit, as in this particular case. The things I have been saying here can certainly be extended to other inorganic substances. We have to go into the details, however. This way of bringing pathology, physiology and therapy together calls for dedicated study of the world inside the human being and the world outside. We may call phosphorus and sulphur combustible. Combustible substances—if we now really extend our contemplation—prove to be the ones that act very much in a way similar to the one just described for phosphorus. Their action is such that they are, in a way, restoring the emancipated I scaffolding to I activity.

Certain salts where the principle which is not combustible dissolves in water and separates out again when the water cools act in the opposite way. The action of these salts, carbonates, other salts, is such that they cause the element of mind or spirit and soul, and especially I activity, to connect too closely with the scaffolding, not separating the scaffolding off but in a way pushing the mind and soul element too firmly into it. They may be used medicinally when something has made the connection too loose. We are thus able to say: If we understand what a substance that we introduce into the organism brings about in it, if we understand how it influences the whole organization, we also understand how we can counteract some process or other that has become abnormal and needs to be counteracted.

With certain processes, for instance the one behind tuberculosis, called consumption in the past, soluble saltlike minerals are particularly effective. For tuberculosis demands that we counteract a process in the human organism which is the opposite of the process which occurs when salt dissolves in a solution. Extending our insights to the whole of essential human nature takes us into the human being's relationship with his whole outer environment.

Other examples can illustrate what I've been saying—I can only give some instances in this talk which is altogether aphoristic. Let us take examples—one can take them from anywhere, really, but let us take examples from a field which can at the same time take us into the whole relationship between mind and soul on the one hand and the physical on the other. The functions of the neurosensory system mean that we are conscious from waking up to going to sleep. We can say, therefore, that the head system reflects our conscious life. The system of metabolism and limbs is not a reflection in the same way of conscious life. We are moving around in the world with a conscious head and unconscious limbs, as it were. Our limbs only grow conscious when touched in some way, or are subject to injury and the like. We are thus able to say that for the head, the neurosensory system, consciousness in the waking state is the norm, and unconsciousness is the norm for the opposite system.

In a way it is however possible to generate a kind of consciousness for the system of limbs and metabolism artificially. It is done with massage, for instance. For what is massage? External measures are taken to make conscious what otherwise remains unconscious. One can improve inadequate connection between mind and soul on the one hand and the physical on the other by giving a massage. Let us assume someone was pathologically organized in such a way that where his mind and soul is concerned he is little inclined to drive this element of mind and soul fully into his system of metabolism and limbs. We support the physical aspect of this system of metabolism and limbs by massaging it, raising it to some degree from being spiritual to a state of consciousness. We support the functions of this system and this leads to an increased flow of the mind and soul element through the system. If we then know how this system of metabolism and limbs works, knowing for instance that the mind and soul element pulsing through arms and hands continues on inwardly and governs the internal human metabolism, we will also know what it means to induce partial consciousness by massaging arms and hands. This helps mind and soul in the metabolic system, but in the metabolic system which brings about digestion by being anabolic in an inward way, taking up physical matter in the digestive process.

We may say, therefore, that when someone is suffering internal metabolic disorders, these being metabolic disorders of a kind where food taken in does not integrate properly or the anabolic processes do not go the right way, in short, inward-directed metabolism is out of order, massaging arms and hands can be a help in some cases (one does of course have to have detailed knowledge to diagnose this correctly). This is because you are supporting the activities of mind and soul by the degree of conscious awareness arising on massage. Massaging legs and feet will have a different effect. The mind and soul element present in legs and feet is organically connected with eliminatory, degrading processes. If the digestive problems are such that eliminatory processes do not proceed in the right way, massaging legs and feet may be some help in the right circumstances.

You see that by using the science of the spirit to bring light into the field of medicine we are not acting in random empiricism, as evidence presents itself, but can quite deliberately work to influence the relationship between physiology, pathology and therapy in the various areas. As I said, I want to tell you these things merely to cast light on the directions to be taken. And I know full well how much they will take you aback, for it is of course not possible to go into every detail.

Take a condition, for instance, that may also prove to be a major headache for physicians—diabetes. We must again consider the relationship between mind and soul—the conscious mind and soul imbued with I on the one hand, and the physical vehicle for this I activity on the other. Something very different arises here from the first situation I spoke of today. Let us assume this I activity gets excessive in the human organism. It goes beyond its boundaries. Abnormal eliminatory processes like those seen in diabetics may then occur. We thus have excessive I activity in the organic sphere itself. The I is entering too deeply into the organic sphere, bringing out the phenomena one gets with diabetes.

Once again we may turn attention away from the processes within the human being and direct it to the surrounding world. Plants grow in that world, and this morning we saw how in a way they develop a process going from below upwards which human beings develop going down from above. The hypertrophic I activity influencing the organism in diabetes does indeed go in a direction opposite to that of plant growth. If we find the appropriate function in a growing plant, we may be able to establish a relationship between the process which in diabetics acts downwards from above and in the plant works in an upward direction. We merely have to say to ourselves as we look at the plant that it is a life form, and also physical; it grows, reproduces, and therefore has an etheric body. It also has an etheric body from the spiritual-scientific point of view. But it does not achieve inner mobility of soul, and therefore does not have astral quality; nor does it have I activity. But it does grow towards I activity, towards astral activity. Human beings develop in a downward direction what the plant develops in an upward direction.

When we are able to observe what is really going on in the plant as it grows in the direction which is the opposite in human beings, developing the I from above downwards, we find that something arises in the plant which can indeed have an inner connection to this inner I activity because it also has something to do with combustibility. I spoke of combustible substances before. Now we see combustible, volatile substance close to combustibility develop in the volatile or essential oils of the plant. When we see volatile oils develop in certain plants the kind of view to which I have just been referring shows that this is an activity opposite to the one performed by I activity pressed into the human organism which leads to diabetes. We can then combat diabetes by treating the individual concerned in the right way with something which is the opposite in the world outside.

It must be done by truly working in the opposite direction in this case, which means that we put the volatile oils or the actual plants containing the oil into baths and let the people bathe in them. The powers which the plant develops in its volatile oils then act inwards from outside to counter the powers that cause diabetes. We are able to help people in this way, with exactly such baths.

I am giving just a few examples, for there are many one could give. I did present many to the medical specialists in spring.[16] Here I am merely giving them to show the principles, but you can see that medicine is gradually made rational, giving examples, and truly seeing the process in the inner human being, seeing the process in the natural world outside, and seeing how the two processes either support, sustain or counteract one another. A process in the human organism can thus be brought to a halt, and it is possible to work towards a cure. Taking the approach further we can advance in gaining insight into the physical human being and his relationship to the human mind and soul. As you know, the problem of heredity plays a great role in modern scientific medicine. But it is treated in a highly abstract and superficial way. Only very little connection can be established in modern science with the processes that really go on in the human being. For human beings are indeed created out of the whole rest of the world which belongs to them as both the earthly world and the world beyond earth. I want to speak of something which has to be gained from a rich field of anthroposophical research, but here I would merely wish to give you a result.

Human beings have been created to be different. We find, for instance, that the female organism is made to be such, let us say, out of nature or the cosmos, that the forces are more to the fore which are less bound up with the forces of earth, as it were. The female organism has a powerful extraterrestrial element to it. The forces which predominate in the male organism are more connected with life on earth. This does not mean so much in everyday life, but it does play a role in procreation. The forces active in the female organism that play a role in procreation are really and truly a transmission of the extraterrestrial aspect in the whole of essential human nature. The principle which brings human beings down into the earthly world is mainly organized in the male organism. Let us consider the aspect of human beings which really is in them because of their earthly environment. The most obvious part of it is I activity. I activity actually gives human evolution on earth its full meaning. We have to find our way from other worlds into the earthly world so that we may fully develop I activity in mind and soul. I have shown you how this I activity is bound to the scaffolding of powers mediated by the blood. We would therefore have to say that the principle which is predominantly organized into the blood, acting predominantly towards I activity, is in procreation brought about by the male individual. The element which mainly organizes the extra-terrestrial in us and must first be imbued with I activity comes more from the female side.

We find thus the male and female principles working together in this way in procreation and can only gain the right ideas about heredity by realizing this. First the female seed, the ovum, is touched by the male influence. And this ovum has a degree of independence in the female organism. Considering the fully grown female organism we have to say that the extraterrestrial element is above all active in the rest of the female organism. It is not involved in the part of the female organism which provides the occasion for developing the ovum, especially after conception. The ovum therefore, having gone through conception, has a degree of independence and where the offspring is concerned independently transfers that which it signifies as mediator of I activity. Knowing these things we can apply the knowledge so that phenomena in the outside world come to meet one as if to illustrate the things we have first gained in the seeing mind. With the seeing mind we gain the insight that something from beyond this earth is indeed anchored in the female organism, that the earthly principle, which is particularly attached to blood activity, is mediated by the male organism, that this mediation gives the ovum a degree of independence, so that after insemination it develops apart from the rest of the extraterrestrial female organism.

Such a process, perceived in mind and soul, provides the background when we want to explain a remarkable condition such as haemophilia. The strange fact emerges that there are people whose blood does not coagulate properly and they may bleed to death with just a slight injury, often discharging much blood though there is no obvious injury. This haemophilia has a most peculiar characteristic. Men born into haemophiliac families will not develop the disease if born of women from non-haemophiliac families, but when women coming from haemophiliac families have descendants these do not themselves develop haemophilia but their male descendants do. The disease thus passes through the woman. This makes us aware of the ovum's independence to which I was referring. An external phenomenon serves as an illustration, as it were, for something we have gained in the seeing mind.

Today I have presented some things more or less in anecdotal form that point in the following direction. I have shown you how with the seeing mind one can see into essential human nature in real terms, into processes of anabolism and catabolism, processes of gaining health and falling ill that are really in constant interaction, with the balance needing to be found between them. I have shown you how with the seeing mind we can discover human interaction with the surrounding world, and how in this way a bridge can be built from physiology and pathology to therapy. And in the end I wanted to show you by means of a particular example—I chose the extreme instance of haemophilia and heredity with haemophilia—how looking at the natural world in the right way in situations where nature reveals her open secret we get an illustration of the things which we first perceived in spiritual science. So the objection cannot exist that it is not possible to see into the spiritual world, or words to that effect, that there is no way in which anyone can look for proof of anything which spiritual scientists maintain. That is indeed not the way things are. The point is that we can accept the spiritual-scientific results, I'd say, without being dogmatic about it or belief in authority, and on the other hand also without predetermined scepticism, full of prejudice. We simply take them in. We do not immediately say: I believe them, but we also do not reject them out of hand. We take them and test them against the reality of the world we live in.

If you apply in life what supersensible vision brings down from the spiritual world—what at first seems paradoxical and often even fantastic to you—you will see that it is confirmed in life, in the points that matter. You will find that empiricism is everywhere providing confirmation for the things discovered in the science of the spirit. People may make the excuse today that they cannot see into the spiritual world and therefore reject the insights into this world. They are like someone who sees an iron shaped like this [drawing, Plate 4, left] and says: I shoe my horse with it, it's a horseshoe. And someone else tells him: It's a shame to shoe your horse with it, for it has magnetic powers, it's a magnet. And the response is: I don't see any magnetic powers; for me, it's a horseshoe.

The situation is that the spiritual is present in all things material, that we are living in an age where this spiritual element must be sought. Someone who wants to research, to question matter without looking for the spirit is like the person who uses a magnet to shoe his horse, not knowing how things should be used exactly in the material world. The things I was able to say today to round out my lecture are aphoristic and lack completeness. The aim was merely to show the direction that needs to be taken especially in the study of medicine in future. For the study of medicine is intimately bound up with the social sphere. The human world can only gain social health if spiritual insight is brought into our social views, and in the same way medicine can only grow sound if the seeing mind is brought to it.

You see that we are not dreamers in any field. And the last thing we want to be in any field is amateurs. This is serious research, but research where the principle has been developed that is widely used today. When a hypothesis is set up somewhere one says it is useful for reviewing the phenomena. People are even thinking up such hypotheses or lines of thought in mathematics. The underlying principle in the science of the spirit is that we must not shy away from anything that is necessary for progress in human life, we must not hesitate to use all our powers to meet that need. We clearly perceive the signs of the times in the course of human evolution today, telling us that the old principles will no longer take us forward.

This Dornach has come into existence only because the old principles will no longer take us forward and we want to look for the new principles. We have specialized enough. Now we must bring the individual specialties together again. Perhaps this course will show you that there is a centre where the powers of mind must arise that will bring the individual specialties together. For this it will, however, be necessary to abandon the easy ways people are looking for today. But the fruits will above all go in the direction of human progress. It is exactly because of this that I would have liked it very much if specialists could also have said the things that may be said here in spiritual-scientific terms. And so I was not at all happy that when it came to a most important field, the field of medicine, I had to take over myself. But since that is the way things developed, there was nothing else for it, and you have to accept it.

What needed to be said here above all, presented by a specialist or someone taking a general view, would have been to show that even in this difficult field of medicine progress is possible only if the science of the spirit helps to make things fruitful. I'd say it would have been very clearly evident if in this field, too, someone had spoken who out of the traditions of our time, of everything which our age can provide for the medical profession, could on the other hand also have shown himself to be open to the science of the spirit. It is possible to be at the very height of modern medical science, official medical science, and yet be such a good spiritual scientist that one would think one could bear this medicine of today only if one can bring in the light of spiritual science. I do not know if this could be sufficiently evident to you from the fact that I had to take the place of the medical professional. But I hope there will be other occasions when one can show how it also grows perceptible to our age through external circumstances that medicine, too, can only be taken into the future if the spirit enters into it in the way intended or at least endeavoured here at this Goetheanum, with the spirit of Goethe brought into medicine.

II

ANTHROPOSOPHICAL BASIS FOR THE PRACTICE OF MEDICINE

LECTURE 5

You'll have to excuse me a little today for I have only just arrived, with an exhausting tour behind me, and basically will probably not be able to give a proper talk until tomorrow.

I would, however, like to give a kind of introduction today to the lectures I'll be giving here. It was not my original intention to speak at this medical event, for in my opinion ideas for medicine and natural-scientific thinking that result from the anthroposophical method of investigation should be taken up by people who are qualified in the field concerned. With any findings made in anthroposophical spiritual investigation relating to medicine and for example also to physiology, it is only possible to make suggestions which must then be taken further empirically. It needs this empirical work to form a valid, convincing opinion about the matter in question, an opinion of the kind needed in the field of therapy.

If I now give these few lectures after all, it is at the special request of our physicians here, and I'll endeavour to touch on the particular aspects in these days that enable the actual anthroposophical element to cast its light on the field of medicine. I will attempt to show that the opinion we can gain concerning the human being both in sickness and in health can be enriched and deepened with the anthroposophical view. In this introduction I may perhaps draw your attention to how this anthroposophical view should really be taken today—that is in the historical present. People easily confuse the discipline here called anthroposophy with earlier, traditional ways of considering humanity. I won't say a

word about them, nor criticize them, though it has to be said that the
views I represent have a very different basis than the mystical, theosophical, gnostic *etcetera* views that have become traditional in the course
of human history. I only have to stress the main point to show clearly
and radically the difference between the views represented here and
those earlier ones. Those earlier views are wholly based on human
thinking at a time when there was as yet no natural science in our sense,
and my views are based on the fact that they are arising at a time when
natural science has been developed and has even achieved a certain if
only temporary perfection. We must always think of this when we want
to grasp the whole meaning of the discussions, a meaning present in
anything that can be said and explored from the anthroposophical point
of view in the many different branches of human knowledge and skill.

   You all know—I need not go into detail—that in those earlier days
when the view of the supersensible world was free from natural science
(to our way of thinking, of course) there were also many supersensible
views in medicine, views about the human being that do not arise in the
way which we really consider to be a matter of course in empirical
science today. We need only go back to the time of Galen[17] approximately, and if sufficiently open-minded, we will everywhere find views
on the human being that provided the basis also for medical thinking.
Those views, considering the human form, the form of the organs, and
the functions of the human being, did in their way connect the things
which we today gain in empiricism with thoughts on supersensible
elements. They seem—as one will easily think—to have placed the
supersensible in human nature, but for them it was bound up with
human nature the way colours, forms and inorganic forces are bound up
with things in the outside world. Only prejudiced people will today
speak of those past times in the development of human medicine as if
views were childlike compared to modern ones. Historical texts are as
inadequate as possible particularly in this respect, and for someone who
enters a little into the historical evolution of humanity and does not take
the point of view that perfection has now been achieved and all that
went before was foolishness it will, of course, be clear that our present
level is again only relative and we certainly must not merely look down
on earlier times—as is evident even when we look at the successes. Yet

no one—irrespective of the approach he may be using to any branch of modern science—should fail to recognize the achievements of science in more recent times. If a way of looking at the human being in sickness and health that is in accord with the spirit, to use the Goethean term, is to find any kind of confirmation today it must not work against natural-scientific research but solely with natural-scientific research.

You will therefore not expect me to enter into any kind of polemics about natural-scientific views. Quite the contrary, I would stress from the beginning that this cannot be the case for a quite specific reason, on principle. You see, looking back at those earlier views in medicine we find that—although they were not as foolish as some might think today—they did lack the element which we have gained from natural science today. The reason why it was lacking was simply that human powers of perception were not at all such in those earlier times that things could be seen as we see them today in an empiricism based on the senses and given more power by instruments. The insights we gain through empiricism today are something of which we may say: The physician of old—forgive me for putting it like this, I might just as well say: The physiologist or biologist of old—saw something that was very different from what people see today. We could actually speak of the medical mind having a different orientation in those earlier times that really came to a radical end with Galen.

Galen did not see his four elements of the human organism—black and yellow bile, phlegm and blood—the way people see them today. He saw things differently, in such a way that as he described it and if one understands his words—we do not usually understand them as they have come down from earlier times—it's like a mist today. He saw this mist as a reality, not seeing phlegm as we know it today in his 'phlegm' but something that was not only fluid filled with life but also fluid filled with soul. That is what he saw. He would see it as clearly as when we say it is something red or blue. He thus saw something for which the modern scientific mind is no longer organized; on the other hand he did not see the things that we really have in mind scientifically today. One might say, let us assume, someone whose eye is not all that abnormal is using glasses and this means clearer outlines than he would perceive normally. And with modern empiricism, things that were blurred in the past but seen in mind and soul have vanished and instead we have the sharp outlines of present-day empiricism. People did not have those in earlier times. They would therefore also treat the sick out of a kind of instinct, which by the way was bound up with powerful development of human compassion. Physicians of old always entered into the patient's sickness with feeling, wearing them down at times. They treated them out of this. And they did not see the sharp contours we have with our empiricism based on the senses today.

The process leading to this empiricism has its foundations in human evolution and because of this we cannot simply get rid of it and go back to the old ways. We would need to acquire some kind of atavistic abilities to have the kind of thing naturally which the people of old had in all spheres, including the medical. Today we grow into our civilization simply because of the nature of our primary school education—I won't even mention higher education—and it is therefore impossible for us to see what people saw in the past. We cannot do so. If we were able to see things the way the people of old did we would be thought to be psychopaths today, not very bad ones but at least not quite as we should be. And that is not entirely wrong. For everything of an elemental nature today—well, let's call it clairvoyance—has something psychopathic about it. We have to be clear about that. But what we can do is to develop the inner capacities that otherwise lie dormant in the soul and so work our way up to seeing the spiritual element in the soul, just as the eye has worked its way up in the course of phylogenetic evolution from seeing things blurred to seeing sharp contours. Today we are able to develop powers of a seeing mind.

I have described the development of a seeing mind in *Knowledge of the Higher Worlds*[18] and in other books I have written.[19] When people develop such powers they will at first see a world which they did not see before, but one which encompasses a kind of spiritual cosmos beyond the cosmos we perceive with the senses today and the discoveries made and calculated in astronomy. A cosmos is added to the one we perceive through the senses which is wholly subject to natural laws. This is a spiritual cosmos. If we then pursue the things we can find in the spiritual cosmos we also find the human being in it. We grasp a spiritual universe, filled with soul, and as part of this universe filled with spirit and soul we find the human being. In ordinary natural science we start with the simplest creature or the simplest form of life, the cell, and then move up to complex elements, ascending from something which closely resembles simple matter that is physically differentiated, to the highly complex human organism.

Working in a serious way with the science of the spirit we start at the other end, as it were. We go down from grasping the spiritual in the universe and see this as the complex form. We see the cell as the simplest thing in the organism. From the spiritual-scientific point of view the universe is the most complex and where otherwise we make our own elements of insight complex to go from the cell to the human being we now simplify the things given in the cosmos more and more and this brings us to the human being. We take the opposite route, that is, we start from a point that is the polar opposite. Yet when we work with the science of the spirit today we do not initially and basically come to the regions that lie within our present-day evidence-based empiricism, for instance. I must really take care that no misunderstanding arises in these fundamental points. So I have to ask you to forgive me for being pedantic about some terms. It would be a massive error if someone were to think that it is pointless to apply evidence-based empiricism in physiology, in biology, what need is there of specialist knowledge; you develop spiritual abilities, look into the spiritual world and gain a view of the human being in sickness and health, establishing a spiritual medicine, as it were. Some people do this, but they gain nothing from it, except perhaps that they complain about empirical medicine but are in that case complaining about something they know nothing about. So there can be no question of drawing a line against the usual evidence-based empirical science and establishing a science of the spirit out of some cloud-cuckoo-land. That is not our attitude to the empirical sciences, that is, science called empirical today, though I'd prefer to call it evidence-based empirical science. That is not at all the case. Doing spiritual-scientific investigations you will not, for example, arrive at the same result as when you work with a microscope. You may certainly call someone a charlatan who wants to make you think that one will find the same through the science of the spirit as one does under the microscope. For that is not how it is. The things arising from empirical studies in the present-day sense are there. To make science complete in any particular field, also in terms of spiritual-scientific anthroposophy, it is not permissible to clear the evidence-based empirical findings out of the way, for we must indeed take them into account. Someone who is an expert, if I may use that term, in anthroposophical spiritual science will never find anything other than that to work in that science we are even more obliged to consider evidence-based empirical findings and the phenomena of the world.

The science of the spirit initially provides guidelines for empirical research, directives which show that when something is in a particular location in the organism we must also consider the nature of that location. Some will say that a cell is a cell, and that empirical observation must also show the distinctions between cells, be they liver cells or brain cells. But that is definitely not the case. You see when I pass a bench on a walk I take at nine in the morning there are two people sitting on it side by side. I look at them, form an opinion about various aspects relating to them. At three in the afternoon I walk that way again, and the two people are again sitting there. Well, the empirical facts are at first sight exactly the same in what I see, apart from subtle differences. But it may be that one of those people has continued to sit there for the six hours, and the other went away immediately after I walked past, has only just returned and went a long way in between. This will greatly change the picture and has nothing to do with the facts initially presented to my senses. The same facts present at nine in the morning and three in the afternoon. But the evidence of the senses must be judged in its context and in its elements. And there it is very much a matter of understanding, for instance, in how far a liver cell has to be judged in a completely different way from a brain cell, let's say, or a blood cell.

Only if it is correct, for example, that there was one original germ cell which was fertilized, and the whole organism can be explained as due to simple division of that germ cell—only if that were the case could we simply treat the liver cell in the same way as the brain cell and base ourselves wholly on the evidence of our senses. But if it were not the case, for instance because compared to a brain cell a cell in the liver relates differently to forces outside the human being, outside the human skin, simply because of its location, we cannot simply consider what happens in continuation of the division and the resulting location, but have to relate the brain cell to the universe in a totally different way than we do the liver cell.

When someone looks at a magnetic needle and finds that it points from south to north, north to south, and then insists that the forces responsible for this are in the needle itself, one would very definitely not call him a physicist today. As a physicist one relates the magnetic needle to something called the earth's magnetism. People may have all kinds of theories, but the direction of a magnetic needle cannot be ascribed to forces within it; the magnetic needle must be related to the universe.

When someone looks at the organic sphere, relationships to the universe are as a rule extraordinarily subordinate to him. But if it were to be the case that the liver, for instance, would have a totally different relationship to powers of the universe that are outside the human being than the brain, we would not be able to arrive at any kind of explanation for the human being by today's route of factual empiricism. In that case we'd only arrive at an explanation of the human being if we were able to say what share the whole universe has in configuring the brain and configuring the liver, just as the earth has a share in determining the direction of the magnetic needle.

Today we are studying the aspects of the hereditary stream, let us say. We go back to the ancestors or to the present time, we go to the descendants, doing so in the succession of animals, in the succession of human beings, consider what we find in that way—we must, of course, have the necessary knowledge—but we are only considering whatever the immediate events tell us, considering them in their inner human aspect, as it were. We don't ask if it might not be that the fertilized ovum in the human organism is merely given opportunity to let powers from the universe influence it in all kinds of different ways. Nor do we ask if it is perhaps not altogether so that the configuration of the fertilized ovum cannot be explained if we stay inside the human being. Surely we must relate it to the whole universe. In official science the powers influencing us from the universe are secondary. You will say: Yes, but science takes us to a point today where we do not come to ask such questions; it is out of date to relate the human organs to the universe.

And it is indeed something out of date the way it is often done. The fact, however, that we are altogether and on the broadest base not encouraged to ask such questions is merely due to our education in science. This is such that we are kept at the level of this merely evidence-based empirical science, as it were, and therefore never think of asking questions of the kind which I have been putting here, initially merely hypothetically, as an introduction. It really depends on raising questions how far we get in gaining insight and how far we progress in human activity in all areas. When no questions are asked we are really living in a kind of scientific fog. We obscure our view of reality itself. And then it happens that we will really only see how limited our vision is when things no longer fit in with our thoughts and ideas.

I do however think that this feeling which I am thus referring to may really be most prevalent in present-day medicine. It is the feeling that things are really going very differently in human beings than they ought to if following the often rather straight theories, theories by the way on which treatment is also based. One then gets the feeling that surely it must be possible to use some other approach to the issue. I really believe that the things which need to be said here can mean something to hardly any expert in the field but to those who follow developments in healthy and sick individuals and see how the views generally held are too glib and never get anywhere near the complexity of things.

Let's be honest for once. Let us consider how in the whole of the nineteenth century scientific and practical thinking did in all spheres always produce something like an axiom. It's enough to make one despair how this axiom-like thing is always flung at one. People would always say that explanations should be as simple as possible. And people did make their explanations as simple as possible. Well, when things and developments are complicated it is prejudice to say that explanations should be as simple as possible. It needs an effort to go into the complexities. Enormous damage has been done in this respect, I'd say, in the whole of human nature where knowledge and practice are concerned because people would proclaim again and again: Explanations must be as simple as possible.

Everywhere, on the smallest scale and the largest, nature is not simple but tremendously complex. And we can really only get anywhere near nature if we know from the start that even the seemingly most perfect views relate to reality the way photos of a tree do that are taken from one side. I can photograph the tree from many different angles. The photos may differ completely from one another. The more photos I have the sooner will I come close to the reality of the tree in my idea of it.

With regard to theories and views the present-day opinion is that one particular theory is true. Any other theory one may have is then wrong. But that is exactly like the situation when someone photographs a tree from one side. He then has that photo. Someone else photographs the tree from a completely different angle. The first person shows him his photo and he says: That's wrong, completely wrong, only this one is right. Meaning that his view is the right one. That is more or less how people have been in dispute over materialism, idealism, realism and all kinds of things. The battles fought in this sphere are no different from the seemingly commonplace example I have been giving you. I would therefore ask you from the start not to take the things I have to say here as if they were materialistic, idealistic or spiritualist, but merely as intended to approach reality in accord with human powers of vision. We can sometimes achieve a great deal with materialistic ideas when we want to control the real world, providing we are also prepared to marshal the opposite aspect. If we are not in a position to tell the aspects apart, well then we get human views that are more or less like having all kinds of different photos taken on one and the same [photographic] plate. Many of the things put forward today do look as if photos from all kinds of different angles had been taken on one plate.

Now you see if we make the powers which I said are latent in the soul active, using the means I discussed in my book *Knowledge of the Higher Worlds*, we do indeed go beyond the ordinary level of insight—pursued with special care in the most recent phase in biology—to the insight in images which I described. A further level is inspired insight, and the highest level to date, if I may use the term, is intuitive insight, truly intuitive insight. With insight in images I get images of the reality, knowing full well that they are images, but I also know that they are not dream images but images of the real thing. Insight in images does not yet give me that reality, but I have images of something real. With inspired insight these images gain consistence, as it were, something is alive in them; I know more thanks to the images than the image as such is able to give. I know from the images that they refer to a spiritual reality. And with intuitive insight I am within this spiritual reality itself. That is the progression. You will find everything that can be said about these three kinds of insight in the book to which I have referred on several occasions.

Initially these three kinds of insight, which are beyond the insight into facts apparent to the senses, give us insights into spiritual worlds—a spiritual universe and the spiritual human being, the human being in mind and soul. Initially it is not insight concerning empirical research findings we have in, say, biology today. But the application of the special state of soul into which we enter with image-based insight, inspired or intuitive insight to the study of the human being is something else.

You see, we contemplate the structure of the human brain, for example. This is something worthy of note, not so much to physiologists and the medical profession but to those who are called psychologists. Psychologists are a group apart within our civilization, for as you know they have managed to have a science with no object—psychology without soul, without psyche. For psychologists the structure of the brain is worthy of note. Take a psychologist, for instance, who has actually come from wholly empirical science. People did not know how to get anywhere with philosophy in most recent times, for they could not tell if a philosopher knew something or not. It was clear that natural scientists always knew something, and so natural scientists who also had an interest in philosophy were given chairs of philosophy in more recent times. With natural scientists it is a matter of course that they know something, for in philosophy you can use lots of words but in natural science you can't be airy-fairy, saying you've seen things under the microscope or through a telescope or on an X-ray. This will be evident when checks are made. In philosophy it is not so easy today to check if someone is being airy-fairy. Consider how Theodor Ziehen[20] talks about the structure of the brain. Something really interesting happened to me in this respect. Maybe a story will help to make it clear. I attended a meeting once—many years ago—where a physician spoke first about the structure of the brain, explaining it in relation to the inner life, his point of view being one it would be fair to call materialistic. This out-and-out materialist explained the structure of the brain pretty well according to the present state of knowledge, and related the inner life to the structure of the brain. The chairman at the meeting was a Herbartian and he construed for himself not the structure of the brain but life in ideas, as the philosopher Herbart[21] once did. And he said that it was remarkable how a physiologist, a physician, makes a drawing of the brain, drawing figures. When I as a Herbartian, he said, draw the complex associations of ideas, meaning just a depiction of linked ideas, not of nerve strands connecting one nerve cell with another—when I as a real Herbartian who is not concerned with the brain draw my ideas of the way in which ideas are linked and so on, doing so in a wholly symbolic form, it looks very similar to the physiologist's drawing of the brain's structure.

The similarity has its reasons. As scientists have progressively established the structure of the brain in natural science, it became more and more evident that the external structure of the brain corresponds most beautifully to the structure of our life in ideas. Everything we find in the life of ideas may also be seen in the structure of the brain. It simply is—please take this with a grain of salt—as if nature herself deliberately made the brain a sculpted image of our life in ideas. Such things really strike one when one reads what someone like Meynert[22] has written, for instance. It is now a little out of date. Meynert was a materialist but an excellent brain physiologist, psychiatrist, and one would like to say, 'Yes, he is a materialist, but the things he gives us as a materialist are an excellent payment on account for the things we also discover if we don't bother with the human brain at all but merely consider how ideas link up, separate, and so on, merely wanting to draw these symbols.' In short, if anything is liable to make us into materialists, the structure of the brain would be particularly apt to do so. We certainly have to say that if there is such a thing as mind or spirit and soul, it has found an adequate reflection in the human brain, so that we are very close to saying, 'Well, why do we need spirit and soul in order to live in ideas? If we were also to ask for a soul that is able to think! Since the brain is such an accurate reflection of mind and soul, why should it not also be able to think?'

You must, of course, take all these things with a grain of salt. My intention is merely to give you the meaning of this whole dispute today. The human brain can certainly make us into materialists, especially when we go into more detailed research. And the secret which governs it all, the background to it all, will only emerge when we gain the power of insight in images. For there you see images, images of things truly spiritual, images one has not seen before. I'd like to say, however, that those images are reminiscent of the images taking form in the human brain out of nerve cells and nerve fibres. In answer to the question as to what this insight in images, which is of course wholly in the super-sensible sphere, really is, I'd say this. To give you symbols for this insight in images, the way a mathematician does with the symbols for mathematical problems, I might also say: Imagine that we perceive more in the world than we do through the senses by rising to images that present a reality, just as the human brain presents the reality of the human soul. In the brain, nature herself presents as images real to the senses something which insight in images really provides at a higher level.

With this we enter more deeply into the human constitution. In the days to come we'll see that we always arrive at a possibility not to see this marvellous structure of the human brain in isolation. But, I'd say, when we see a world, a supersensible world up above by means of vision in images, it is as if part of this world had come to realization down here, with an image-based world presenting itself to us in the human brain. In fact, I do not think that anyone can speak adequately about the human brain who does not see its structure as a presentation in images of our soul life. And it is this which takes us again and again into a dilemma when we want to get to the soul life from the physiology of the brain. For if we want to stop at the brain, we simply don't need the soul life. The only people who have the right to speak of soul life as compared to the structure of the human brain are those who know this soul life in another way as well, not only the ordinary way of this world. For when you get to know this soul life in the spiritual world, it is adequately reflected in the structure of the human brain, and anything which the supersensible organ of the soul is able to produce by way of ideas the brain is able to produce as well. The brain is a reflection, an image, even in its functions, and no one can prove or disprove materialism on the basis of brain physiology. That simply cannot be done. If human beings were nothing but brain, one would have no need to discover that they also have a soul.

Let us now turn to a function other than forming ideas. This will just be an introduction to a subject matter which I'll be presenting over the next few days. Let us turn to the breathing process. I am treating it as a function here. Call to mind the respiratory processes and human awareness of them. You will not arrive at something like life in ideas. Saying, 'I have an idea; it reminds me of another which I had three years ago. I'll link the one with the other . . .' you will indeed have sketches, especially if they cover a number of ideas, that are very similar to Meynert's drawings showing the structure of the brain. You will not be able to do this when you relate the nature of the breathing process to the human organism. You'll not find the same kind of adequate reflection in the structure, differentiation or formation of the organs for the respiratory process as you do for the process of forming ideas in the brain. This you cannot do. In the respiratory process we have something which cannot be adequately reflected in the human organism the way our life of ideas and of sensory perception is reflected in the human organism, with the life in ideas, in perceptions, also adequately reflected in the structure of the brain. But when we rise to inspired insight, that is, come to perceive how with insight in images we first have images and then reality enters into them with inspired insight shining through them, I'd say: If we learn thus to look into the supersensible world and the images are saturated for us with spiritual reality, then we are suddenly in something supersensible which is wholly similar to the relationship between the respiratory process, the structure of the lung, the structure of the epidural space or spinal canal, with the thrust of the breath penetrating to the brain. In short, when you advance to inspired insight you find the principle which takes you to the whole significance of the respiratory process just as insight in images takes you to the significance of the brain's structure. You are then able to say: Where the brain is insight in images brought to realization, everything connected with respiration is an inspiration brought to realization, taken down into the sense-perceptible world. All that someone who is looking for inspired insight is doing is to enter into a world which in that case is spirit and soul but lies before us here in the sense-perceptible world when we study the whole of the respiratory process in its significance for the organism.

We thus really need insight in images to understand the structure of the brain and inspired insight to understand the breathing rhythm and everything connected with it. Everything connected with the breathing rhythm is therefore something entirely different, relative to the universe, from the structure of the brain. The latter, I'd say largely reflects the spiritual in its external three-dimensional form. And so we need not advance far into the supersensible world, only as far as insight in images which comes right next to ordinary insight and we will gain understanding of the brain's structure. You won't find the respiratory process with insight in images; you need inspired insight and have to move higher up in the supersensible world.

And you see we have to go farthest in the supersensible world if we want to understand the metabolic process. Essentially this metabolic process is the most mysterious element in the human being. We shall see in the days to come that we have to think very differently about this metabolism from the way one does today in empirical physiology based on sensory perception. The changes gone through by the physical matter placed on my tongue, to the point, let us say, where it makes something happen in my brain cell—these changes cannot be discerned with mere empirical research but only with intuitive insight. With this we penetrate from merely looking at the object into the object itself. And human metabolism is indeed such that compared to the element of mind and soul which creates an image of itself in the brain, otherwise remaining outside it, influences the breathing rhythm, entering into it and filling it with spirit and soul, but always withdrawing again, the human spirit and soul enters completely into metabolism, actually vanishing into it. We won't find it again. Nor will we find it empirically.

Take a look at Theodor Ziehen's book, how well he describes the structure of the human brain. You can indeed analyse the powers of memory so well, also symbolically, that you will be able to demonstrate matching physiological and anatomical forms in the brain. Things got awkward when Ziehen came to the feelings; he therefore did not refer to feelings as something independent, but only to ideas with a strong feeling element. Psychologists no longer refer to the will at all today. Why? It's perfectly natural that they don't. Now if I want to raise my arm, that is, perform an act of will, I first have the idea; then something goes down into the sphere which is completely 'unconscious', as it is said to be today. Everything that cannot be observed in the soul but is nevertheless believed to exist is put into this reservoir. The whole of it then goes down into the unconscious mind. I then look at the way I move my hand. But between the intention and the accomplished fact the act of will taking place goes wholly down into the material aspect of the physical organism. Intuition allows one to follow this exactly. The will goes down into the inner nature of the organism. The act of will goes as far as metabolism. There is no act of will in physical human beings on earth which cannot with intuitive insight be traced to a particular metabolic process. Yet there also is no will process which is not reflected in a process of decomposition or dissolution, call it what you will, in the metabolic sphere. To be able to unfold, the will first gets something which is there somewhere in the organism out of the way. It is as if I must first burn up something in my arm when I need it to express my will. Something must first be got out of the way. In the next few days it will become evident, I know that it is utter heresy in natural science but it will show itself to be the truth, that something must first be put out of the way. Physical substance must first be destroyed so that the will may have a place. The element of spirit and soul must occupy the place made free by destroying some physical material. That is the essential nature of intuitive insight. You will not be able to explain metabolic processes in human beings unless you look for them with intuitive insight.

All the functions to be found in human beings really consist in these three: the neurosensory process, the rhythmic processes—breathing and the circulation of the blood—and the metabolic processes. The human being thus is really insight brought to realization and made physical, i.e. what we see initially when looking at it from outside or investigating by dissection. Limiting ourselves to the human head we come to realize what is really going on in the head if we know that there is such a thing as insight based on images. Looking at the rhythmic human being—

what is really going on there becomes evident if we know that there is inspired insight. Looking at the metabolic processes—we realize what is going on there if we know what an intuitive insight is. The reality principles in the human being thus lie one in the other. Look at the organs, for instance, that are wholly organs of the will and only intuitive insight will make it possible to understand them.

For as long as we apply the one, unvarying form of gaining insight to the human being we will not discover that this human being is in fact something different from what we ordinarily feel him to be. As you know, it is known in modern physiology that the human being is largely seen as a column of water. No need for me to tell you. But if you now consider in all honesty if the fact that the human being is a column of water is taken into account in physiology, or if people do not after all think of nothing but sharply outlined solid forms in considering the human being, if you ask yourself about this you will say: Little regard is given to the fact that essentially human beings are fluid, with solid forms merely included in it. The human being is also made of gases, however, air, and finally also in the main of warmth.

Ordinary study gives me a good grasp of the solid element in the human being. Just as I get to know the nature of red mercury sulphide (cinnabar) in the laboratory, so I can get to know the nature of solids by physico-chemical investigations of the human organism.

I cannot do this with regard to fluids in the human being. The fluid organization is constantly being organized and de-organized in human beings; it cannot be drawn the way I draw the stomach or the heart. If I draw these organs as if they were solid, it is, of course, easy to discuss them. But that is not how things are when we really take this fluid organization seriously. In the fluid sphere something is all the time developing and disappearing again. It is as if the heart were always developing and disappearing again, though not at great speed. To approach the fluid human being we need insight based on images.

As to the gaseous, aeriform part of us, we do of course know the great significance of the functions in the aeriform part of the organism; we know that aeriform substances in the organism move from everywhere to everywhere, and how everything is in circulation in that sphere. But when one sphere of the aeriform influences another it does so exactly according to the pattern of inspiration. We are only able to gain an overview of the aeriform element in us if we work with inspiration.

As to the sphere of warmth in the human being, try for a moment to understand that man is something quite special because human beings are warmth structures, with warmth and coldness in structure in all kinds of different places and in all kinds of different ways. You have to be right inside the way human beings live in their own warmth with their I. You have to enter into this with intuitive insight.

If you consider the human being as a whole, not as a combination of solid, sharply outlined organs but as a whole, you may truly say that we have to go in from different angles. Driven to gain insight in images, by inspiration or intuition we come from the brain to the other organ structures, and the same applies when we consider the different states of aggregation in the human being. You see, when you consider the solid structures, the actual solid bodies in the human being, these hardly differ from such as are found outside the human organism. But the fluid elements and the gaseous elements differ greatly, and the warmth element even more so. We will talk about this in the days to come. But the organs only gain their proper significance for our insight into the nature of the human being if we broaden our approach to the human being.

Physiology that is purely based on sensory perception and empiricism barely allows you to trace the functions of the human organism beyond the progression of chyme from the intestinal villi into the lymph vessels. That is as far as you can still get in today's sensory-experience-based empiricism. Beyond this, people are really fantasizing. All ideas on what then happens to the material we take in from outside—for instance what happens in the circulating blood—are basically mere indulgence in fantasy in modern physiology. Something like the involvement of the kidneys in the human organization, for instance, can only be grasped if we consider the descending processes and not only the ascending processes which today are almost the only ones considered important for the human constitution. A long time ago I told a friend: Considering the unfolding of the human germ from fertilization to birth is important, but it is equally important to consider the organs that lie around the germ and are later cast out. We will only get a complete picture when studying cell division if apart from this ascending process we also follow the descending process. For we do not only have this descending process next to us, as it were, in the embryonic period but we have it in us also in later life. We need to know for every organ in how far there are ascending processes in it and in how far descending processes. Descending processes are as a rule connected with increased conscious awareness. For a clear mind we actually need descending processes, decomposition, destruction, clearing away matter.

It is the same with the eliminatory processes. The kidneys are organs of elimination. The question is, however: If in the sensory experience of empiricism they are initially organs of elimination, do they not also have significance for the human constitution? Is there not something other than this eliminatory function, something which makes the kidneys more important in building up the human being? If we trace the functions further and move, say, from the kidney to the liver, we have the following interesting phenomenon. The kidney ultimately discharges matter to the outside; the liver secretes to the inside. The question arises as to what it means for the relationship of the liver process to the kidney process that the kidney relatively discharges its secreted products to the outside and the liver to the inside. The human being is thus communicating with the outside world in the one case and with itself in the other. This gradually guides us to full insight into the human organism. But we must, of course, make use of the insights sought along the routes I was able to refer to briefly as an introduction today. I intend to take this further in my next lecture and show how these methods lead to genuine understanding of pathology and therapy and how far we have guiding principles for empirical research, the method recognized today, which we certainly do not want to touch in any way. We merely want to show how it is really only given its true value if we are able to establish such guidelines.

I am not in the least keen to do anything against modern natural-scientific research. On the contrary, I would like to show that tremendously rich resources still lie in this natural-scientific medicine to provide better insight than is gained with present-day methods and above all from the present-day point of view. The natural-scientific approach is not to be given a bad name but rather given the right foundations. Given such a basis out of the spirit it will gain its full significance. I'll continue with this tomorrow.

IF I were asked to organize the study of medicine for people who come to it directly and want to complete it in the course of some time, I would have to start—once the necessary knowledge of natural science has been gained—with a look at the different human functions. I would have to start anatomically and physiologically with the digestion of foods from mixing with ptyalin and pepsin to where foods are taken up into the blood, and then, having discussed the whole act of digestion in the narrower sense, move on to discussing the system of heart and lungs and everything connected with this. Then I would have to discuss everything connected with the human renal system. This would have to be considered in conjunction with the whole apparatus of nerves and senses which does not at all relate to the renal system in the way suggested on the basis of today's accepted knowledge, and then come to the system of liver, bile, spleen. In following this cycle we would gradually gain an overview of the way things are arranged in the human organism. We need this to develop what needs to be developed with the anthroposophical science of the spirit. On the basis, I'd say the illumination, of the results of empirical studies based on sensory experience, we would arrange them in the order I've just given, and then be able to move on to the therapeutic field.

Now you can imagine that a few days only allow me to touch lightly on such a vast, comprehensive field. Our professional medical friends can only touch on things lightly in the whole of this week of medical talks, and it will therefore be necessary for me to say a great many things that are based on a way of treating the empirical data which is not customary today but nevertheless arises of its own accord, I think, for anyone with the relevant present-day knowledge in physiology and also therapy. Some things will of course have to be put in a different way from the usual, but there is really nothing which cannot be made to be in some kind of harmony with today's empirical knowledge based on sensory experience and taken as a whole. Everything I will be able to say will be aphoristic and basically merely state the ultimate aim. Our starting point would, however, be present-day empiricism based on sensory experience, and the road in between would really have to be produced by the efforts of our medical friends to the widest extent, for this road in between is extraordinarily long and absolutely necessary simply because of the way things are today. The things we can present here today will essentially never be given full recognition unless this road is taken at least for the most important phenomena. Nor do I think that it is as difficult as it looks today. The effort must simply be made to bring the preliminary work—already available—sometimes extra-ordinarily good but not taken to its culmination the way it is today— into the context of the kind of general view I am attempting to indicate here.

Yesterday I attempted to show you how we can approach the human being by broadening the usual way of gaining insight, as it were. If you take into account what I have just been saying I may also be permitted to add the following. You may initially find it most objectionable when people say in the field of anthroposophy that one must differentiate the human being, as he presents himself in the physical world, into a system organized etherically, a system—please don't take umbrage at the words used, they merely serve to give us a terminology—a system organized astrally and the one which characterizes the human being as an actual I system so that he may develop that inner combination of soul qualities, inner soul which we do not see in animals, a combination which on the one hand appears because human beings are able to bring together their inner experiences in one I point, if I may call it that. From that point their whole organic activity radiates out, in a sense, at least in the conscious state, and this is on the other hand reflected in the fact that during their development on earth human beings relate differently to sexual development, or the development of generations, than the animal organization does. Basically the animal organization is such—there are, of course, always reasons for exceptional development—that it culminates in sexual maturity and there is then a certain decay which may not be very radical after the first period of sexual maturity, but there is a degree of organic decay. In human beings on the other hand physical development takes a certain upswing with sexual maturity. Externally, empirically, if we take all factors into account, there certainly is a difference between man and animal.

You may say that it is really an abstract differentiation to speak of physical organization, etheric organization, astral organization and I organization. Various people have raised that objection, especially from the philosophical side. One has the functions of the human organism and differentiates between them—differentiation need not always have a factual basis—and believes one is dealing with an abstraction. That is not the case. We shall see what lies behind it in the course of these days. It is not just a longing to have things in schematic form which is behind it, for it is actually the case that when we speak of the human physical organization this includes everything in the human organism which we are able to treat the way we do in our laboratory experiments and investigations. We cover all this when speaking of the human physical organization.

Yet when we speak of the human etheric organization we are not in a position to treat our way of thinking with regard to this etheric organization which is incorporated into the physical organization by stopping at the ideas and laws we discover in our laboratory experiments and observations. You may think as you will initially about the etheric organization as it presents to supersensible investigation. But without the need to go somehow into the mechanistic or the vitalistic method, it is nevertheless evident—it would be subject to long discussions that would be part of the curriculum of which I spoke before—that the whole etheric organization, which you merely have to think of as a structure of functions, intervenes directly in everything that is fluid by nature in the human organization. We must therefore limit our physical way of thinking to everything which is solid in the human organization, essentially the solid state of aggregation, and only manage to cope with the human organization if we consider the fluid element in this organization not merely as fluid, as we have it in the inorganic natural world outside, but as a fluid element that is fully enlivened, as living fluid. This is what we mean when we say that the human being has an ether body. And we need not go into hypotheses about life but merely take what we mean, for instance, when we say: The cell has life. We need not go further than that, irrespective of whether we are mechanists, idealists or spiritualists. If we say the cell has life—as an out-and-out empiricist would also say—it is directly evident, with the method to which I am referring, that the element which is fluid by nature in the human being has life. This is the same as saying: The human being has an ether body. We therefore have to see everything solid as embedded in fluid. This immediately gives us the contrast. Everything known by way of laws and ideas in the inorganic world is also applied to the solid parts of the human being, and not only the cells as the smallest organisms found in the human being are believed to have life but the totality of fluid elements in the human being is considered to be full of life.

What is more, when we then come to the gaseous element in the human being we find that everything of that nature is in a continuous exchange process. We will have to make it clear during these days that the exchange is not merely inorganic, nor is it mediated merely by the solid organs. The human organism has its own laws to govern the swirl of one into the other in the internal exchange of gases. We have inner laws relating to the solid element, reflected in the relationship between kidneys and heart, and we also have to accept a set of laws within this organism of gases or air, if I may call it that, which is not limited to the laws of solid physical organs. The laws which directly govern the organism of gases or air are in anthroposophy called the astral laws for the human being, the astral organization. They would not exist in human beings if these had not brought the aeriform organization into their solid and fluid organization. The astral organization does not intervene directly in the solid and fluid elements; it acts directly on the aeriform organization, and the latter does indirectly intervene in all kinds of ways in the solid and fluid organization. An organized astral organization thus exists within the airy human being, if I may call it such. This gives the airy organization a particular inner form which is, of course, fluctuating.

We simply move up through the states of aggregation and say to ourselves: Looking at the solid human being, we need to assume nothing but a physical organization. Looking at the living fluid present throughout the solid physical organization we have to assume something which is not limited to physical laws, for there we come to the etheric organism which is a system complete in itself. In the same way I call something 'astral organization' which does not intervene directly in the solid and fluid organism but in the first place in the gaseous organization. I do not call it 'astral laws' but 'astral organism' because it is a system complete in itself.

And we arrive at the I organization in the same way. It only intervenes directly in the differentiations between temperatures in the human organism, so that we may speak of a warmth organism, a human being of warmth. The I organization influences this human being directly; being supersensible it effects the differentiations in temperature and above all also perceives them, lives in them. There the I organization lives directly; it does so indirectly in the rest of the organism in that the warmth influences all gaseous, fluid and solid organization.

Thus, you see, the human organism gradually becomes transparent. But everything I have said so far is such in physical human beings on this earth that it is also reflected in the physical human being. Looking at the organization which we may, in a sense, call the most volatile, the I and warmth organization, we see that it has an indirect influence on the gas organization below, on the fluid organization and the solid organization, and the same holds true for the others, so that a solid organ system, initially capable of being established in external anatomy, reflects how this whole differentiated system influences the human organization as we know it from empirically established facts based on sensory experience. We can thus always refer to organ systems where only the solid, physical system relates directly to its laws, the fluid does so indirectly, the gaseous even more indirectly and the element of warmth as the most remote but nevertheless relating through intermediaries.

All the things I can now only refer to briefly as in thoughts to aim at can always be proved by means of extended empiricism, simply from the evidence of our senses. Time is short and so I can only give you thoughts to aim at.

If we take the human organization anatomically and physiologically we can first of all consider the route taken by a food until it arrives at the intestinal walls with all the complicated organs in that location and is taken up into the lymph and blood channels. We are thus able to follow digestion or nutrition in the widest sense as far as uptake into the lymph and blood channels. Initially we limit ourselves to this field as we use a method of study generally applied in natural science today, though it is not entirely mechanistic, and manage reasonably well. A completely mechanistic view will not quite take us to our goal in this field either, for the laws we observe outside, in the laboratory, and characterize as inorganic laws in natural science, do after all come into play in the digestive tract, i.e. in the living organism. Life takes them in from the beginning, when ptyalin is added. Yet if we take account only of this, that external inorganic laws are as it were immersed in the life of the digestive tract, we can certainly manage for such a limited field providing we stick to the things which can be observed within the human physical organization. But we must in that case be clear in our minds that there remains a residue of nutritional activity, digestive activity, that nutrition is not quite finished when the intestinal wall has been passed, and that we need to bring in other methods of study, as it were, for what follows.

For the limited field we'll manage reasonably well if we first consider all conversions that take place by analogous methods, I'd say, like anything we get to know externally. There, however, we find something which is not easily acknowledged in modern science but is nevertheless a truth which does certainly emerge from modern science. It would now be up to our medical friends to follow these things in a purely scientific way and then to show that it simply emerges from the empirical facts based on sensory experience that with foods taken in, ptyalin and pepsin added and so on, the foods are prepared in such a way that they first lose every trace of their old existence in the outside world. You know, we take in foods from the mineral sphere—you may not like to use the term 'food' for this, but we can understand one another when I want to use some term or other—we take in food from the mineral, vegetable and animal worlds. The food we take in has gone through the mineral, animal and vegetable organization. The food most similar to the human organization is the milk which the infant is given by his mother. He receives it as soon as it has left the human organization. The process which takes place in the human organization when food is taken in is that it is taken into the different glandular products and essentially every trace of its origin is removed. We might even say that the element which makes it possible for us to let a purely natural-scientific, inorganic way of looking at things develop is something in which the human organization comes to our aid. Truly the chyme or partly digested food comes closest to external physical processes when it moves from the intestine into the lymph and blood channels. Human beings remove all the external properties of the chyme. They want to have it as similar as possible to inorganic organization. This is what they need, and they differ in this from the animal world.

If you study the anatomy and physiology of animals you will find that animals do not remove the constitution of material that passes into their body to the same degree. It is another matter with their products of elimination. The matter which passes into the body is more similar to its outer organization in animals than it is in humans, that is, more similar to the vegetable and animal nature, continuing on into the bloodstream according to its external constitution in its inner laws. In human beings the organization has advanced so far that human beings have made the chyme as inorganic as possible when it is allowed to pass the intestinal wall. There the purely physical human being is really present in the region where the chyme passes from the intestine into the organization of heart and lung, if I may put it like that.

This is the point where the approach we have been using here must for the first time turn into heresy for official natural science. For if you take the whole heart and lung tract—meaning the vascular system—if you take this whole tract, it is this which really changes food that has become wholly inorganic, if I may put it like that, into something that has life. The human organization cannot survive unless it gives itself the quality of life. In a wider sense—again we need not go into the inner nature but only the things we are always talking about in physiology— this is similar to the moment when we see the inorganic parts, say of protein, transformed into living protein, dead protein into living protein. Time being so short, we cannot in view of the present situation in theoretical science look at the way plants produce living protein. The fact is that in human beings the process in which protein is given life comes when the chyme has been made as inorganic as possible. It happens through the system of heart and lungs, with all its appendages, of course. We are thus able to say: The system of heart and lungs exists to take the element which is physical system into the etheric organization. As human beings—it is not at the same level in animals, where it is much less clear-cut—we thus have a process of vitalization, catching the inorganic and taking it into the organic, into the vital sphere in a process taking place in the system of heart and lungs.

This process could not happen in our physical world if certain conditions were not met in the human organization. You see, what I am now presenting to you as a transformation of chyme into an etheric organization, capturing and taking it into an etheric organization, cannot really happen without further ado within the laws that apply on earth. Angels can do it, but if they did the spirits who did it would have to do it by flying around having a mouth, an oesophagus and finally a system of stomach and intestines. Then that would cease to be and vanish into the etheric. So we would have digestive tracts floating about, borne by invisible etheric angelic spirits. The process I have been describing could not at all happen in the physical world without further ado; that would be impossible. It is only made possible in that the whole etheric system is forcibly taken down into the physical, made part of the physical, and this happens due to oxygen being taken up in respiration. So human beings are not angels now but able to walk about on earth in physical form, walk about because their angelic nature is made physical as they take in oxygen. This projects the whole—but in real terms— into the physical world, with the whole taking place as a physical system. Something that otherwise could only be wholly supersensible by nature performs this function as a system of heart and lungs.

We thus come to see that just as carbon is the basis of animal, vegetable and human organization—the human organization as well, except that it is not as solid as in the plant—in that it fixes the actual physical organization, so does oxygen relate to the etheric organization in so far as it comes to expression in the physical realm. Here we have the two substances which essentially constitute protein in vitalistic form.

But we have been using an approach that might equally well be applied to the protein cell, the cell itself. We merely extend the approach that might be used for the cell and really should only just begin, by taking not a microscopic view of the human being but a macroscopic view as we look at the processes that are the link between digestive tract and the tract of heart and lungs, seeing how they are inwardly connected, how an etheric organization intervenes and is fixed physically by taking in oxygen.

Now you see that this would only give us an entity that would exist in the physical world as having a digestive organization and an organization of heart and lungs. We have not reached the point where it is an entity with soul. This would nevertheless only be able to function in the supersensible sphere, and it is our task to show how into this whole, where the human being is a solid and fluid entity, comes the principle that makes the human being sentient, entering into his solid and fluid organization to make man a sentient entity with soul. We must be able to follow the ensouled before we can see the human being as an ensouled entity. By connecting the etheric organization in the physical body with oxygen we now have the whole organization in which oxygen plays a role within the human being.

The ensouled organization cannot develop unless there is a direct point of attack for the gaseous human being which continues on into the physical organization. This is something still very remote from present-day thinking. Just think—I now have to draw your attention to this— just as thanks to the organization of lungs and heart, oxygen intervenes in the etheric, so the astral intervenes in the human organization via another organ system. This astral element also needs direct access to a physical organ system. If I draw a diagram of this physical organ system, the process I am referring to does not come from those physical organs but from something connected with these physical organs in gaseous form, from the gaseous organization therefore which is connected with these solid organs. The development of astral and organic powers in the organism radiates out from this. The physical organ itself only develops on the way back thanks to its own radiation. First the gaseous organization radiates out, making the human being into an ensouled organism, ensouling all organs, and then radiates back again by a roundabout route, so that a physical organ then also develops because it is now also involved in the human physical organization. This is the renal system which is generally seen as an apparatus for elimination. It is secondarily an apparatus for eliminatory processes, as I will show today or tomorrow. I still have to speak about the relationship of renal eliminations to the higher kidney functions.

Apart from being a physical organ for elimination—and of course playing a part in vitality—the kidney in its gaseous basis is the the astral organism's organ for outward radiation, entering into the gaseous and from there directly into the fluid and solid elements in the human organism. The renal system is thus something which from its organic basis fills us with powers of sentience, ensoulment and so on, and thus fills us with an astral organism.

Let me tell you that if you know the details concerning renal function available in evidence-based empirical science—knowing it merely from books does, of course, always make it difficult to get a clear idea—and if you bring a certain instinctive inner vision to anything you have seen and observed in such functions, you will today have the possibility to discover the relationships everywhere between inner, sentient experience and renal functions; it is merely that the eliminations are but secondary indications of the source from which they are eliminated. This source has come into existence through the renal functions. In so far as the functions are the basis of the sentient system this is also reflected in the different kind of elimination.

If you need to broaden science there I would recommend that you look for people who are a bit more sensitive and able to tell you certain things on examination, for instance how elimination via the kidneys changes to a marked degree when they are thinking, depending on whether they are thinking in a room that is cold or one that is warm. Such purely empirical facts, which you must vary the way one does in modern science, will show you the outcome. With strict, systematic investigations you will see the difference in eliminations via the kidneys when thinking in a cold or a warm room. You can also arrange the experiment so that you ask someone to think—think logically—and place a warm cloth on his head. Study the renal elimination, and then, as he thinks the same things, put cold compresses on his feet. You can thus do wholly evidence-based, strictly empirical studies and they will give you the proof.

Today we are not getting enough investigations of this kind, the reason being that people feel disinclined to go into such things. Nor do they go into allantois and amnion when studying cell division, investigating the embryo. These organs, which then drop away, are also studied, but to get to know the whole of human development one would have to study the appendages much more thoroughly during embryonic development than the developments due to division of the germ cell. So once again we need to establish everywhere the starting points for investigation of the right kind. Such investigation will show something of tremendous significance, for it alone shows the road we must follow to really understand the human being as a giant cell that is not visible but invisible.

Today we do not describe the things we do describe of the human being by starting from the cell, for microscopy does not make us do this. The strange thing is that when one goes to the microscopic level with the methods to which I am referring we get all the good results obtained in the school of Hertwig, for instance. You reach a certain point up to which you can study the cell under the microscope; but you cannot go beyond this and study the complex processes of life. Ordinary empirical, evidence-based science comes to a halt here, but you can take it further in the science of the spirit.

You now look at the whole human being, and the small point of the cell continues on for you for the whole human being. And you discover how the purely physical organization, I'd say, intervenes in everything connected with the structure of carbon, and the transition to the etheric organization is then connected with the structure of oxygen. Now when you move on to the renal system in series of exact experiments you will in the same way get a connection with nitrogen, and you have now included carbon, oxygen and nitrogen in your study. The trace of all the roles played by nitrogen as the body is astralized can be easily followed in the metamorphoses of uric acid and urea, though these must be studied in series of completely exact experiments. In everything you'll find in those exact series concerning the secondary secretion of uric acid and urea you will get confirmation that this points to quite specific things that show how the human being is fully astralized in a process coming from the renal system. This will also be evident from other things that play a role in renal function, including pathological states— to which I'll briefly refer tomorrow—when blood cells of one kind or another are found in the urine. The renal system simply lets the astral organization radiate into the human organism. We must not consider the physical organization but the gaseous organization connected with it, and nitrogen again plays its role, so that the whole would otherwise be supersensible, just as we would be etheric if oxygen did not come into it. Nitrogen ensures that human beings can walk on this earth, can be earthly human beings. Nitrogen is the third element to connect with it.

One feels the need all the time, on the principles of spiritual science, to work towards a continuation of the methods used in anatomy and physiology. This is not because of some fantasy, as you can see from the things arrived at in the first place. The strict demand is: Approach the renal system, investigate urea and uric acid secretions and so on as exactly as possible—more exactly than is done anywhere today—under different astral conditions, investigate the whole systematically and step by step you'll find that what is said in this way is proved. And it is only with this that you are able to look into the constitution of the human organism.

We are thus able to say that through the renal system everything human beings receive with their food intake is captured in the astral organism. We only need now to get it into the I organization. Everything is initially taken into this through the liver and gall bladder system. The principle found in the warmth structure and in everything by way of warmth structure in the liver and gall bladder system radiates out in such a way that the human being is filled with I organization, an organization which is altogether bound to the temperature differentiations in the whole of the organism.

You truly can organize your methods of experimentation as accurately as possible in line with what I am now saying. For in the first place: look at lower animals, where there is no suggestion of an I organization, from the point of view of the soul. You do not find a developed liver, nor bile acid in the process. Phylogenetically these things only develop in the order of animals when things go in the direction of an I organization. The development of liver and gall bladder is entirely parallel to the level of I organization which an entity gains. You can of course also set up physiological series of investigation, though these need to cover also the different stages in life. You will then see how such I organization as there is in the human being is connected with liver function. You merely have to study pathological states, like certain childhood diseases that are fatal, and you will discover that certain soul organizations—not in the direction of sentience but in the direction of the I—are connected with the secretion of bile. You'll find that there an enormously fruitful series of experimental methods opens up; some of them it will be possible to put together from what evidence-based empirical science has to offer; they merely need to be developed.

You'll see that in the same way as the physical organization is connected with carbon, the etheric organization with oxygen, the astral organization with nitrogen, the I organization is connected with hydrogen. You will be able to incorporate all temperature differentiations—I can only refer to this briefly—in the particular function that hydrogen has in the organism, of course always in conjunction with other substances. Moving up from the sensible to the supersensible but grasping this supersensible by considering its physical representatives, we reach the point where we can take the whole human being as a highly complex cell, as it were, a cell which is ensouled and filled with the spirit.

You see, here again it is really only a matter of taking the trouble and not simply leaving our marvellous natural-scientific findings at a particular point but to take them up, follow them and take them further. The way I see things and with my experience of life I am convinced that if you were to sit down today and simply go through the empirical material available in conventional science, putting things nearest to hand together with those most remote, considering how things are connected, you will come across every single thing I have been saying here. I am absolutely convinced that all the occultists you study and altogether people of the kind one calls 'occultists' today will not help you. You will have much more help with what is meant here if you really follow the empirical facts presented in conventional natural science. Natural science itself makes you acknowledge things which of

course can only be seen supersensibly but from which you get the idea
that we must follow the empirical facts in the one direction or the other.
You'll discover the methods for yourselves, the facts will make you
develop them. There is no point in complaining that you make someone
prejudiced with these regulative principles or that they are suggestive.
Things arise from the subject matter itself, but the facts which arise are
complex. To pursue the matter further you'll need the following.
Everything you get to perceive of the human being in this way then
needs to be investigated in its relationship to the outside world.

I'd now ask you to follow me in a brief train of thought. It is meant to
be more an example but will put you in the way of how to proceed
there. Let us take an annual plant rising from the ground in spring and
going through its annual cycle. Relate the phenomena you observe in
the annual with other things you are able to observe. Above all
something like the way farmers dig trenches of a certain depth to store
their potatoes through the winter, putting the potatoes into them so
that one will have them for the next year. They will not be fit for
consumption if stored in the ordinary kind of open cellar. You know
that all series of experiments in this area let you experience the outcome
of interaction between exposure to the sun on the one hand and the soil
on the other taken down to a deeper level in the winter months to
follow. Temperature conditions and the powers of light are at play in
the soil; the dynamics are below the earth's surface in winter, so that we
really have the after-effects of summer down there in winter. Summer is
above ground, all around us. In winter the potential powers summer can
have come into play underground. The consequence is—I have to take
great leaps, of course, but empirical observation will easily verify this—
that the plant in growing from the soil in its year is at first really
growing with the powers which the sun has given to the earth the year
before if not earlier, for the plant takes its dynamics from the soil. These
dynamics taken from the soil can be traced as far as the ovary, as far as
seed development. We therefore only have a genuine botany that is in
accord with the whole physiology if we take account not only of the
dynamics of warmth and light and of light conditions in the year when
the plant is growing, but starting from the root base ourselves on the
dynamics of light and warmth at least in the year before. We can trace

this as far as the ovary, so that we have something in the ovary which happened the year before still active from the year before. If on the other hand you study the foliage, and even more the sepals and petals, you will in the leaves find a compromise, I'd say, between the dynamics of the year before and the dynamics of the current year. The leaves have in them the element pushing up from the soil and the influences of the environment. In the petals the current year finally shows itself in its purest form. The colours and so on in the petals are not something old—they are of this year.

You cannot study an annual plant by only considering the current situation. Just follow the consecutive structural situation over two years—now in time—to see this. But the things that the sun tells the earth, as it were, persist for much longer. Run series of experiments on how good the plants still taste to creatures such as the grubs of may-bugs and you'll see that you need to relate the things which at first you consider to be of this year in the plants with sun conditions from the year before. You know how long those grubs need before they show themselves, enjoying the plant once they have gone through the larval stage.

All these things need to be exactly investigated. Only guidelines can come from the spiritual world. You then find that the structures of substances found in the petals and leaves, for instance, are greatly different from the structures of substances found in the root or even all the way to the seed. The difference is enormous. And this makes the difference if you make a tea, let us say, from the organs of the flower or rather the leaves, or chose to make a decoction of roots or seed. You will find that this difference underlies the other differences—the difference between the action of a tea made from petals and leaves or of a decoction made from the roots or seed. This is how you relate the human being in his organization to the environment, and are able to verify everything you find there in purely physical, sense-perceptible terms. You'll discover, however, that irregularities in translating the chyme into the etheric organization, for instance, as it takes place through the system of heart and lungs are influenced by foliage. Everything connected with the digestive tract is greatly influenced by what we get when we make a tea of petals. A decoction of root and seed influences the activity which follows—into the vascular system and as far as the nervous system. This gives you the rational connection between the functions of the human organism and the sphere where our armamentarium may be built up.

In the afternoon I'll go on to show you the inner connection between the different structures of the plant we are able to identify and the human neurosensory organization and digestive tract organization.

IF we manage more and more to see the human organism in the way which, sadly, I have only been able to refer to briefly, things grow important specifically for judging the human being in sickness and in health, for the full value of some aspects is not generally apparent. To this day, people pay extremely little attention to the principle which I have tried to call 'the threefold state of physical human nature' in the appendix to my book *Von Seelenrätseln* [extracts in *The Case for Anthroposophy*].[23] Yet very much indeed depends on people attaching the right value to this threefold state of the physical human being when it comes to the element of pathology and also to medical treatment.

The threefold nature of the physical human being means that everything that is neurosensory system has to be seen as mainly located in the head, but that this head organization is also spread out over the whole human being. Everything we have to call neurosensory function in the human skin, for instance, and indeed in the whole human organization is certainly part of it. But we cannot arrive at a well-founded view unless we first lift the neurosensory system out of the whole rest of the organization, doing so theoretically to begin with.

The second system I distinguished is the human rhythmic system. It includes everything in the functional sphere that is subject to rhythm, primarily of course the respiratory system in conjunction with the system of blood circulation, in a wider sense also the rhythm which applies at least in the main to human beings even if they may break it up in many ways. This is the day and night rhythm, the rhythm of sleeping and waking, and furthermore anything else that is rhythmic, including food intake, and so on. People do, of course, break the last of these, and the results of this have to be balanced out in a certain way using regulators existing in the organism. We must thus consider the rhythmic human being to be the second element in the human organization, and the metabolic organism as the third. I include the organism of limbs in this, for the functional processes due to moving our limbs are closely bound up with the metabolism in general.

Considering this threefoldness of the human being we come to see that the human organization I spoke of this morning, which is above all connected with the I, has a certain relationship to the metabolic human being, but this is in so far as the metabolic human being extends over the whole human being. The rhythmic human being has a certain relationship to the system of heart and lungs to which I referred this morning. And I also spoke of renal function this morning, arising from the renal system, having a certain relationship to the human astral organization. In short, the threefold human being has a certain relationship to the individual levels of supersensible human nature and hence also to the individual organ systems, as I showed this morning. But we must take a closer look at these relationships if they are to be of real value in gaining insight into the human being in health and sickness, and it will probably be best to start with the rhythmic human being, the rhythmic organization of the human being.

This rhythmic organization is very often not properly valued for one quite specific property and that is the relationship between the rhythm of the blood circulation and the breathing rhythm. In adults it is almost four to one. This is of course an approximate, a mean ratio, and it is the very fact that it is specific to the individual which reflects something of the measure of health and sickness in the human organism. This ratio of four to one in the rhythmic human being really applies also to the whole human being. We certainly have a ratio of four to one with regard to the development of the metabolic human being, which includes the human being of limbs—I say 'metabolic human being' to simplify things—and the neurosensory human being. Again this is something we can verify empirically from the evidence of the senses. The relationship goes so far that we may indeed say that everything by way of processes connected with human metabolism goes at approximately four times the speed of everything the neurosensory organization contributes to the human being's growth. We can actually say that the second dentition, with the second teeth permanent in the child, reflects what is happening in the human metabolic system due to the fact, as it were, that this metabolic system is all the time knocking against the neurosensory system, but that everything which then continues on from the human metabolic system towards the middle—the rhythmic system—relates to everything that extends from the neurosensory to the rhythmic system in a time ratio of four to one. Putting it accurately it is like this: We are able to see the rhythms of the neurosensory system continuing on in the respiratory system, and the rhythms of the metabolic system continuing on in the circulatory system.

We can say that the metabolic system is sending its influences up, as it were, into the rhythmic human being, that is, the third principle in the human organization into the second principle, and in everyday life this is reflected in the rhythm of the blood circulation. The neurosensory system sends its influences into the respiratory system, and this is reflected in the breathing rhythm. In the rhythmic human being, where we are able to observe the four to one ratio—about 70 pulse beats to 18 breaths—we have the neurosensory system and the metabolic system knock against one another in the ratio of those rhythms and, as I said, we can observe this also at any stage in life if we observe how absolutely everything that happens in the human being coming from metabolism knocks against anything coming from the head system, the neurosensory system. It is an extraordinarily important relationship. We can indeed say straight out: In the child's second dentition we have the metabolic system pushing up as far as the head but in such a way that when the metabolic system comes up against the neurosensory system, the latter is initially predominant.

This will be clear to you from what follows. We are able to say that when children get their second teeth at around the age of six, metabolic system and neurosensory system knock against one another in such a way that the activity of the neurosensory system is dominant. What results from the collision—these are the components, as it were, coming from the neurosensory and metabolic systems—is the situation which then leads to second dentition.

At the stage of life when sexual maturity develops we see metabolic system and neurosensory system knocking against one another again. Now, however, the metabolic system dominates. In the male gender this is reflected in the fact that even the voice, which up to this time mainly reflected the neurosensory system, changes because the metabolic system comes up, as it were, and makes the voice duller. We can understand these effects if we observe how much there is in them on the one hand of emanations that have their origin in the renal system, as mentioned earlier today, in the liver and gall system and on the other hand those that originate in the head and the skin organization, that is, the very basis of the neurosensory system. It is an extraordinarily interesting relationship, something which takes us to the deepest depths of the human organization, as it were.

We can really think of the development, the configuring of the organism proceeding in such a way that emanations coming from—let us say—the kidney and liver system are met by the form principles of the head system. To draw a diagram of what happens there we would have to do it like this (drawing). We would have to say: Emanations of this kind come from the liver and kidney system—not only upwards but in all directions, of course—and have the tendency to act in a semi-radial way, but the form principles coming from the head blunt them everywhere. So the shape of the lung can be understood if we think of it being fully formed out by principles coming from the liver and kidney system, but these are met by principles coming from the head system that round them off. The whole human form arises in such a way that we think of radial form principles coming from the kidney and liver system and being rounded off by principles coming from the head system.

This gives us the extraordinarily important fact, every detail of which can be proved empirically, that two power components are involved in organizing the human being, especially in their growth—the powers coming from the system of liver and kidneys and those that come from the neurosensory system round off the forms the others are configuring, giving them a surface. Both components impinge on one another, but not in the same rhythm; the rhythms in which they impinge differ. Everything coming from the system of liver and kidneys has the rhythm of the metabolic human being. And everything coming from the head system simply has the rhythm of the neurosensory human being. This means that when the individual is ready in his organization to get his second teeth in about his seventh year he is in his metabolic organization, everything coming from the system of kidneys and liver and is impinged on, I'd say, by the heart rhythm, made subject to a rhythm which relates in a ratio of four to one to the rhythm which comes to meet it from the heart. It is only in their twenty-eighth year that human beings are as far advanced with regard to their head organization as they were at the age of seven years with regard to their metabolic organism. This means that the sculpting, modelling principle advances more slowly than the radial principle which does not sculpt. It takes four times as long. Because of this we are by the end of our seventh year about as far with regard to the principle coming from our metabolism as we will only be in our twenty-eighth year with regard to the whole of our growth situation in so far as it is subject to the neurosensory system.

Human beings are thus complex creatures, with two streams, two movement streams, active in them that are subject to completely different rhythms. And we are thus able to say that second dentition, for example, arises when the principle connected with the metabolism impinges on the slower but more intensive sculpting principle. The sculpting element thus preponderates in the teething process. At the time of sexual maturity the metabolic element is to the fore. The sculpting element withdraws, as it were, and in the male gender this is reflected in the well-known phenomenon.

Other things in the human organization are also connected with this. One is that the potential for ill health is greatest in the years up to the second dentition, and this in such a way that the greatest potential for ill health exists in the very first stage of life. People's inner disposition for ill health largely ceases with the second dentition. I found I had to study this relationship very exactly because we had to develop our system of education. You really cannot establish a rational system of education unless you base yourself on this knowledge of the human being in health and sickness. The inner nature of human beings is such that they are really at their healthiest in the second stage of life, from the second dentition to sexual maturity. There follows a stage where they will easily fall ill. But falling ill in the first stage of life, up to the second dentition, is essentially very different from falling ill once sexual maturity has been achieved. These two possibilities of falling ill are as different, I'd say, as the second dentition and the breaking of boys' voices.

In the first stage of life up to the second dentition everything in the child comes from the neurosensory organization, going to the outermost peripheries of the organism. Everything really starts from the neurosensory organization. This is still predominant at the second dentition, and the pathological phenomena in the first stage of human life arise from it. You will be able to form a complete opinion, if I may put it like that, of these pathological phenomena if you say to yourself as you consider the matter: It is perfectly clear that the principle radiating from the system of kidneys and liver is blunted, in a way, blunted as the sculpturing principle of the neurosensory human being comes in. The dominant influence with the sculpturing principle is something connected with the human I organization and astral organization, as referred to earlier in these lectures.

You see, it is strange that earlier I had to say that the I organization comes from the system of liver and gall, that the astral organization comes from the renal system, and that I now have to say that everything connected with the I organization and the astral organization comes from the head organization. We'll never manage to cope with the enormous complexity of the human organization by just taking a linear approach, saying that the I organization comes from the system of liver and gall, the astral organization from the system of liver and kidneys, and sticking with this. We have to realize that in the first stage of life, up to the second dentition, these principles radiating from the system of liver and kidneys are blunted by emanations from the neurosensory system, and that it is this blunting which matters. The emanations coming from the system of liver and gall and from the renal system oddly enough prove to be a counter-flow—not directly moving up from below but moving from above downwards in a counter-flow. The whole childhood organization really has to be imagined like this: The astral rays out from the renal system, the I organization from the liver system, but these emanations are of no significance. Instead the liver system is, as it were, reflected by the head system, the renal system is reflected by the head system, and it is only the reflection into the organism which shows itself to be the active principle. You therefore have to say to yourself: How do I look at the child's astral organization? I look at the actions coming from the kidney as they are reflected back by the head system. The actual physical system and the etheric system act upwards from below, the physical organization with its point of origin in the digestive system, and the etheric organization in the system of heart and lungs. These act upwards from below, and the others down from above in the first stage of human life. And the rhythm which relates to the radiation from above downwards in a ratio of four to one is acting into the radiation that goes upwards from below.

It is a pity that one has to be so brief, but this truly informs us on developments in childhood. If you want to study the most striking childhood diseases, these can be divided into two groups, and studying these you'll find that on the one hand they are due to the principle radiating down from above meeting the one radiating from below upwards in rhythms in a relationship of four to one, but balance is not achieved. And if the principle with the four-rhythm, radiating from below upwards, does not want to be part of the nature of the individual, though the inherited rhythm of the head organization is really all right—the rhythm that is one in the ratio—then all the diseases develop which we know in the childhood organism and which nevertheless are metabolic diseases. But these are metabolic diseases arising from a damming up against the neurosensory system, so that the metabolism cannot rightly adapt to the radiation coming from the neurosensory system and we get for example—I can only give examples—the strange blood disease in children which makes the blood kind of purulent. We also come to all other childhood diseases that may be said to be metabolic diseases.

If the metabolic organism is adapted to the child's individual nature and above all if hygienic conditions are reasonable, so that the children are well adapted to their environment, that is, are given the right foods, but due to hereditary conditions of some kind the neurosensory system which acts downwards from above and the influences of which take the emanations from the system of liver and gall and the renal system along with them is not in order, all the spasmodic diseases of childhood arise of which we must say that they are due to the I organization and astral organization not being able to enter properly into the physical and etheric organization.

The diseases of the childhood organism thus arise from two opposite sources. But it is always the case that we can only cope with these diseases in the child's organism by directing our attention to the head and the neurosensory organization. Basically we must also configure the child's metabolism so that it adapts not only to external conditions but also to the neurosensory organization. In that first stage of life up to the second dentition we need to develop thorough insight into the human neurosensory system, practical insight, and really see to it that everything radiates out from the head organization, except that the metabolism may put itself forward, being in good order, and the head organization being too weak from hereditary causes.

In the second stage of life, from the second dentition to sexual maturity, everything radiates out from the rhythmic organism itself. And the human astral and the etheric organization is then of the essence. Everything the respiratory system and the circulatory system perform as their functions radiates into the astral and the etheric organization at that time. These systems can be kept in order from outside and because of this people are at their healthiest where their own organization is concerned. But we can easily ruin the health of primary-school-age children by putting them in poor hygienic and sanitary conditions. We cannot really take care of them from outside in this way in the first stage of life. Knowing full well, having gained real insight into essential human nature, that basically we are responsible for the causes of disease which arise between the seventh and the fourteenth year of life means that we carry enormous responsibility for the medical aspect of education. Genuine understanding of essential human nature tells us exactly that basically the causes for disease evident between the seventh and fourteenth years in life are our own fault. It is exactly at school age that human beings do not really depend on themselves but adapt to their environment in their breathing, taking in air, something which metabolism brings to expression in the circulation. Metabolism is always connected with the organization of limbs. If we don't let the children do proper physical exercise, properly move their limbs, we breed causes of disease in outer terms. This gives us the basis for the study of a real, proper primary school education. All conditions, also during lesson times, must be such that this is taken into account.

You see, this is not done in our time. You may realize this if you consider the following. In experimental psychology, as it is called, which in a way is something magnificent—and I am well able to appreciate its importance—among the sins committed is the sin of saying: When children attend these lessons, they get so tired, and when they attend these other lessons, they tire in this other way, and so on. Conclusions are drawn from this as to how to arrange the curriculum—according to the states of tiredness observed. Well, the question is put in entirely the wrong way; it has to be put differently. From the seventh to the fourteenth year, we are, thank heaven, only dealing with the rhythmic human being who in principle never tires. If it were to tire, the heart, for example, would not perform its movements when we sleep for the whole of our earthly life. The movements of breathing continue and never tire. So if someone says he must take account of serious or slight tiring observed in the experiment he would have to conclude that he has really made an error when that happens. It must be our ideal not to influence primarily the head system between the seventh and the fourteenth year but rather the rhythmic system. We do this by giving our education artistic form. That is how we influence the rhythmic system, and we shall find that we are actually correcting the things which modern research establishes as children tiring with the wrong kind of teaching. It is possible, for instance, to influence the breathing movements, albeit slightly, by wrongly burdening the memory, and this will show itself later on in life.

The opposite is the case when the child has reached sexual maturity and after that. Then possible causes of disease appear in the human beings themselves, in their own organism of metabolism and limbs. This happens because the foods taken in make their own laws apply, and we then have the activity of the physical and etheric organism predominant in the human organization.

In the child's organism we thus have the I organization and the astral organization acting via the neurosensory system; from the second dentition to sexual maturity the astral and etheric organization is predominantly active, but from the rhythmic system. After sexual maturity the physical organization and the etheric organization are mainly active, and this from the system of metabolism and limbs. And we see how pathology absolutely confirms this. I merely have to list the typical diseases for the female gender; we see how after sexual maturity the actual metabolic diseases come from within the human being, so that we are now able to say that metabolism predominates. It is the principle which coming from the metabolism overcomes the neurosensory organization instead of establishing real harmony with it. In a child we have false dominance of the neurosensory system in childhood diseases before the second dentition, then the period of health between the second dentition and sexual maturity, and after that predominance of the organism of metabolism and limbs with its faster rhythm. This faster rhythm is then reflected in everything connected with deposits developing in the metabolism simply because the sculpting organization from the head pushes itself forward come what may.

I am very sorry indeed that I can only present these things cursorily and aphoristically. I do however want to give at least the main conclusions which are that we can actually see from it all that the functional aspect of the human being must be considered primary and that the development of form and deformation must basically be coming from this functional aspect. Outwardly this is evident in that the plastic, form-giving process is particularly powerful up to the seventh year. The organs are developed so far in their sculpted form by principles coming from the neurosensory system that we are able to say, for instance, that the work done in forming the teeth up to the second dentition will not be repeated later. But all the work done by the metabolism in penetrating the organism really enters onto a completely new track when at sexual maturity part of the metabolism is given over to the sexual organs, and the metabolism is altogether given a different constitution.

It is extraordinarily important for you to follow up the things I have mentioned so briefly, doing so methodically and in every detail. The results are put in a proper scientific order by bringing them together with things like those I gave at the end of this morning's session, relating them in turn to world activities outside the human being.

It is possible to deal with everything that radiates out in this complicated way from the renal system, the liver system, simply by provoking changes in there from the outside. We can deal with it by taking account of the things we observe in the plant's growth principle, I'd say more from the preceding year or years, and the growth principles arising from the immediate present. Let us go back to the plant. From the root up to the ovary, to seed development, we really have something that is old for the plant, from the year before. And in everything that develops especially around the petals we have the present. We have to see the combined activities of present and past in the development of the leaves. Past and present unite as two components producing a result. Now in nature everything relates to everything else, just as everything relates to everything else in a complicated manner in the human organism, as I have shown briefly. We have to get to know the ways in which things are connected. Everything is mutual relationship in the natural world, and if we want to trace the relationships evident in the plant, where things are less complicated, we find the following. We find everything which in an earlier, instinctive medicine—which we do not wish to return to, I merely want to mention it so that we understand each other better—was called phosphorus-like, sulphur-like in the parts developing as something belonging to the present, to today, in the flower, leaving aside the ovary and stigma. Making a tea from these parts of the plant, thus also taking out mineral activity, we get the phosphorus-like, the sulphur-like principle. It is quite wrong to think that those earlier physicians saw phosphorus and sulphur as the elements known to us in modern chemistry. No, they saw it in the way I have just described. A tea made accordingly from, say, red poppy petals would in terms of that earlier medicine be considered to be something phosphorus-like, sulphur-like.

If I use the green leaves, on the other hand—a big difference, of course, if you take pine needles or cabbage leaves and make a decoction—you will have what in the old style was called mercurial. That is the mercurial principle, not mercury as we know it today.

And everything connected with the root element, the stem and seed quality was considered saltlike in the old medicine. I am merely mentioning this to make things clear. Today, with our natural-scientific insights we cannot pick up those earlier insights, but we do need to have experimental series to show how on the one hand, let us say, a decoction of some root or other acts on the head organization and therefore also on childhood diseases.

We shall have a tremendously significant regulative principle if we simply do experiments on the actions of anything we obtain especially from the root element, and also the seed element of plants on the childhood organization up to the second dentition. We will then have medicines for everything that is similar to the things that must be acquired from outside—essentially all diseases that are in the main acquired between the second dentition and sexual maturity have to be acquired from outside—that is, at least medicines that act on what is coming from outside, by making preparations of the green leaves, the foliage. That is the mercurial in the earlier sense and it is indeed present to a greater degree in mercury, though it is not identical with it. The fact that mercury is a specific for something very much acquired from outside, that is, for certain venereal diseases, is certainly connected with this. Everything by way of venereal diseases is essentially merely the potentized continuation of conditions that may develop in an extraordinarily mild form in the second stage of life. Yet by nature even venereal diseases are merely a potentized form of what can be acquired from outside from the seventh to the fourteenth year, exactly up to sexual maturity. These do not turn into venereal diseases because up to this age people aren't yet sexually mature. Otherwise various diseases that can potentially be acquired would offload themselves very much on the sexual organs. Someone truly able to observe this transition from the eleventh, twelfth into the thirteenth, fourteenth and as far as the fifteenth, sixteenth year will see how something which before appeared in a completely different way takes the form of abnormalities in the sex life. And then, of course, come the human diseases that may have their principal seat in metabolism, in so far as the metabolism is bound up with the physical system and to the etheric system—diseases that must be considered in connection with activities bound up with the principle that lies in the actual flowering parts of the plant.

Much of this may seem sheer fantasy when it has to be as briefly presented as I had to do here. But they are verifiable in every detail. Our difficulties in really presenting these things in official medicine lie in the fact that initially it all seems difficult to see clearly because we have to reckon with the kind of complication in the human organism which will have attracted your particular attention when I started to speak today; I had to characterize it in such a way that apparently it did not agree with the things said in the morning. The explanation is that emanations from the organization of liver and kidneys will first present in their counteractions. It is then something of importance for the I organism and the astral organism. This comes up most powerfully there. In a similar way, however, the circulatory rhythm and the breathing rhythm work both together and against one another in the middle human being. There, too, we therefore have to look for some things that come from the blood rhythm, first in the counter-stroke of the breathing rhythm and vice versa.

If you bring the things I am now saying together with the things I said this morning, for instance, that the human I organization really lives in the human being of warmth which then penetrates the human being of air, the gaseous human being, and if we consider an influence like that coming from the I organism and from the astral organism, then in physical terms we have something which predominantly acts from the warmth organization and the gaseous and the aeriform organization. But we have to see this in the early childhood organism. We therefore have to see the origin of childhood diseases by studying the warmth organization and air organization. And the effects on the warmth organization and on the air organization which we see if we now use preparations made from roots or seed arise because two polar opposite modes of action impinge on one another, with the one exciting the other. Root or seed preparations we introduce into the organism excite everything that arises from the human warmth organization and from the air organization. This is merely to indicate how, if we consider the actions that go from above downwards, as it were, have from the very beginning a warmth and air vibration established in human beings which is strongest in childhood, though it is not a vibration but an organic structure operating in time. And the actions going upwards from below in the physical and etheric organism are the solid and the fluid organization. Both are in interaction because the fluid and the gaseous organizations interpenetrate in the middle, as it were, thus producing an intermediate stage in the states of aggregation. Thus the intermediate aggregate state familiar to you between solid and fluid in the human organism results from interpenetration. In the same way we must look for an intermediate stage between fluid and gaseous in the living, sentient human organism and then again for an intermediate stage between gaseous and warmth quality.

You see, everything which thus comes to expression in the physiology, I'd say, has its significance for pathology and therapy. I think you'll agree, as we consider the human being in all this complexity, that the situation is such that one organ system is all the time pouring its actions into the other organ system. If you now consider the whole organic effect that comes to expression in a sense organ, for instance, let us say mainly in the ear, the following is the case. The I organization, astral organization, etheric and physical organization are acting together in a particular way so that the metabolism penetrates the neurosensory element, and this is made rhythmical through and through by the breathing process in so far as it influences the organ of hearing, is fully organized, given rhythm by the blood rhythm in so far as this enters into the organ of hearing. Every organ reflects in a particular relationship the situation I have tried to show you in a threefold and a fourfold way—the threefold human being, the fourfold organization to which I referred—to make it transparent to you.

Ultimately, however, everything is in metamorphosis in the human being. What we see here in the region of the ear, for instance—why do we call it normal? Because it presents the way it does present so that the human being may arise, and arise in the way he goes about here on earth. There is no other reason for calling it normal. But when these special conditions—which in the case of the ear are above all configuring things because the ear is in the periphery of the organism—act in such a way that, let us say, metamorphosis makes a similar relationship, similar interrelationship with all these different aspects that arise somewhere in the inner organism, arise instead of the interrelationships which are appropriate in that particular place, something comes in just there which really wants to be an ear. Forgive me for being so sketchy, but one can't put the things I want to say in any different way when one has to be so sketchy. Let us say it comes up in the region of the pylorus instead of whatever was meant to develop there. In this way, a pathological metamorphosis proves to be the origin of tumour development. All tumour developments, including carcinoma, are in fact displaced attempts to develop sense organs. So if you have such a pathological development and rightly understand the human organism you'll discover the degree of involvement of the warmth organism and the air organism in the child's organization, and indeed the embryonic organization, to let those organs develop. They can only develop in the right way through the warmth and air organism in that the fluid organism and the solid organism counteract them, and a resultant arises of components. This means that we need not consider this relationship between physical organism in so far as it comes to expression, for instance, through the metabolism and the sculpting, form-giving organism in so far it comes to expression in the neurosensory system. We have to see, as it were, how the principle which carries matter radially emanates from the metabolic organism, and how matter is sculpted, given form, in the organs by the principle coming towards it from the neurosensory system.

Considering this we ask ourselves how we can really get at such a tumour development. We can only do so by saying to ourselves: The relationship is not right between the physical and etheric organism on the one hand, in so far as it is reflected in the emanating metabolism, and the I organism and the astral organism on the other, as they are reflected in the warmth organism and in the air organism. In thus referring to the outermost limits we must above all consider the way in which the metabolism relates to the warmth organism; in the case of a tumour we can best do this if it is inside, though it is also possible if outside—I'll talk about these things tomorrow, particularly in the therapeutic part—by enveloping the tumour in a mantle of warmth. We merely have to succeed in enveloping the tumour in a mantle of warmth. This causes a radical change in the whole organization. If we succeed in doing this, then—put in a primitive way—we will also succeed in dissolving it. This is achieved in a real way if such medicines are used appropriately, I am sure, as your medical friends have told you about, if they are given by injection. Having discovered the specific action on one organ system or another you can be sure that in every case a Viscum preparation, the way we use it, will create a mantle of warmth around the abnormal organ in question—for that is what a carcinoma is. You cannot use the same for a breast cancer, a cancer of the uterus, or of the pylorus. You have to study the route taken by the effect produced by the injection, but you'll never achieve anything unless you bring about a genuine effect. And this effect becomes evident in that the temperature rises. The injection thus has to be followed by a febrile state. You can be sure of failure from the beginning if you do not produce a fever.

I wanted to give you the principle so that you may see how things depend on a ratio, but that ratio should only be a regulative principle. You will see that everything said to be due to those regulative principles can be verified in the way in which facts are altogether verified in modern medicine. Nor do we wish to claim that these things should simply be accepted without being verified. But the situation is that anyone who takes a real interest in these things will be able to make strange discoveries.

Everything I have been saying today—the sketchy presentation may prove somewhat confusing but it will be clear if you give the matter some thought—you will on the one hand find substantiated in a strange way if you take the right facts on the one side, which are recorded in the literature (these things are recorded somewhere or other which will truly bring you close to the picture painted today), especially if you relate this to something else, if you relate it to the many references to be found in the literature. You will get as far as this but no further.

You will thus certainly find confirmation from two sides in existing medicine that the result is as I have sketched it out for you. I'll now permit myself to add some aspects of treatment tomorrow, and then some of the things which perhaps are not quite clear because of today's sketchy presentation will become clearer.

Lecture 8

ALL I can do, really, is to give you some of the methods, with a view to therapeutic aims as they arise from spiritual-scientific studies. It will, of course, not be possible to go into detail, time being short. However, I think that for starting the work that needs to be done with the aid of spiritual science in the medical direction it is above all important that the points of view emerge fairly clearly. I may say that with regard to individual special aspects these points of view have been applied with great care in making our medicines. It may not be immediately obvious how these more general points of view can be developed in specific instances, but I will endeavour, particularly in discussing the methods today, to point out some things that will at least give you thought also in this direction.

It will not be possible to understand the human organism in health and sickness—or rather, for today's purposes, in its state of health and gaining of health—unless you take account of the fact that 'normal' functions essentially are but metamorphoses also of those we must evoke in order to meet pathological states. We must always take into account that the human organism is inwardly filled with processes which are not the same as the processes in the outside world. Let us first of all take into account that everything people take in from outside, from the plant world, for instance, must first be processed in the digestive tract itself so that the human being may then enliven it further. Vitalizing, enlivening must be the human being's own activity, and the human organism simply could not exist if it did not perform this activity. Now we must clearly understand that the earth's plant cover is essentially going through the opposite process from the one inside the human being. When we refer to 'vitalizing' on the route which human food follows through the organism, on an ascending curve, as it were, a curve rising from essentially inorganic matter to vitalized, live matter, from there to what can be the vehicle for sentience, and finally from there to what can be the vehicle for the I organization, that is, when we speak of food being processed until it is also taken up into the astral organism, the vehicle for the world of sentience, we have to speak of the progressive enlivening of matter taken in as food.

In plants, the opposite is the case. Initially there is essentially a process of devitalization in all peripheral organs as the plant develops from below upwards, calling forth the leaf process and the corolla process. The vital principle is retained for the seed only. In the plant which we are first addressing—for when we address the seed in the ovary we are really already addressing the next plant which is still to develop, that is, we are addressing something saved for the next plant—we do not have a vitalizing process going up from below. The vitality is sucked out of last year's summer warmth stored in the soil, out of last year's power of sunlight. The greatest vitality is in the root element. We have a gradual devitalization process from below upwards, and when we come to the petals, especially petals containing much volatile oil, we also have the most powerful devitalization process in those plants. We have a process which is very frequently, for instance, connected with genuine processing of sulphur which is then found in material form in the volatile oil or at least close to the volatile oil in the flower. The sulphur really brings the process about, taking the plant into the volatile inorganic sphere, I'd say into the kind of inorganic quality that still has the organic, live quality adhering to it. It is extraordinarily important that we clearly understand what we are actually introducing into our organism even as we introduce the plant. The plant is going through a process which is the opposite of the process in the human organism.

If you base yourself on this as you focus on the actual disease you'll have to say to yourself: Plant nature—and this also holds true for other substances in the outside world, and to a much higher degree for animal nature—is the opposite of the human organism's tendency to evoke one process or another. Looking in an unbiased way at human nutrition we cannot but say to ourselves: With every food we are actually introducing something into the human organism which needs to be thoroughly reversed. Essentially, taking nourishment is always a first step towards poisoning ourselves. When we speak of actual poisoning we have to be clear in our minds that this is merely a metamorphosis— greatly tending to be radical—of something which happens a little bit when we are altogether taking food into the ptyalin, let us say. And the further stages of digestion, especially in the renal function of which I spoke, absolutely are always a process of detoxification. We are thus simply going through a rhythm of mild poisoning and detoxification when we eat our daily bread and digest our food. This is the slightest metamorphosis of something which is then enhanced when we introduce medicines into the organism. It is of course utterly senseless to fall into raptures about 'non-toxic medicine'. It is nonsense because the question can only be: How do we enhance something which is already happening in ordinary digestion by introducing something which is more foreign than ordinary nourishment to the human organism?

We need to understand the human organism really well to be in a position to appreciate the value of an external medicament for this organism. Let us take something which is really always present in the human organism as a medicinal agent—the iron in our blood. This is really always playing the role of a medicament, protecting us from the tendency to fall ill which we have in us. I'll start by putting this the most primitive way. As you know, if the brain, weighing 1500 grams, were to rest on the base of the brain, the vessels in the brain base would, of course be squashed. The brain does not rest on that base but actually floats in the cerebrospinal fluid. Due to the law of buoyancy it loses as much weight as the displaced fluid weighs, so that the pressure the brain exerts on the brain base is only about 20 grams and not 1500 grams. This is a fact of principal importance for it simply shows that gravity is not the effective principle behind functions of the brain such as I activity. This I activity and largely also idea-forming activity in so far as it is not will activity—I am now definitely referring to the physical correlate, brain activity—does not rest on the weight of the physical matter involved but on buoyancy. It depends on the force that seeks to remove matter from the earth. With our I and our thoughts we are not living in gravity but indeed in buoyancy. Here this is particularly apparent as we consider the matter in this way.

The principle that applies to the brain does essentially also apply to many other things in the human organism. Above all it applies to the red blood cells which contain iron. These float in the serum and each of them loses as much of its weight as the displaced serum weighs. Consider this: If we altogether live in buoyancy in our souls, what it means for the whole way we feel and altogether live the whole of life in the human organism if we have a greater or smaller number of red blood cells containing iron inside us. In other words, if we understand in a given case that what is happening in the blood simply due to the buoyancy of those blood cells is not in order, we will know that we must supply iron in some way and this will make it possible for the iron to unfold its activity properly in the blood and not to be used in some other kind of way.

In spiritual-scientific terms this means that we are dealing with the iron level in the blood as far as the relationship of the etheric to the astral organism is concerned. If you understand how heart and lung function transfers everything taken in by the human being into vitalization, that renal function then takes it into the astral organism, you will not be that far away from realizing that this needs balance. When etheric activity or astral activity gets too powerful, and there is no balance, the whole organism must fall into disorder. The way of producing this balance, giving the organism the possibility of transferring just as much of the food into renal function as is necessary, is to regulate the iron level in the blood. Since you give either gravity or buoyancy to the actual dynamics in the blood, depending on how you regulate the iron level, you are regulating the whole blood circulation which in turn influences renal function, and in transmitting iron or taking it away you have a major regulator for the blood circulation function, that is, the interrelationship between the human etheric and astral organism.

Let us now apply this by considering something specific. Let us assume we detect flatulence, wind, as a first symptom in the human organism. I am choosing the most primitive things here so that we may understand one another. What does flatus mean to someone who fully understands the human organism? It means that there are air organizations in the person in which the astral organism is strongly present, which do not dissolve rapidly enough. This is an effect of the astral organism which is active in the gaseous, the airy human being. Activities of the astral organism are present in the individual which do not develop and dissolve in the regular way but accumulate. We then have a preponderance of astral organizational activity coming to physical expression in the aeriform human being. This is what we have if there is flatulence. Being too powerful, astral activity affects all our sensory functions, especially the functions of the head. Because astral activity does not spread properly through the organism but congeals, it does not act properly into the metabolism but rebounds onto the neurosensory system, being more closely related to it. And we will very soon find that the neurosensory system is not functioning properly either, or at least assume that we have a syndrome partly consisting in that the neurosensory system is also not functioning properly. At this point I have to say something relating to a neurosensory system that is not functioning properly.

A lot of mischief goes on in physiology where the neurosensory system is concerned. Forgive me, there is no ill intent. You have to take everything with the familiar grain of salt, of course. If I am too compromising we'll understand one another less well. Permit me therefore to put things in radical terms. Seen from the supersensible point of view, if we consider any function which we are able to demonstrate empirically, using our senses, it will from such a higher point of view be the sense-perceptible reflection of something which exists in the spirit. The whole human organism is the sense-perceptible image of something spiritual. However, interaction between spirit and soul on the one hand and the physical, organic element in the human organism on the other certainly is certainly not as easy to comprehend as we tend to imagine for the neurosensory system. The reason is that if we consider only the human physical organization things are not the way one would like to assume with the physical organization a whole, as it were, excepting the nervous system and the senses, and the nervous system is embedded in this structure and functioning separately to serve only the psyche. It is not seen in such radical terms, of course, but if we then base our practical considerations on our theory of the physical, then this is pretty well what we get. This is why there is hardly any possibility of forming a sensible idea on 'functional diseases', as they are called today, nervous disorders, and so on. There is not anything in the human organism that is not part of the whole organism and interacting with other organs. There is no separate nervous system so that the organism takes care of itself, with the nervous system embedded in it—who knows by which divine spirit—so that it may be a soul. Look for proof—you'll find it in a trice. Primarily the nervous system is the origin of configuring, rounding powers in the human organism, as I mentioned yesterday. The shape of your nose, the shape of your whole organism, is essentially configured from the nervous system.

The renal system sends out the powers of matter radially and the nervous system is there to give the organism its forms both inwardly and outwardly. Initially it has nothing to do with the psyche; it configures, shapes the human organism inwardly and outwardly; it is the sculptor. In the early stages of individual human development a particular part of nerve function separates off. The organism does not use it for its own configuration, and the psyche adapts to this part—secondarily—gradually adapting more and more. If one notes how a piece of the nerve process is torn out in the early years of childhood and how soul life adapts to these configuring principles, one will then have the actual empirical state of affairs. There truly is no question of the nervous system needing to be incorporated into the organism by some council of gods and has to be the basis for life in the will, in feelings and thoughts. There is simply no question of this. The life in senses and nerves is born with a kind of hypertrophy, some of this is taken out and soul activity then adapts to this saved part, whilst the primary function in the neurosensory system is configuration. All organs are configured from the neurosensory system.

If you wish to verify this empirically start with the senses located in the skin, spread out over the whole skin, with the sense of warmth, the sense of touch, and try to see how these senses cause the whole modelling of the human organism, whereas other senses configure to the form of specific organs. Even our ability to see depends on some of the configuring power originating in the visual tract to develop the cerebral organs being left over, with the soul qualities we develop in our power of vision adapting to it.

We must first see things properly in this area. Otherwise we won't be in any position to understand the human being properly, for we simply won't know that with metabolism in progress day by day, year by year our organs must in the first place be provided all the time with the principle sent out from the kidneys with the radial principle and that the organs must then be rounded out, modelled. Throughout life this comes from the nerve organs which extend from the senses to the inner human organism. The psyche simply adapts to this one organ tract, and this allows higher sensory functions and the forming of ideas to arise. This will demonstrate to us that when on the one hand we have flatulence in the syndrome and with this establish that the astral organization is too powerful, this excessive power of the astral organization moves things towards the configuring power of the senses, so that towards the periphery and upwards in the human organism it is not only that astral activity is dammed up and pushed together but these bubbles of gas which really want to turn into organs are rounded off. In other words, over-powerful renal function means that the attempt is continually made in the upper human being to hold the I organization back in the upward direction from letting anything entering into the organism via the blood remain behind in the given way. With the complex of which I am speaking we will therefore frequently see spasms associated which are due to the fact that the astral is not entering into the rest of the organism in the right way. When it comes to a halt up above it will not enter into the rest of the organism. We note spasmodic phenomena in the rest of the organism, always due to the fact that the astral is staying behind. It stays behind in this case, and when we inwardly look at such a syndrome, initially with the help of the supersensible, we can relate the things we see outwardly to what we have seen inwardly.

Consider, the astral is up above held back and this causes the whole metabolism to be drawn upwards. The astral body will then not provide properly for the renal organs and above all the stomach. The stomach, getting too little from the astral organization, defends itself. Outwardly you'll see colics and gastric spasms. Or characteristic spasms will develop in the sexual organs because they are not fully and properly organized by the astral or periods are delayed or stopped because I activity is held back up above.

We now ask ourselves what we can do about such irregularities. You see, it is really best if we understand that the magical names we give to diseases actually only serve as labels for conventional communication and what matters is that we do indeed everywhere see what individual symptoms come together and actually group together and one into the other. We must, however, be able to rate these symptoms. Consider, therefore, that we now look to the function which is attached, as it were, to a flower that contains sulphur. What I want to say is that when we have a flower that contains some sulphur this means that a very powerful process is going into the inorganic, with the organic still attached to it. If we now introduce such a flower or even just the sulphur produced from such a flower into the human organism as a medicine we are above all calling on everything that happens in the digestive tract to be more active. We call on it to be more active. The plant is essentially going through a devitalization process, as I said before, which has to be reversed. A tea of flowers containing sulphur stimulates the stomach and particularly also intestinal activity. As a result, the irregularity which has developed in renal activity is indirectly challenged to react strongly, and it is possible for us—perhaps only temporarily, for the things that act in this way are generally only temporary, but if we help the organism for a time it will in most cases come to help itself—to balance out this delay or stoppage in the upward direction by means of powerful downward counter-pressure, calling the astral organization back into the digestive tract again, as it were, and this is evident in that the colics and stomach cramps disappear. This will only rarely be enough on its own, however. It may be enough when the gastric spasms are mild. We should never overstimulate the organism when a gentler medicine will do, never use a more powerful one.

Let us assume we have a syndrome of the kind I have been describing, and as the disorder is severe we first want to direct our attention to the fact that powerful renal activity is making demands on an excessively active astral body which exerts a powerful influence on the sensory organization, weakening and undermining it in a way. It is not, in fact, undermined as sensory organization, but the influence of the astral organism is so powerful that the configuring power of the neurosensory organization is drowned out just by the astral organism being active. The sense organs or the neurosensory organization altogether is not less active but it is not active in its own true function as neurosensory organization. Instead it is, as it were, assuming the organization of the astral organism and functions in the way the astral organism itself functions, that is, it does not perform its sculpting action in the right way. We have to use something that will get the astral activity out of the neurosensory organization. We can do this in no other way but by using something which acts on the neurosensory organization, which after all relates to the outside world most of all and as an organization is also in the human being most related to the inorganic.

The physiology of the senses is in a happy position because many things in the sense organs can be explained in inorganic, that is, purely physical or at most also chemical terms. Consider how much in the eye is sheer optics. You can make nice drawings if you take the eye to be a kind of camera. I merely want to indicate here how we relate to the outside world especially through our sense organs, how we have bays in our sense organs through which the outside world extends into us particularly through the inorganic.

If we need to support this specific activity of senses and nerves we can do this very well with a principle which is introduced into the human organism as silica, for silica has an affinity to this inorganic element in the periphery. We drive the astral organization out, as it were, with the principle which exactly in everything that underlies silica moves so extraordinarily powerfully to the inorganic also externally. If you find silica in a flower you'll always discover that the flower grows spiny, that it moves strongly towards the inorganic. In this way we can relieve the sense organs on the one hand with this silica principle and on the other by providing the organism in such a state with more sugar than it usually has. Sugar also is a substance processed in the human organism in a way where the process is closest to the inorganic. Everything introduced into the body as sugar will also relieve the sense organs. If you are also able to do so, you can support this further by introducing alkaline salts. These relieve the nervous system in particular of astral activity. These things need to be demonstrated in series of empirical experiments.

Spiritual science thus makes it possible to arrive at regulative principles, for in the activity which develops as we gain in intuitive insight, for instance, we see the after-effects of sugar quite specifically in the parts of the human nervous system that go from the central nervous system to the sense organs; seeing the after-effects of silica, we see that it actually tends towards the peripheral quality which develops in the senses. These things can be verified, checked. Medicines simply made of alkaline salts which powerfully relieve nerve functions of astrality, made of sugar which of course must not be given in the usual amounts but in unusual ones, to which I will refer in a minute, and silica are all effective when the syndrome to which I've been referring is present to a high degree.

The substances to which I have just been referring are best made into medicines by simply making a suitable decoction of chamomile root. You might think it strange that I am referring specifically to the root, but the points of view cross and we have to understand that when the symptoms are powerful we have least need of sulphur or anything taken from the floral organization. What we do need is something still very vital in the plant, so that a long road must be followed to make the counteraction strong enough. If we introduce the characteristic substances contained in chamomile root into the digestive tract in suitable dosage the counteraction is not strong enough in this case to make vitalization occur at the transition from intestine to blood. Instead the principle inherent above all in sugar and silica and also in the alkaline salts is simply pushed through unprocessed. This gives renal function the opportunity to take it up into its radiations so that renal function makes the substances thus received act towards the neural and sensory functions. This relieves neural and sensory activities of the astral functions concerned.

If we understand such things, actually see how to proceed with treatment in such a way and this is the healthiest way of working, such a course of events can teach us a great deal. We can then easily be guided towards other things. We can see, as it were, how something taken up into the human organization is transformed there, how renal function then comes into play which really takes up what the blood channels bring to it and lets it radiate out, how sculpting activity then acts back on it; how this sculpting activity is produced in pure form by silica, sugars and alkaline salts. One would like to say that from the super-sensible point of view, seen intuitively, silica, alkaline salts and sugars create a kind of human phantom. We have something like a phantom before us when we envisage the creative powers of these substances. For they are above all sculptors, have sculpting in them. Gaining this insight this becomes clear to us even at the level of external physical con-figuration.

The powerful effect of silica is in the first place due to the fact that silica tends to occur as long crystals in the inorganic field. We would not be able to achieve what it is possible to achieve with silica using other substances as these tend to form more rounded rather than elongated crystals. One might be able to cure a hedgehog with them but not a human being, the growth principle of the latter tending towards elongation.

You have to have a feeling for this artistic tendency in nature which configures the organism mainly out of neural and sensory activity, or you will not be able to find rationally the connections between outside substances and processes in the human organism. But there is such a rational treatment where one simply sees both what is going on outside and how it is broken down in the human organism where renal activity can radiate it out and it can be taken over by the sculpting activity of the neurosensory organism.

Let us take some other example. Let us assume that instead of excessive overpowering kidney radiation we have renal function that is too weak, that is, too little of the food substance is absorbed into the astrality. Everything I said about the previous syndrome comes from action into the astral organism being too powerful. The astral organism is active in the upper human being and holds back from digestive activity, heart activity, lung activity. Mucous congestion develops alongside this syndrome and so do other things which you can easily establish. So that is the situation with excessive astral activity.

Let us assume we are dealing with the opposite, with astral activity that is too weak. Renal activity is not radiating enough and the human astral organism actually is not in a position to provide what it is meant to provide for the configuring power, striking into it. The configuring power cannot work its way in as far as the astral organism. That organism does not adequately reach the periphery and there is therefore no lively contact between configuring power and the power of circulating foods, matter, the distribution of matter. The matter is distributed but not utilized by the configuring power. The modelling, sculpting power is reduced, matter is left to its own life, the astral body stays too volatile, does not properly enter into the processing of matter. You see, we may also look at such a thing as a syndrome. What will it be like, this syndrome? Well, above all the matter in the blood channels is not taken up properly by a weak renal function, that is, an astral organization functioning at a low level, so that the astral organization is not working adequately. The matter drops down, as it were. Haemorrhoids develop, heavy periods develop. There is no contact, and the metabolism deteriorates in itself. When this situation exists in the organism, a kind of occult febrile condition may very easily develop, and even intermittent fevers.

Now, you see, it is like this: How do we deal with such a syndrome? The activity of the astral organism is too weak. We have to stimulate renal function so that it allows sufficient matter to be absorbed into the astral organism. Something arises here to which I referred earlier. The best thing is to establish a balance between etheric and astral organism. This will simply give us the right transition to renal activity from what enters into the system of heart and lungs from the digestive tract. We get a kind of balance, but we can actually regulate it in very many cases by regulating the iron level in the organism. The iron level regulates the circulation in that it now actually provokes powerful inner renal activity. This can be demonstrated in physical terms as a change in urea elimination through the kidneys and also in the sweat on the skin. It will certainly be possible to demonstrate this. In very many cases we must, of course, understand that this balance is always extraordinarily unstable and the medicinal agent in question, which is already in us, really helps only in the grossest cases.

Yet whilst things which in some way contain sulphur are helpful in the digestive tract, and substances such as silica and alkaline salts are mainly helpful in the neurosensory system, which we now consider to be the configuring principle, it is the pure metals which serve to regulate the balance between gravity and buoyancy in the right way. We merely have to try and see how we must use them in order to maintain the upset balance in all kinds of different ways, starting with iron. Sometimes it will be gold, sometimes copper, depending on the nature of the syndrome. But when we are held fast here by the type of illness in the human organism, pure metals will allow us to achieve the most important results. And if it is a matter of the interrelationship between form-giving and deformation being such that there is too little form-giving and it becomes organic, if initially this relationship between system of lungs and heart on the one hand and renal system on the other is not in order, we will actually do best with iron if the situation truly is such.

If it is such, however, that long-term disorders in these processes have caused organs to be deformed, with the sculpting activity unable to get down to these organs, that is, when organs have become deformed, have suffered from lack of sculpting activity, then we must use mercury, let us say. Mercury has inherent powers of form, the drop form retainable in the metal, which means it acts particularly on the lower organs in man. We can also establish certain connections between metals and the organs of the head if attacked and deformed, let us say, when the nervous system itself has been impaired. In this case it is, however, best not to depend wholly on establishing a stable balance as against a fluctuating balance. This is extraordinarily difficult. It is the way it would be with highly sensitive scales. We try everything to get the beam to balance, but it is really difficult. We will find it easier, however, if we do not just fiddle around with the beam but with the scales. We can achieve the state of balance by supporting the iron action, for instance, by introducing something containing sulphur into the digestive tract and give it the counter-effect with alkaline salts in the neurosensory organism. We then have iron effective in the middle, rhythmic human being—it will then disperse most beautifully—and potassium and calcium or alkaline salts active in the neurosensory organism, and the sulphur quality in the digestive rhythm. In that way we manage better to establish the balance.

It is most remarkable that we have the opposite situation in the leaves of certain plants. If you process the leaves of *Urtica dioica* in the right way, for example—they have to be the leaves of the ordinary stinging nettle, *Urtica dioica*—you'll have a medicament consisting of sulphur, iron and the necessary salts that act in this way. You merely must be able truly to see together the devitalizing power in the plant and the vitalizing power in the human organism. It is actually the case that the whole sulphur process in the *Urtica dioica* root is gradually moving towards the inorganic. The human organism goes in the opposite direction, converting the sulphur via protein to such effect that it will gradually put the digestion to rights. The iron in *Urtica dioica* acts in a direction from the leaves that *Urtica dioica* throws apart also in the seed and hence also in next year's leaves the very principle which in the human organism brings together the rhythmic process.

It is the opposite process in *Urtica dioica*. The attack coming from the leaves of this plant is a destructive element that must indeed be overcome if the rhythmic process in the human organism is to be put in order. And again, the alkaline salts in the plant are least transformed into inorganic matter and therefore have the farthest to go, going up to the neurosensory organization, easily so, for as we know renal function is asleep and suppressed with the syndrome under consideration. In the human organism we truly have a distribution which is the opposite of that perceived in an outward form in plant development. But it certainly is not necessary for us to limit ourselves to medicines based on plants; we can also make synthetic medicines by putting the substances to which I have just been referring together in suitable dosage and cure patients with these.

These things can indeed gradually make therapy into a rational science and an art or skill, for it will not be wholly a science any more than you can be a sculptor without also being an artist. You may know a lot about how to handle the trowel, shape the clay, but something always results which is also artistic. We also cannot achieve therapy without this. We have to have it in hand—a mental or spiritual hand, of course—to establish the dosage. This is something which does not suit a great many people who want to make medicine into a pure science, but that is the way it is.

Let me suggest what may also happen by means of an example. It may be the case that appropriate combined activity of the inorganic produced in the human organism in preparation for organizing things on the one hand and intervention of the ether body, of heart and lung function on the other, is disrupted. This disruption becomes more and more likely the older a person gets. The digestive tract and the vascular system are not working together as they should. We must then above all pay attention to the consequence—an accumulation of metabolic products. If the business does not spread through the organism as it should we do of course have to deal with a massing of metabolic products. We enter into the whole field of metabolic diseases, from the mildest to the most severe forms. And we have to understand that kidney function is then also out of kilter, which is because it is not provided with anything to emanate since it is all dammed up before this. And we are dealing with highly complicated forms of disease in that case. On the one hand digestive and renal activity are not providing what is needed to have material for their sculpting activity, and on the other hand deterioration of sculpting activity means that the organic balance is upset from the other side so that sculpting activity is gradually also lost. The metabolic products spread out in the organism, and the power to get them into sculptured form, to use them as creative material, gradually ceases altogether. We then have the metabolic diseases that are really difficult to treat and have to be treated by trying to take everything which may be said to be related to the process of becoming inorganic, that is next door to the sulphur-like, phosphorus-like principles in flowers or connected to the volatile oils and make it take effect in the digestive tract and then also in the cardiopulmonary tract, so that we bring about renal activity in the organism and so assist the sculpting powers. With this disease it is of the greatest importance to be able to get at the digestive tract.

Renal function and the production of sweat are polar opposites in some respect, intimately bound up with each other. And when renal function is not properly occupied by the things that I have been characterizing sweating activity will also regress. And this is something which merits special attention. Wherever sweating is not in order, renal function will also be out of order. Generally speaking, reduced sweating activity means that renal activity is like a machine that has nothing to process and yet goes on working. The materials coming from food have been dammed up before this and spread in the human organism in the wrong way. If we manage—with courses of sulphur given externally or internally—we can influence this from either side since we can act via the skin as well as via the kidneys to stimulate the digestive tract so much that it will on its own part stimulate cardiopulmonary activity so that renal activity takes in the material again, receives it so that it does not get held somewhere else but is pushed into the renal activity, then we may indeed manage to get control even of metabolic diseases.

With all this we must, however, clearly understand that in the human organism we are truly dealing with something that does not want to be fully healed, I'd say, but merely wants to be stimulated to heal itself. This is enormously important. In sickness, the human organism really wants to be stimulated to heal itself. To make the cure a lasting one we really have to limit ourselves to providing the necessary stimuli. A cure that seems to proceed smoothly will more easily lead to relapses than a disease that is stimulated to heal. The organism has initially got used to the healing process and continues with it by its own activity. In this way it connects much more closely with the healing process until the reaction comes up again. Initially, however, there is a kind of habituation. And if we adapt to the healing process in our organism for a time, that is the very best way of healing. For the organism then truly takes up the healing process that has been placed in it.

All I have been able to do in this way is to make some suggestions as to method, but you will see that it is a matter of being really serious now in letting spiritual science cast light on physiology, pathology and therapy. The human being does not exist in isolation but is part of the whole cosmos, and if you have some process or other that takes a certain direction in the human being, say in an ascending curve, we must look for the descending curve outside the human being. We will be able to have a balancing effect on curves that rise too strongly, and so on. Medicine demands that in a sense you do already know the whole world. I was of course able to give you only a tiny segment but this tiny segment will make you aware that you'll need to get to know *Urtica dioica, Colchicum autumnale* or any other plant in a very different way from that generally required today. You have to see, as you look at the plant, where it seeks to go in its descending trend.

So if you come to *Colchicum autumnale* you have to perceive that first of all the season when the plant appears has some significance for the whole structure. It establishes a certain relationship to devitalization. The colour of the flower and the season indicate that very slight devitalization occurs in autumn crocus. If you then do your experiments as to how *Colchicum autumnale* might help, you'll find that the organism has to make efforts that go a long way up to effect the opposite, vitalization—that is, to kill the plant off first and then bring it to life again, to put it in primitive terms. And the whole process goes all the way up to the human thyroid. And you can now do series of experiments to see how *Colchicum autumnale* becomes a medicine for goitre.

Honestly, there is no question of complaining wildly, in a dilettante way about modern scientific methods. No, it is a matter of indicating directions that will really lead to a more practical utilization than just trying things out. I do not in the least want to say that trying things out may not also take one to one's goal. It does also lead to goals. But many things escape us altogether. Above all much escapes us of what we can learn from nature. It truly is good if we can synthetically produce a preparation of iron, sulphur and alkali if we know how nature herself brings them together synthetically in a certain way, so that we may also learn extraordinarily much for synthesis if we understand what is going on in the natural world outside.

It would indeed be fascinating to go into detail about various aspects. I think our medical friends will have done so for one thing or another in their lectures. Some of it may also be found in our literature. Some other things are such that I would hope to see them soon in our literature. For I am convinced that when these things are properly presented in our literature people will take the standpoint where they say: Well, to be a physician I must be able to heal, and so I'll also turn to something which at first goes against the grain; if it helps I'll not be able to reject what is written in that literature as well.

And so I think it would be good for us to have, as soon as possible, a literature covering the science of the spirit and the science based on the evidence of the senses. This will help us so that the opinion will be: Yes, it does help, and so it cannot be such dreadful nonsense after all. And I am quite convinced that once the matter has really got going the opinion will be: It helps! And that is what I would wish to rely on. Try it, and you'll see that it helps. And it will also be of some importance, for among the things used in official medicine are many, after all, that do not help. And the struggle between things that do not help and those that do will be where that must take place which we do so very much desire to see from the point of view of spiritual science.

LECTURE 9
ON EURYTHMY THERAPY (GIVEN IN
THE MEDICAL WEEK)

STUTTGART, 28 OCTOBER 1922[*]

I'VE been asked also to say something about our eurythmy therapy. Essentially I presented the empirical material for this eurythmy therapy in the last medical course I gave in Dornach, and there is hardly any need to go beyond what was said then. Used as intended the therapy can indeed be of far-reaching significance. Today I would prefer to speak to you about the whole meaning and significance of eurythmy therapy.

As you know, it has in a way evolved from a pure art which did initially develop as an art form, and in some respects the art of eurythmy must provide a kind of basis for real insight into eurythmy therapy. Perhaps the clearest way of putting it is that I try, first of all, to show the difference between eurythmy as an art form and eurythmy therapy. Generally speaking, the basis of eurythmy is that we can metamorphose the processes that develop in the human organism when we speak, doing so in a particular direction. As an art, eurythmy therefore truly is a form of visible speech. We have to understand that there are two components to human speech. One arises from a particular way of using the plastic, sculpted, apparatus—after the earlier lectures it is reasonable for me to speak of a 'plastic apparatus'—a layer of the nervous

---

[*] German notation is used for eurythmy vowels in this chapter. Thus A stands for ah, E for eh, I for ee, O for o, and U for ooh.

system that lies further in. The sphere of ideas comes into this. Essentially the ideation apparatus continues on in a rather complicated way in the speech apparatus, going as far as the build of the nervous system, and the one component of speech arises as this radiates out further, I'd say. The other component actually rises up from the human metabolic organism. In a way we have dynamics arising from the human metabolic system meeting with dynamics coming from the human neurosensory system. The two meet in such a way that the metabolic system initially metamorphoses in the circulatory processes and the principle of ideation, coming from the neurosensory system, metamorphoses in the respiratory system. The two dynamic systems then encounter one another in the respiratory and circulatory systems. With the aid of the speech organism the whole is transmitted to the air and the human astral organism is then also able to pour itself into the movements created in the air. Speech arises, if we consider the outermost periphery of the human organism, as it were, by embodiment of the ideation principle on the one hand and of the metabolic principle on the other, a metabolic principle which in terms of the soul is in fact the will principle.

We thus have everything which in the soul comes to expression in will, and physically is reflected in the metabolic system in so far as the nervous system has a part in the will—it has a part in so far as metabolism takes place in the nervous system, not as neurosensory function. So the will principle, which comes to physical expression in the metabolic system, and the ideation principle, which I'd say comes to physical expression in a section, a layer, of the neurosensory principle, come together in a 'resultant', as it were. They then come to physical expression in ordinary speech sounds or in song. It is something different with song, but it is indeed something similar.

In eurythmy, we exclude the principle of ideation as such as far as possible and let the will principle take effect. With this, ordinary speech sound metamorphoses into movements of the whole human organism. We thus enhance the one component, which is the will principle or the metabolic principle, weaken the ideation principle or neurosensory principle, and eurythmy will be the result. This truly enables us to create human movement correlates for individual sounds, be they vowels or consonants. Just as a certain form and movement given to the air corresponds to an A or an L, so can an outwardly visible movement correspond to an A or an L. This is a movement, movement structure, I'd say, which sensible and supersensible vision has taken from the human organism. It obeys the same laws of the human organism as speech sounds do, but is a metamorphosis of speech and orientated more towards the will principle. The whole alphabet can thus be put together also in this language; every element of language can be represented in this eurythmy.

When eurythmy is performed as an art, human attention and all processes in the human physical, etheric and astral organism that support attentiveness turn to the sound in question, the word configuration or the artistic configuration of a sentence, metric configuration, poetic configuration and so on. In the art of eurythmy, human beings are wholly given up to the artistic configuration of speech sounds. As they are of course following the configuration of language, they are, in performing the art, given up to the outside world. And just as we don't hold on to an A in a word, or to an L, but these things are passing, so we are in the art of eurythmy dealing with something which may certainly proceed within the normally functioning human organism. With ordinary eurythmy as an art form there is no other physiological consequence but that ordinarily the eurythmy will energetically harmonize the human functions, doing so in so far as they are a complete whole in the human organism.

We are thus able to say that providing any excesses are avoided in performing the art of eurythmy, this activity also has a general health-giving effect. But everything conducive to health can also make people ill if it is overdone, and it is also possible to overdo eurythmy as an artistic activity. Professor Benedikt,[24] the famous neurologist and criminologist who did not like the anti-alcohol movement, would stress again and again that many more people die of water than of alcohol. Statistically this is true, for inappropriate excessive intake of water causes many different health problems. To the degree to which it is meant to be done, eurythmy—from the artistic point of view it will anyway result in a certain state of satisfaction or dissatisfaction in the human organism—can generally speaking only be health-giving.

As far as eurythmy therapy is concerned, the quality which lives in the devotion to configuring speech sounds, words, sentences known in eurythmy as an art form is reflected inwards. It is reflected inwards even by the fact that in eurythmy therapy the sound A, let us say, often has to be repeated a number of times. This is something totally different from moving from an A sound to an I or the like in performing the art. We need to look into the actual healing process which may come with eurythmy. I must not fail here to voice a certain concern which is indeed likely to come to mind with things like this. Laymen and amateurs are apt to take hold of such things. I have, however, stressed from the beginning that eurythmy therapy must really be given by the physician or at least by someone working very closely together with a physician. The reason is that things developing on the fringes of what is intended for medicine in spiritual science must be regarded in the same way as is the whole attitude to medicine in the science of the spirit.

It truly is the case that in spiritual science relating to the field of medicine one does not work towards the kind of thing I came across on an occasion 20 years ago. People attended anthroposophical meetings who, well, called themselves naturopaths, and I was given a paper on one occasion that really contained only the same thing said repeatedly in different ways: 'All healing consists in harmonizing what is inharmonious in the organism.' This statement was presented in all kinds of ways through six pages. Now there cannot be the least objection to this statement, but it is a matter of being able to do it in a wholly specific way in the individual case. It gets to be a problem for people with the kind of attitude expressed in the last sentence: 'Everything written in this paper shows that we can abandon medicine which is so tremendously complex and limit ourselves to harmonizing the inharmonious, and this'—as it literally said—'is intoxicating in its simplicity.'

I cannot offer you such intoxicating simplicity. In the science of the spirit the aim is to take medicine not to such an intoxicating simplicity but in fact to a greater complexity, as you will no doubt realize from what has gone before. With the science of the spirit, you'll have to learn more, not less. As to less need to learn, well, that's the hitch, but things will get clearer, giving you a good overview, and learning will thus get more interesting. People who have been thinking that healing is to be made easier with the science of the spirit will realize that this is not the case even from just listening to what I have been saying here.

I'd say that this also holds true for eurythmy therapy. It is certainly the case that eurythmy therapy should not be given without a sound diagnosis, and it certainly is the case that it should only be practised in full collaboration with expert medical knowledge. We are here truly dealing with the application of tremendously fine and detailed knowledge of the human organism.

Even with ordinary speech, metabolic activity and plastic, form-giving activity coming from the neurosensory system come together in the human organism. The 'resultant' of the encounter discharges in the movement of air which relatively speaking proceeds separately from the human organization, speech thus coming free of the organism. Because of this, everything created in eurythmy therapy is reflected back into the organism and we therefore have the following. Imagine you are, for instance, bringing an A movement together with an L movement. In the first place, you ask for the movements to be repeated, so that the matter does not discharge to the outside but the repetition pours into inner processes of the human organism. But by always letting the vowel or the consonant quality act together in the A movement or L movement you have always taken the human organism into function, which means that the metabolic human being and the neurosensory human being are working together. Yes, the activity of the neurosensory system is generally reduced in eurythmy, but the two components are nevertheless working together in this specific relationship, with neurosensory activity reduced and metabolic activity increased by the eurythmic movement. And by letting an L movement, for example, be done repeatedly we have the metabolic human being coming up against the neurosensory human being when we associate the L movement with an A form. We may say, therefore, that the repeated excitation of necessary forms or movements involves the whole functioning of the human organism being taken along. If you ask for a consonantal movement to be done, for instance, this will initially act by unloading all its power, its inner dynamics, on the process of inhalation, and you therefore really have the whole process of inhalation in hand. Depending on the consonant you excite, you'll have the inhalation process in hand. You strengthen this process of inhalation with every consonantal activity.

Perhaps you know from what has already been said of eurythmy therapy that here movements are somewhat modified from the way they are given expression in eurythmy as an art. We are able to say that when you do an A or an L, the movement is always connected with strengthening or reducing the thrust applied when one inhales. You have to take into account that this involves inhalation in its totality. When we consider inhalation we must first follow the route it takes, spreading at first in the middle part of the human organism and then continuing via the spinal canal to the brain. Brain activity is essentially a coming together of refined breathing activity and neurosensory activity. No brain function exists that can be considered in isolation; it is always the resultant of neurosensory activity as such and breathing activity. In studying all cerebral processes we must always also consider breathing activity.

With the excitation of certain consonants, of the different consonants, you actually are in a position to influence, by the roundabout route of respiration, human plastic, form-giving or modelling activity in a truly striking way. If you grasp the human organism artistically you merely need to know, in the case of a child, for instance, who is just developing his permanent upper teeth:[25] How are they created out of the modelling activity that moves downwards from above? They are created in that with the upper teeth the modelling activity acts above all from front to back. How are the lower teeth produced? For the teeth in the mandible, the modelling activity acts from back to front. To sum up the activity which comes into play when teeth develop: The upper teeth are formed from front to back, which means that the posterior aspects are generated, the anterior surfaces set off.* The lower teeth are created from back to front. That is how the forces work together.

If you find that the child has teething problems you can simply support teething in the maxilla by asking him to make an A movement; you can support teething in the mandible by asking him to

---

*The German original is not clear here. The 'set off' is a literal translation of *abgesetzt*, but it may also be 'set/put down', or also 'offset'. Translator.

make an O movement. You will actually have the modelling powers in hand by using certain influences. Yet to provide this modelling activity altogether with sustenance you must focus mainly, as it were, first on supporting the thrust of inhalation, adding to the modelling activity brought to bear by the A and O movement in this way the element which arises for you from the whole constitution of the individual. Let us say someone has weak peristalsis and tends to be mildly constipated. At the time of life when the teeth develop intestinal function is also very much connected with dental development, and we have to discern where the origins are of irregularities in dental development. If you assist the breath as it passes through the vertebral canal to the brain and then encourages from there the modelling powers which we get in hand through vowel movements, you can if you have this situation before you ask the child to make an L movement. You merely have to study eurythmy therapy and the diagnosis will show you how to use it. It should not really be used unless there is a diagnosis, otherwise there is the danger of doing entirely the wrong thing. But the point is that we must, I'd say, awaken a feeling for the artistic element in the dynamics of the whole human being. You have to develop an intuitive eye for the artistic element. Let us assume a child just beginning to teethe evidently has problems; he or she shows signs of being unwell or the like that should not be there. You then find that intestinal movements are inadequate, irregular. You begin with L movements in preparation. Doing the L movement for some time meets the element one has guided towards the form-giving centre by letting the child make A or O movements. For the vowel movements influence exhalation. The vowels begin their action even in the brain. The stream of the breath is active in the brain. And everything which in a comprehensive, total sense is connected with inhalation comes to expression in the consonants. It can be supported and promoted by consonantal eurythmization.

Everything connected with exhalation can be supported by doing vowels in eurythmy. But when you do that—you have to assess the repetitions which must be done depending on whether force needs to be applied—the modelling element is then working directly together with the outward-radiating element. If you are dealing with some renal condition, for example, you may say to yourself: 'The renal condition[26] is at a certain stage, let's say an early stage. The moment I ask for certain movements to be made, A* movements, for instance, I help the renal condition in an early stage. But if it has existed for a long time and inadequate function has already led to deformation, I must first prepare the field by using consonants in eurythmy and follow this with vowel eurythmy. I can thus use the vowel element to act on form-giving principles to counter the deformation which has developed.' In short, it has to be done as untheoretically as possible, but wholly from insight into the human organism in health and sickness to discover what I have given in the rules which I presented then in Dornach, rules that have been passed on to you.

If heart and lung function is suppressed, for example, and this also affects the kidneys, you do very well with B or P movements, especially in the early stages. You can see from this that one really has all function in hand with this, and that everything depends on understanding that in every individual human organ one has a kind of centrifugal dynamics, plastically rounded off by dynamics acting from outside in, not wholly centripetally therefore but such that they may be called centripetal, dynamics with an influence on every human organ.[27] We will alto-gether only be in a position to do proper physiology when we are able to consider every single human organ in its polarity. For we have these polarities, centrifugal and centripetal dynamics, in every human organ. And for everything that sculpts, models, the distribution and differ-entiation of states of warmth in the human organism play a major role, as does the air status. With everything centrifugal, radiating out, everything in the human organism coming from the individual dynamics of the substances of the world plays an important role and everything develops as the individual vitality of external entities is overcome in the human organism. These two dynamics have to be regulated one against the other, and we may hope that eurythmy therapists will be trained who will develop a really subtle feeling for what may happen in the individual case. Here in particular extra-ordinarily much will depend on an artistic state of mind.

---

* Another person's notes have S here, not A.

If you also consider that the whole system of eurythmy therapy can be further supported by the essentially therapeutic element, this gives us two factors that work together. We may say to ourselves that something acts particularly on the heart in one way or another, and you specifically support this with a eurythmy therapy exercise. The two things will help one another, and this opens up truly great prospects and can have an extraordinarily great future. Just think of how much of an effect there has been in some respects with massage being used. But this scrabbling about on a person really is—I don't want to say anything against it, I am not denigrating it, I recognize it for what it is—but it has little significance compared to the kind of massage you apply when you get all the organ systems which are working together there to move differently internally simply due to the factors of eurythmy therapy. You are inwardly kneading the whole organism through and through, and this involves activity in the etheric, in the astral and the I organism. We may say, therefore, that the quality we can fairly acknowledge for massage is in an infinitely powerful way made inward with this eurythmy therapy.

In fact we will also only come to understand the healing consequences of physical training (PT) when we consider the similarity between free exercises and eurythmy exercises. The healing element in PT is but a secondary analogue to the principle that applies with eurythmy. In Dornach I said that if one gets people to do E exercises in rhythmic sequence in a particular way, as we demonstrated on that occasion, extraordinarily much can be done to help children who look weak, children who perform their bodily functions weakly, to gain health, gain the strength they need. But it is absolutely necessary to take the whole human being into account with such things. It happens again and again that this is not done enough, yet the whole human being must be considered. I know this is a commonplace, and you'll say: We know that. But in practice it does happen again and again that this is not done. How often do we hear someone say: This person's heart is not functioning properly; we must do something. Yes, but if we consider the whole person we have to say: Thank heaven that he has such a heart, for his organism would not tolerate a normal heart. When someone has broken his nasal bone, for example, one has to say that fate has been kind to him, for if he were to inhale the air through fully developed channels this would be too much air for his organism to cope with. We must always consider most carefully what lies behind things in the organization as a whole.

When you get someone to do the I movements in a certain way, these I movements will above all harmonize association between the left and right sides of the human organism. I movements can be helpful with any asymmetry developing in the human organism. Even with a squint we can get very good results in eurythmy therapy by using I movements very carefully. With a squint, I would advise you not to proceed the way you would if someone's walk is asymmetrical, for example, or they may use the right and left arms too asymmetrically. Instead let them do I movements just with the index finger, repeating this as often as possible through the day. You may see good results with this in growing young people, especially if one gets them to do it with the big toe as well. And you'll see the best results if you can get the patient to do the movements with the little toe. Asymmetries relating to vision will respond particularly well to these eurythmy exercises done in the periphery. Conversely, when there is need to deal with some kind of awkwardness in walking, it may give good results to ask the individual—in a way that will not be harmful to him—to do I movements with the eye, so that you let him do I movements with the line of vision, the line of sight. We can actually establish a kind of law here: Everything abnormal in the lower human being is normalized by a balancing action done in the upper human being and vice versa. If there is uncertainty in standing, which again may be due to a number of causes, the U forms are particularly important, though you must make sure that the U form is done completely, with the limbs concerned truly put together so that the one feels the other; this is particularly important, for this alone makes the U form complete. In eurythmy as an art form this need only be hinted at; in eurythmy therapy it must be done so that the one limb lies against the other. Properly done it results in 'standing to attention', with the legs pressed together. This is an extraordinarily beneficial exercise for people who have a little bit of twitching in the head.

When there is need to do eurythmy therapy especially with children who are on the stout side, the O forms are particularly suitable. All these forms, if they are to be effective in eurythmy therapy, must involve a definite awareness of the muscle system in question. If you simply do the O form the way many eurythmists do it, this may be sufficient for giving an indication in stage performances but will only prove effective in eurythmy therapy if you actually feel the muscles through the whole length of the arm as you do the exercise. A loosely flung form does not have the effect. The whole muscular system must be felt in every detail; then you have the appropriate effect in eurythmy therapy. It is particularly important for you also to pay attention to supporting the eurythmy therapy exercise in its continuation into conscious awareness. So if you do the O movement the way I have just shown this also involves projecting strongly into the conscious mind. If you have a stout individual whom you wish to treat with O forms, tell him: 'As you do the O forms, think of how stout, how broad you are.' You are literally focusing his mind on the problem to be corrected. Doing so, you are essentially supporting the real intention, which is not at all under-estimating the conscious mind as a factor in the therapeutic process.

I think there will be some problems with the orthopaedic surgeons with regard to this, when one is paying attention to such things. Most successful in the field of their activities they are still firmly resolved today to see the human organism as a kind of mechanism and treat it accordingly. Apparatus is applied with the aim of keeping the person concerned aware, conscious of the matter all the time, an example being that I consider that someone should straighten his shoulders and apply bandages to give him the actual feeling that the shoulders need to go back and the matter does not remain unconscious. In that case conscious awareness is an excellent therapeutic factor. This is something which in eurythmy therapy, too, leads to things being brought very much to awareness, as I said earlier, and such concentration greatly supports the eurythmy therapy.

A particularly important thing I want to tell you is that all E forms essentially have a regulating action when the influence of the astral organism on the etheric organism is too great or too weak. In all the cases where we can say the activity of the astral organism is excessive or too little we can often do a great deal with E forms, repetition of E forms. E forms will be able to help with the two syndromes I discussed in the earlier session today.[28, 29] This thing I have been saying will be the case especially when the astral organism is influenced by the etheric organism, that is, when it is too weak, letting itself be influenced by the etheric, when an irregularity in the astral organism of the head makes it too strong. The opposite may be the case when the etheric is too much under the influence of the astral; that is the case when the astral comes to expression most powerfully in the intestinal organization, so that one gets diarrhoea whenever one feels even the slightest bit of fear or anxiety. In that case U forms will be particularly helpful.

Yesterday a question arose which I wish to consider briefly in conclusion. It was whether we may ask individuals who are pregnant or have a pelvic disease to do certain eurythmy therapy movements. Examine the rule given in Dornach and you will certainly be able to obey it. Although you have to see to it that the pelvic region is left in peace during pregnancy or in cases of pelvic disease, it has to be left in peace and must not be irritated by eurythmy therapy. Although it is left in peace, exercises can certainly be done with the arms, also sitting down, lying down, leaving that which must have peace fully in peace, or with the head. And you'll still find enough in the information given to intervene with eurythmy in all cases. Of course, if the individual concerned is completely unable to move, eurythmy would be the greatest help of all, for instance with symptoms of paralysis; but the situation may be that he cannot do the exercises. As you know, such symptoms of paralysis are essentially due to abnormal functioning of the astral body which is not intervening in the etheric and physical organization, and in that case one can achieve a great deal with E movements. A most helpful E movement—for pelvic disorders as such—is an artificial squint, not overdone but done with due care. It is absolutely true, therefore, that those somewhat decadent yogis who focus on the tip of the nose when doing certain exercises are really intending to evoke the most harmonious function of their pelvic region, knowing only too well what pelvic activity means also for 'spiritual work' as these people call it. It is thus reasonable to say: These things are such that something done even in jumps by someone whose pelvis is sound, can simply be replaced by a more subtle eurythmy therapy done with the arms, the fingers and even the eyes when it is necessary. Whatever the circumstances, a pregnant woman, for instance, must not be encouraged to jump about in eurythmy therapy exercises. That will not do, of course.

You see, in this case, too, it truly is not a matter of wanting some kind of universal panacea, to be acquired in half a day. No, eurythmy therapy, too, has to be acquired by making serious efforts, and it is in fact necessary to acquire it through practice. Almost every time when your instincts to heal have made you use the eurythmy therapy exercise a little bit you will gain greater ability. It is absolutely true that practice will be particularly useful for making progress in eurythmy therapy.

Well, I wanted to discuss eurythmy therapy with you in this more theoretical way because everything was said at that time in Dornach, with our medical friends passing it on, so that you can always have it, also because I wanted you also to understand the whole physiological and therapeutic meaning of eurythmy therapy. On the other hand we must not overestimate it. Eurythmy therapy will be an extraordinarily important aid in many cases, but we must not overestimate it. And we have to understand that intoxicating simplicity really does not get us anywhere, and that just as cancer cannot be cured by that 'intoxicating simplicity' any more than it can by 'harmonizing disharmony', so a broken leg or arm cannot be cured with eurythmy therapy exercises. We must be clear about this. Our aim with the science of the spirit is not to increase amateurism and lay medicine, but to add to expert medical skills.

Forgive me for stressing this over and over again but to avoid mis-understanding I wish to stress again and again and most specifically that the methods are not part of a lay opposition to conventional medicine, as is often the case with fanatical movements, but take full account of the present status of medicine, seeking merely to take it further along the road on which it needs to go, for the simple reason that it is not true to say that human beings are merely what they are said to be in modern physiology and anatomy. They are this, but they are also something else. They must also be perceived in their mind and spirit. Strange ideas like those repeated by people again and again today will then disappear, ideas that the brain is a kind of centre of telegraphy, with the 'sensory' nerves going to it, and will nerves coming from it. The whole does not at all agree with the facts, as you have seen from today's lecture. In the neurosensory system we are dealing with modelling dynamics; and something is wrested from these to which the mind's activities then adapt. A great deal needs to be done to restore to a sound physiology what has been taken from it by seeing the physical organism as a correlate for the mental functions. Something physical does exist for every one of those functions during human life on earth; but nothing is used for the mind which does not on the other hand have much greater significance in the interaction with other organs for the bodily organization. Nothing is used purely as an organ for the mind. The whole of our soul and spirit has been wrested from the bodily element, is taken from that element. And we must not speak of separate soul organs. All we can say is that soul functions are differentiated out from the organic actions and specially adapted to soul activity.

We have to grasp, in all seriousness, what is really taking effect in the human physical organism and not take such a superficial view of the whole nervous system solely as something put in to serve the inner life. If we do this we can hope to understand the human organization wholly. The human organization must be thus fully understood to provide a basis for a physiology and therapy that is working in the light and not merely trying things out in the dark. This is what I also wanted to say at the end so that you do not go away misunderstanding this, and that you will be able to counter the misunderstandings which will come up again and again.

Criticism was launched into the world with 'intoxicating simplicity' against our cancer medicine, for instance, when in fact people had no idea what kind of insight had led to it; they construe some easy analogy and think they can reject the medicine by rejecting that easy analogy. One condition for being true to the spiritual-scientific side of medicine is that we correct misunderstandings a little. For people will find that when they can no longer spread misunderstandings there will be precious little for them to say, for opposition consists mainly in spreading about misunderstood ideas about the whole of anthroposophy. Just try and find out how many opponents have anything to say that is not a misunderstanding. I must say, I often read articles or books by opponents, and if it did not give my name I could just as well connect it with something else. It really has nothing to do with what we are doing here, but concerns itself with completely different things. It really surprises me sometimes. I would like to discover where the matter to be refuted might be found; it certainly is not here.

Things are done here in medicine just as they are also done with reference to theology. You come up against the same thing. You may for example tell a truly learned theologian: 'We say the things you are saying about the Christ, but something else as well.' He won't be satisfied with our saying what he is saying and something else as well. He'll say: 'You must not add to this.' He will not criticize something that goes against his word but something which he is not saying at all. He criticizes it simply because you're saying something about something he knows nothing about. We must not fall into this error in medicine. We have to look at things carefully and not say anything against them, but here, too, we have to add many different things from an insight into the human being in sickness and in health which has quite a sound basis by now.

III
ASPECTS OF THERAPY

Lecture 10

It is good to know that you have already stated what you would like us to consider, and we'll start with those requests. I hope the three sessions at our disposal will permit us to cover it all. In these few sessions I would wish to talk to you truly as things arise from anthroposophy, so that we won't concern ourselves with the current terminology of another field but concentrate on the subject matter as requested, the way it can arise from anthroposophy.

The first question raised, and other things can no doubt also be covered by this, at least in principle, was about syphilitic conditions. So far we have not said much about these. They have to be carefully distinguished from all kinds of sequels, concurrent phenomena, and so on, and really point most intensively to the organism's behaviour in sickness. The luetic or syphilitic phenomena are a significant issue in medical theory and practice, for without doubt—let us speak without any prejudice, you will see that we do not wish to stop at prejudices for this reason—mercury treatments are the specific for them. Yet it is exactly the study of mercury treatments which will help us to realize how the problem may be dealt with in a more appropriate way.

Essentially every illness is due to lack of harmony in the way the three systems in the human organism work together. The study of these systems—the neurosensory system, the rhythmic system and the system of limbs and metabolism—is much more important than even physicians think today. Just consider what this harmonious interaction rests on. In the system of metabolism and limbs we have an activity of the human organism that proceeds above all in conjunction with the etheric body. But the other aspects of the human organism also have an influence on each of the systems. Thus we cannot say that the two aspects of the human organism, the physical and the etheric organism, are acting together in the system of metabolism and limbs; they are merely the principal agents. The others have an influence—the astral body and the I organization. In the organization of the head, that is, in the whole neurosensory organization, the situation is that the I organization and astral organization are the main influences, and in a more subordinate way also the etheric organization and the physical organization.

Above all we must clearly understand that the difference between the waking and the sleeping state is that in the latter, with the organism showing a kind of inertia, the activities coming from astral organism and I organism continue on, in a way, activities which in the waking state have a direct influence. They continue as an after-echo in the sleeping state, when the astral body and I organization are absent. Can we understand this? The actions continue on, just as when I give a ball a push and it will roll on even when no longer pushed. And this is how the activities of the astral body and I organization continue to be effective in sleep. It would thus be wrong to say of anything derived from the I organization or the astral organization that they could not be present in sleep. Sleep merely has to end when there is a danger of the astral after-activities or I after-activities coming to an end. That is the moment when sleep must end again and the waking state arise. But these things cannot be taken in the schematic form in which they sometimes have to be presented in anthroposophy to help lay people to understand.

Here we must truly present the facts as they are. All those many questions as to the causes really should in the main relate not to the internal organization of the organism but rather the way things are brought about from outside. This is something we should always know. We should always make the diagnosis such that it is a complete case record. Speculation about causes in the organism does not really help one to find the medicinal agents in the right way.

If I put the question like this, I have to say: What is the actual situation with syphilis? Let us consider syphilis on its own, leaving aside anything which might also be sexually transmitted disease, gonorrhoea, chancres and so on, everything therefore which essentially—we'll consider it separately later—is not connected with syphilis but essentially a different disease. Syphilis as such essentially is due to the human I organization being in demand too much for the system of metabolism and limbs, mainly the metabolic system, therefore. In a way, the human I organization slides down into the pelvic region. And all the symptoms which develop are due to the I organization sliding down excessively into the pelvic region. This gives rise to all the processes reflected in the familiar symptoms, processes resulting in preponderance of the I organization over the etheric organization, which should not be present in this tract in the human organism. The I organization is simply too powerful in the sexual tract. These are the facts. We must first consider these facts and not so much the infection and so on; for the facts are there. And the cure must really be based on these facts.

Let us consider the effects of mercury treatment. What happens in the human organism with any mercury treatment? As you know, this is a very old method of treatment and on occasion extraordinarily useful in treating not only syphilis but also other conditions. But what happens with mercury treatment?

Mercury is one of the medicinal agents that was considered beneficial in times when medicine was instinctive and far-reaching, used on the basis of a certain instinctive insight into the human organism. But what brings about healing when you have to have mercury treatment for syphilis? Exactly as much of the mercury preparation in correct dosage as is introduced into the blood will heal. The exact amount does it. Consider the consequences. In the first place it is not the custom, so far as I know, to give mercury by injection to treat syphilis. People have started to do so in recent years, as the earlier ointment treatments are no longer so effective, or too effective; but all in all even this partial change came about empirically because people realized that the ointment had aspects that lead to problems.

What is going on? If you use the ointment it will essentially lead to partial, and indeed general infection. It is designed for all of it to enter into the bloodstream. But when you apply the ointment, the mercury impulse also follows other lines in the human organism. The part which enters into the blood will cure; any that does not get into the blood but follows etheric pathways, is carried along etheric pathways that run along the nervous system, the nerve strands, for instance, creates problems. All of it spreads the I organization through the whole organism, as it were, and essentially you merely get the problem spread over the whole organism in a different form. The internal processes which prepare for this go on for years, and then all the phenomena appear which are the sequels of the mercury treatment.

We may say, therefore, that the treatment of syphilis with mercury shows the actual medicinal action of mercury. What is it based on? The subject matter can today be spoken of in quite general terms, as I did yesterday in the general lecture.[30] From a certain moment onwards the organic substances are no longer under the influence of the earth's forces but under the influence of cosmic forces acting from the periphery towards the centre of the earth. The point is that from a certain moment onwards everything we receive into the organism via ordinary digestion once it has passed the intestine is under the influence of cosmic powers, powers that round things off, real cosmic powers that round things off.

The I organization mainly lives in these cosmic powers. If it intervenes too much in the metabolic system the I organization simply shows the tendency to atomize, to round off individual elements in the human organism, organizing them, rather than to organize whole body through and through in its form. All the signs of syphilis, all the symptoms of syphilis, result from this partial atomizing, this atomistic organizing process. The I organization intervenes in truly very small systems in the human organism, systems that should be left for the ether body to organize which alone is subject to the peripheral cosmic forces directly and not via the I organization.

Mercury has the peculiarity that introduced into the human organism it is under earthly conditions the substance which for itself imitates the outer form of the cosmos most intensively. The moment we introduce mercury directly into the bloodstream by injecting it, the tendency develops to hand this partial organization, this small-scale atomistic organization over to the mercury. The I organization is then free again, active everywhere in the organism, and able to restore the state of health by reaction.

All this does, however, depend on the patient never having more mercury in him than is absolutely necessary. It is a problem which can never be solved. For when giving mercury treatment you must never run the risk of giving even just a little too much. You must give exactly as much as can be taken up into the bloodstream according to the current status of the disease, for any excess remains as a residue and causes the sequels which are familiar to you.

So you will always find that mercury treatment cures but the patient may often have to pay a truly heavy price for this with the terrible sequels which also look like syphilis but really must gradually and irrevocably destroy the organism. The very fact of mercury being a certain cure shows us that its use is highly problematical.

It was not always problematical. You see, not exactly syphilis but various other conditions were always treated with mercury—we may perhaps talk about this on one of the next days. Mercury actually provoked a quite specific emotive reaction in the sick who were gifted with instinct. The patient would know when he had enough. He would be sated with mercury. The instincts have degenerated now. Patients can no longer provide the standard for what happens to them through mercury. They are no longer sated with mercury but overfed with it. This is generally the situation today. Patients are more than sated with mercury, and the devastating sequels then develop. Just as we can clearly see the action of sulphur and phosphorus in the organism, and what happens in the organism when salt dissolves, though one must always be careful about the dosage, so we can see it in the case of mercury. We know the basis on which mercury acts.

The question is, would it be possible to give such treatment so that it does not harm, even if the dosage is too high, because elimination to the outside would deal with the excess. Mercury has the peculiarity that it is not eliminated to the outside when too much is applied to the body; it is eliminated to the inside. In this respect it was extraordinarily important to me when I was young to see Hyrtl[31] simply take the bones of people who had had mercury treatment at the post mortem, knock one against the other, and one could then see the small droplets of mercury in those bones under the microscope. The whole skeletal system was full of mercury. This is the peculiarity of mercury. It is not eliminated to the outside. The organism takes it up, and in someone who has had mercury treatment the whole I organization is all the time involved in organizing these tiny mercury droplets, mercury atoms, which are present everywhere in the organism, and especially in the calcified parts.

It is fair to say that we must try and find something in the realm of nature that is taken up by the organism when mercury is used and takes the place of the I organization to relieve it and set it free. Yet if you give too much of it, which is inevitable, it must be eliminated not to the inside but to the outside, like anything else that gets digested.

We must find something which in the natural world outside corresponds to I nature and where it may be possible to process it so that it actually enters into the bloodstream, evoking a phantom, as it were, of the I organization in the bloodstream. What we have to do is to put an artificial I into the bloodstream.

Our physicians in particular should do the relevant experiments. You will without doubt see results that will certainly be surprising. Take material obtainable from plant parts that show extraordinary hardening, with the root process applied to the rest of the plant. In the root process of a plant we have an extraordinarily great imitation of the I organization. The flower is etheric in organization. In the parts below the flower the astral organization is playing around the plant. The I organization comes in where the plant is rooted in the soil. In very woody roots which, however, are still part of the plant and have not been separated from the plant and grown inorganic, we have impulses of the I organization.

It will not, however, be possible to take plant roots, extract substances and inject them. The reason is that the plant root does very much contain the I organization, being a phantom of the I organization, as it were, but the impulses living in the root are limited to the neurosensory system and do not act strongly down into the rest of the organization. We may say, therefore, that when the root organization is taken as root only you will hardly be able to produce a preparation for the above-mentioned purpose. There are plants, however, where the root organization has a powerful influence on the whole plant. Such a plant, where the root organization penetrates the whole plant as far as the fruit, is *Astragalus exscapus*, hart's milk vetch.[32] Its fruits look like pods but are rock hard and contain grains. I am referring to something which is completely cornified, as it were. Or take certain types of wood which are in fact used and the action of which is based on the principle I have been presenting.

We have to take the seed grains from a plant such as hart's milk vetch, grind them finely and then treat them with the plant's sap, sap from the flowers and leaves of the same plant. This gives us a preparation that may perhaps be taken to the third decimal. Injected in the third decimal it will introduce this phantom of the I into the bloodstream, and in a case of syphilis that has affected the whole blood we will, under the influence of this preparation, have exactly the same picture as with mercury treatment. We must then ensure that the excess is driven out with hyperthermic baths. We must thus combine two things—injection with a preparation of this kind and then driving out the excess with hyperthermic baths.

Something else will also come out. The harmful substances in the blood of syphilis patients will come out. This must happen through the discharge of sweat. We therefore have to say that sweating is the only way of getting out the things that must be got out. But these must first be held on to, and this can be done with this rounding-off action of the impulses in the hart's milk vetch seeds. So you see, we can really only manage such things by bringing diagnosis and treatment closely together.

Individualization is absolutely essential in medicine. It is easy to observe that with forms of syphilis in particular, the syndrome is completely different for an obese person and a lean one. With an obese person it will be extraordinarily difficult to get the syphilis poison out of the body. I don't know if anyone present today has experience in this. The syphilis poison is harder to get out if the individual is obese compared to someone who is lean. The latter kind of person will have the poison come away relatively easily. With a lean individual you will probably manage well by using the method I have given. You must make sure, however, that there is a reaction, that perspiration is massive; otherwise you will get all kinds of internal diseases as sequels, for the disease process will then not take its course. There has to be a reaction. It may well be that you have to take other measures as well to get the same result with obese patients. It will be a very good thing to turn to something which in nature, too, has come up more into the astral process. It will be a good thing in certain cases where you see no reaction with the usual plant to use plant galls.[33] I spoke of them in a different context yesterday.

In plant galls, the etheric roundness is already there; the gall shows you mercurial nature in the vegetable realm. If you process it by trituration, adding a very small dose of the venom of the wasp which caused the gall to develop in the process, this will give you a very effective medicine which provokes a reaction also in situations where it is difficult to get a reaction.

The situation with us is that we really have far too few cases which we can observe step by step. I would imagine that our friends who are physicians do not exactly consider it to be the ideal to bring syphilis patients into their institutes. But things like this cast a light on the whole of therapy altogether. We really learn something for the whole of therapy from such a treatment, and I am also convinced that once someone has seen how the skin of a patient who has had the injection and the bath looks different when he gets out of the bath. Taking a more subtle look—we might perhaps use a microscope. The skin looks as if it had tiny holes everywhere, like very small pustules[34] almost; we see how the organism is affected by something like this. I believe this is the route to be followed in treating syphilis.

You see, with this disease in particular it is necessary not merely to see to it that one helps the patient and then discharges him, but also that one sees to it that the patient sustains the cure as life goes on. This brings me to a question that has also been asked and will be of great interest to most of you: Meditation to accompany medical treatment— are there any typical suggestions available for this?

I am referring to syphilis specifically in connection with this question, for syphilis is the disease which perhaps allows us to answer it most intensely. It is a fact that a syphilis patient who appears to have been cured—every syphilis patient will at first only appear to be cured, for the disease may recur on some future occasion, and every apparently cured syphilis may come up again at a later time—and this will depend on the individual in question having made his organism altogether into something different from that of someone who does not have syphilis. It is a different constitution, and we must seek to maintain this different constitution for the future, otherwise it will simply prove to be too weak in the face of certain attacks from everyday life, with the syphilis recurring.

We will of course consider the question of meditative treatment only in general terms, but it can be brought in at just this point. With syphilis, the I organization is making itself independent, in a way, something that does not happen with a normal person. The syphilis patient has made this phantom out of his own organism due to the injection, and as a result his I organization will be more independent for the rest of his life on earth than that of someone who has never had syphilis; it is more independent, and this must be taken into account. To cure a syphilis patient permanently you must see to it that he begins to take a great interest in turning some kind of highly abstract thoughts over in his head again and again, meditatively so. You thus have to advise him to think through geometrical or mathematical problems meditatively, over and over again in rhythmic repetition, so that he will never cease really to continue to make his I organization abstract in this artificial way. You have to get his thinking used to this, to develop a certain inner constitution. You will therefore really help him by giving this advice: Every morning, when you've woken up, consider how a small similar triangle relates to a large one. You have the same angles, different sides. Think this very slowly at first—same angles, different sides. Then think it a bit faster, then yet faster, and then think it in a way where you are practically no longer able to see it. After that start to think more slowly again.

Thinking at different speeds, arbitrarily, will get him to provide in the right way for this I organization that has grown independent. This is one such a type of meditation. But wherever you see that the I organization has grown more independent in some healing process or other you can try to make it possible for the patient to continue through life with such a meditation. It is just that it has to be applied particularly strongly in the case of syphilis patients. These patients must really be encouraged to provide for their independent I organization by means of such a meditation done at different beats. Does that make sense?

These things take us to other questions that have been put. We will come back to it all again; I merely would like to have the right context which the matter demands.

Question concerning the root of hart's milk vetch.

They are pods. You open them up and in there are the rock hard seeds which must be reduced to a very fine powder.

Another question that has been asked does not appear to be connected, but inwardly these things are connected. It concerns the development of glaucoma. I think today glaucoma is practically always treated surgically, except perhaps by the homoeopaths; but homoeopathy is not yet rational. It will be necessary to understand the background to a phenomenon such as glaucoma. In a sense, from an organic point of view, in terms of the four levels of human existence—physical body, etheric body, astral body and I—glaucoma is really the opposite of all possible forms of ear inflammation if we consider the total process of the organism. The two things are almost polar opposites. You have otitis on the one hand and glaucoma-type phenomena on the other. If you simply consider the fact, it is like this. Glaucoma involves a powerful activity infiltrating the vitreous body, substantially constituting it. The vitreous body grows too intensive inwardly where its own substance is concerned. This leads to hypertrophy of vitreous body activity, and that is the real basis of glaucoma. But what happens next?

In terms of the general bodily constitution, a sense organ such as the eye is just on the point of being sufficiently independent, objectively separated off from the organism as a whole. If it is separated off a bit more than is the case for normal vision, it will be sick and the organism as a whole can no longer extend its activity to this organ.

It is really most interesting to see, especially with glaucoma, how the etheric body—particularly important for the eye—is present throughout the eyeball, so much so that the physical substance in the vitreous body acts like a physical substance. If it goes beyond the bounds of this it will act too much as a physical substance. The ether body can no longer reach it, can no longer infiltrate it. We have to see to it, therefore, that the ether body comes into play again, or that physical activity in the eye is toned down. It may be commonplace but it is true to say, when something like this happens, that the whole of organic activity in this tract of the human organism is simply too weak, partly paralysed. The activity is too weak and must be spurred on. You can only do this by making exhalation stronger in the human organism than it is in the person with glaucoma at the time when it develops or progresses. If you are able to establish the glaucoma signs and symptoms at the right moment—but the organism sometimes achieves powerful results with regard to such partial diseases—you will get the organism to respond to everything you introduce into it to encourage exhalation, thus stimulating it to increase activity within the head, and you will manage to counteract the activity of glaucoma development. We can achieve this by introducing calcium carbonate from bone ash into the human organism, adding some aerial roots of some kind to it. This gives you a product which regulates respiratory function in the way that is needed in this case.

So I mean to say that if we take calcium carbonate from bone ash and introduce it into the human organism we get the requisite powerful stimulus to exhale. However, to get the organism itself involved and have the activity proceed not sluggishly, without the organism, as it were, we have to combine this calcium carbonate with the kind of impulses found in the roots of plants that climb rocks, roots that live in the open air, so that the root element which otherwise grows in the soil is taken out into the air. This will make these roots such that their impulses do indeed resemble breathing activity more closely and we thus have a possibility of getting breathing activity into us. You feel it then. Breathing activity is otherwise stimulated quite involuntarily by calcium carbonate. But if you add the sap from such aerial roots, you have the urge to breathe in like this added. This urge to breathe in like this then strengthens the whole human organization which you need to balance out what has forcibly left you as the glaucoma developed.

Things like this really show that it is always necessary to consider the whole human being. But the physical body is never the whole body. The physical body is always only a part; it is liver, stomach and so on, and the individual parts are interconnected. The ether body is whole human being to quite a degree, and the astral body is whole human being in a truly magnificent sense. This astral body is, however, organized in a most peculiar way. We might say that the human astral body as far as the diaphragm—those are approximately the outer limits—is some-thing very different from the astral body below the diaphragm. Astral body activity up towards the head, towards the neurosensory organi-zation, is the complete polar opposite in its activity to that active in the system of metabolism and limbs. Do consider metabolism altogether, which essentially proceeds under the influence of the astral body. Metabolism as we usually see it is really an activity of the human organism where it is only the activity that matters. It is really only the taking up and elimination of substances which matters. We might say that food as such, as substance, does not interest the metabolism at all, but only the overcoming of the outward, substantial form of foods and their metamorphosis, not the needs of the organism. Elimination starts immediately in the metabolism itself. Uptake does really immediately become elimination. Only some of it is separated off. And this pene-trates as far as the neurosensory organization. With regard to substance, the neurosensory organization is extraordinarily important, for nerve substance is metabolic substance driven to the very end.

It may seem grotesque, but in real terms it is certainly so that the contents of the intestine are nerve substance that has gone only halfway. Nerve substance, especially of the head, is intestinal content processed all the way, intestinal content transformed by the human organism and especially the I organization. The contents of the intestines have only gone halfway and are eliminated at that point. The content of nerve substance has been driven to the very end, where it is fully used up and then needs to be processed by the organism. In actual metabolism the astral organism performs a function which is completely different from its function in the central nervous system. They are absolute polar opposites. This means that the one stops halfway, and the other is taken all the way. Between them lies a zero point. It is an absolute fact that polar opposition is complete here. If we were to draw the ether body, it would still be as an ovoid. The astral body can no longer be drawn as an ovoid; it has to be two parts, above and below, their mode of action totally different. Unless you see this, you cannot really understand the human being in health or in sickness.

We have to understand that a very different activity takes place in the metabolic sphere compared to that in the nerve sphere. This insight alone makes it possible for us to influence the human organism in a suitable way. If you give preparations made from the volatile oil obtained from a flower, for instance, you do not take them from the lower part of the astral organism into the upper part. They can only be used to evoke some processes or other in the lower part, in the actual metabolic tract. The moment you use anything obtained from the root of a plant, this pushes through from the lower to the upper tract of the astral body, and you have it in there because it acts back again from the head onto the organism. You have it in the whole of the organism.

For you must understand that the ordinary way of looking at the composition of the human organism is really most amateurish. You know, people imagine that when, let us say, after a certain time in life new substance has appeared in some part of the human organism or another this has come about by way of ordinary metabolism. It means that old substance has been cast off and the new substance has come about by way of ordinary metabolism. That is how people imagine it to be. I do not think that people who have studied medicine in some way today have a different idea, that some substances or other which are summarily different after a certain time in life have come to be there in any other way but by metabolism, by an exchange.

That is not the case, however. If after a certain time of life you find a different substance in some part or other of the human organism, it will never have been secreted along the pathways of ordinary metabolism. Ordinary metabolism only provides the substance for the nervous system, only the internal structure of the nervous system, only the building stones for the nervous system. The activities of the neurosensory system, in conjunction with respiration, then make it possible to take in substances from the cosmic surroundings. The substances are very finely divided and integrated into the organism by the neurosensory organization. In material terms they replace everything that has been cast off. For things are cast off much more slowly than you think.

The human body is thus never made up of the food substances. Nutrition merely maintains the activity which must be there to organize the nervous system. Anabolism, synthesis of matter, does not proceed by the route of nutrition, which is purely imaginary, but really comes in from the cosmos. So if you cut off a nail and it grows again, the material of the new growth does not come from the food, the only role of which is to induce the build-up of the nervous system. The new growth in the human being truly is organic matter substantially replaced, taken up from the cosmos.

This does, of course, give one quite a different picture of the way the human being is made up than if one thinks human beings are a kind of hosepipe. Food comes in at one end, exchange takes place in the meantime, and anything which is of no use is separated out. But human beings are not hosepipes. The hosepipe processes happen wholly inside the human organism. The new substance of which human beings are made up again after a certain time of life comes with our breathing and even with subtle absorption into the human organism from the outside world through the senses. The ears are extraordinarily important receptors in this respect, and also the whole sense of awareness, sentience, spread out over the body. Seeing the human being in the right way we thus have to say to ourselves right away that metabolism is internal work in the human organism. The rhythmic organism is also involved in building up the human being, as is the neurosensory organism.

Well, we'll continue with this tomorrow and gradually answer the other problems brought to our attention. Do tell me if you would prefer a different way, for the hours we have are but few. I am sure we'll get to the individual problems raised. If any of you have further problems, please let me have them tomorrow.

LECTURE 11

DORNACH, 1 JANUARY 1924

I have just heard that some confusion has arisen because I spoke of treatment with mercury on the one hand and then of another preparation yesterday. The point is that the mercury treatment was merely given as a specifically effective one, but it has its dangers and can be avoided. Yesterday I thought I had spoken of the hart's milk vetch root preparation as something that fully takes the place of mercury.

Let me go straight to the questions on the old list. We'll still have one more session tomorrow. The new questions include one, I think, that relates to our present subject: How can we understand the effectiveness of Salvarsan in treating syphilis?

Above all we must describe this effectiveness in more detail. With treatments like this you may always have a degree of success, but you also get harmful side effects. It is simply unthinkable to speak of rational treatment with Salvarsan, for the preparation—at least the way it is described—is such that it tears the human bodies apart, tears people apart. Nothing really fits. It may be possible to introduce whatever we want into the body and there may always be a positive result, but it is impossible to say what will come after that—undoubtedly so with Salvarsan, because things are contradictory. We are therefore only able to say: Salvarsan therapy is very much the outcome of present-day thinking. Essentially the situation is such that one cannot give it serious consideration. Perhaps one of you would wish to say something more about this?

Dr Rascher. Would this then also apply to the whole of modern metal therapy, including bismuth therapy?

You know, bismuth therapy is wholly comprehensible from our point of view. It is discussed in my courses. But Salvarsan is not fully comprehensible. It tears the body apart. There may, of course, be bismuth preparations which do the same if combined with other preparations. But the mode of action of bismuth should be evident from our courses.

Dr Noll. Can an antimony preparation be effective in treating syphilis?

Antimony has its sphere of action between the sexual and respiratory tracts. Everything in the human organization that lies between these two tracts can be covered by antimony, the rest of course only in so far as the action of a tract radiates out into the organism as a whole. But it is not really possible to treat anything that is wrong in the sexual tract specifically with antimony. Sequels of syphilitic conditions can be treated very well with antimony, but treating syphilis with antimony from the beginning will definitely not give a complete cure. Antimony relates wholly to the middle organization in the human being, the whole digestive tract, the transition from digestive tract to bloodstream, and of course also the part of the circulatory system which then continues on to the sexual organs. It is, however, distinctly limited to this tract.

Dr Kaçer. The bad effect of Salvarsan is sufficiently evident from the fatalities.

The greatest probability is this: Salvarsan has been used, and not that long ago. The bad effects in their culmination will be evident in five to ten years, perhaps also a period of seven. Unfortunately no case records are produced today. It is after all much, much more important for gaining insight in medicine that case records continue beyond the cure. This will profit us much more than a study of the internal condition of the organism prior to the disease. This may be most important on occasion, but there external things are generally of particular importance in most cases.

This is where I must again and again refer to such cases: Our friend Dr Haakenson[35] brought a patient to me in Oslo. The man had inexplicable skin eruptions. He was about 45 when he was brought to me, and in everyday medical terms presented with symptoms that could not possibly be said to hang together. You see, purely taking this further in terms of the organism you simply cannot find a plausible cause. Physicians are of course largely dependent on what patients tell them. I was able to tell the patient straight off (I'll leave out things that are less relevant), 'You must have been poisoned in some way when you were between eight, ten or eleven years old.'

Gradually it emerged that the man, then 45 years of age, had been thirsty one day at school. There happened to be a laboratory next to his classroom, with a weak solution of hydrochloric acid on the window sill. He drank this to quench his thirst. And the problem he had at age 45 went back to that poisoning.

To understand an illness we must look to this external cause as the most important thing. But afterwards we really must carefully continue to observe the organism after recovery, to see what brings about recovery.

And this would be particularly important with Salvarsan treatments. Here you clearly will not be able to apply what I said yesterday for the treatment of syphilis altogether. I referred to a kind of meditative treatment to follow, using abstract concepts which have to be done at different speeds, increasing the speed and then reducing it again, and most conscientiously. This will allow us to make psychic follow-up treatment (which will take years, however) bear fruit with syphilis—if it has been cured in the way I stated yesterday. This kind of psychic treatment would also be an advantage with the mercury treatment, which I do not, however, recommend. Doing such follow-up treatment with Salvarsan you will probably at a later stage in life get something we can't say is dementia praecox, but something very similar to dementia praecox later on in life. Mercury treatment with non-psychic follow-up will result in psychiatric phenomena because of the things I mentioned yesterday. But because of the tearing apart, it will be found that a kind of schizophrenia will follow Salvarsan treatment, especially if you attempt follow-up treatment in terms of the psyche.

Dr Palmer. *It would be very interesting to hear your views on 'tertiary' syphilis and iodine treatment.*

As to what can be said about this, the important point is that with a highly generalized condition such as syphilis we are dealing in the first place with the actual focus of the disease and anything that emanates from it, and then, however, because syphilis affects the whole human being, reaching up as far as the I organization, we are dealing with the counter-image in the neurosensory human being. Schematically it is reasonable to say that the disease is located in the human being of metabolism and limbs, and has its counter-image in the neurosensory human being, including also the laryngeal tract, for example—everything connected with the differentiating upper respiratory function. These two things are intimately connected. With mercury we act on the actual source and its emanations. With the iodine preparation we influence the upper part. Polar phenomena in the nerves and senses can be paralysed by iodine during mercury treatment. So that is the connection.

Yesterday, as you'll recall, I spoke mainly of two parts of the whole of syphilis treatment. The first is injecting the preparation, the second is the bath treatment to drive out [any excess].[36] This corresponds in a much more natural, rational sense just as mercury and iodine do. So that is the idea. It is altogether the case that treatment generally takes us to treating the two polar opposite organizations so as to balance them out.

Dr Palmer. The gummas would therefore have to be seen as sequels to excessive mercury?

Yes, very definitely so. Are there any more questions relating to this?

Dr Kaçer. How does arsenic act?

Generally speaking, the action of arsenic is essentially to energize the human astral body. That is the basic phenomenon of arsenic action. Arsenic and also its compounds act so powerfully on human beings that we may say it energizes the astral body. If you use arsenic, especially in fluid form, simply as Roncegno or Levico water in suitable dosage, you will always get a response when there is need to stimulate the astral body to produce the impulses which are natural to it.

With every disease of this kind by the way, with syphilis and also other venereal disease, a defect in the astral body is either cause or consequence. It is quite natural for arsenic to have an observable effect in that case, but it would not necessarily cure. It does not go deep enough for us to speak of a cure.

Dr ... Is the situation different for a child with congenital syphilis?

You mean hereditary syphilis? In children the situation is of course completely different. And if you are able to make the diagnosis in good time you will get somewhere, especially with arsenic, but not with Salvarsan. Use the arsenic in its greater dilution[37] and perhaps with added lactic acid or similar to have it act far enough ahead in the body. In this way you'll be able to get very good results especially in children. For congenital syphilis is not really a syphilis. It differs from syphilis in that among the levels of the human organization, particularly in adults, syphilis due to infection acts mainly on the etheric body. The inherited form enters only into the physical body and is not present in the etheric body. By strongly stimulating the astral body with arsenic, you can transfer that to the etheric body and then combat it in an entirely rational way in the physical body. The problem with congenital syphilis is that one has thoroughly ruined an element which is so difficult to access with substances from the earth.

Here we must consider the element which I spoke of in the general lecture,[38] showing it to be subject to the peripheral forces. If you altogether want to have any kind of influence on such deformation and degeneration, damage altogether connected with the peripheral forces, you must also find a way of setting etheric powers in motion.

Now this milk vetch of which I spoke yesterday has the peculiarity that it has hardened, cornified, and therefore does not really have forces that are still etheric flashing around it. If you then obtain these etheric forces in the sap of its own flowers and leaves, the resulting preparation will be as I described it yesterday. This leads to rational thinking on the subject.

Dr Palmer. *Further question about tertiary syphilis.*

Concerning tertiary syphilis, one can only say that to be truly rational one can only endeavour to stop it developing, seeking to deal with syphilis in its first stage. Once it has become secondary or tertiary, the syndrome is very complicated, from the occult point of view, and need not be the same for any two patients. It only looks similar from outside; inwardly it need not be the same. It is therefore extremely difficult to deal with, for you cure it at one end and it breaks out in the opposite sense at the other end. If one has to take a position with reference to this, one can only say that secondary syphilis must of course be treated in the way I said yesterday; with tertiary syphilis one may on occasion still get a cure, but it will always be problematical.

Dr Palmer. Concerning glaucoma process, ear process. The glaucoma process is considered to be a kind of tumour process; ear processes are purulent processes, inflammatory processes, and ear development must be considered to be a tumour development process. Is the polar opposition represented on the one hand by glaucoma and on the other by otitis?

Surely that is obvious? If the eye is normally an inflammatory process, and the ear a tumour process, then disease must be a tumour process in the eye, an inflammatory process in the ear, which is the opposite in each case. It is obvious, as it were, that it has to be this way.

This may be a good opportunity to speak of these polar opposite processes of otitis, and specially otitis media. Otitis absolutely means that the etheric organization is gaining the upper hand in this local tract. This is evident not only from occult observation but simply by looking at the end stage of otitis media, with the organs fusing, and so on.

Looking at the physical organism one will then see that here the etheric body is getting excessively active. One has to know that in this tract an overweening ether organization immediately causes the I organization to be enhanced in this tract, a process which goes down into the subconscious.

So we have a physical development which should not be there and which depends on the I organization. We can best deal with it by getting the breathing process active again. This is possible with medication, so that exhalation comes more alive, giving Levisticum in suitable doses. This gets the breathing process—in the opposite sense to yesterday's reference to glaucoma development—moving. Breathing is more such that the strengthened breathing process goes inwards, whilst it must go to the outside with the Levisticum process. The strengthening of the breathing process thus goes more to the inside. And for otitis, strange as it may seem, eurythmy therapy will prove particularly helpful. It will be extraordinarily helpful to do L, M, S exercises. Everything relating to the ear is really only a localized process for a process in the whole human ether body. Because of this we can influence everything that becomes localized in the ear by helping the breathing—

we only help the breathing with this—in getting the patient to do the L, M, S exercises.

Now there are some other things I want to say.

Dr ... Eurythmy would no doubt have to be different for otitis and for sclerotic processes?

With sclerosis one will above all practise eurythmy therapy based on vowels. With inflammatory processes it has to be consonants, especially L, M, S and such speech sounds.

Other questions have been raised and I'd like to consider them one after the other. The case asked about here, and we do already have some experience with it, is indeed particularly interesting. The question was:

Is it still possible for treatment to be effective with arthritis deformans which has persisted for years?

Perhaps Dr Palmer will be so kind as to give a brief review of our case in Stuttgart.

Dr Palmer. This case which we treated at that time, with the treatment now general knowledge, was one of a fresh arthritis deformans. Mrs X was treated for four or five weeks with phosphorus oil 1% and triturated Stannum 4–5%, and all her symptoms, previously treated at other clinics, disappeared. Apart from the medical treatment the patient also had eurythmy therapy. We used the same treatment in the cases that came to our clinic, but did not, of course, have the same success as in this fresh case. A boy who had developed the condition in his third, fourth year, was also treated with phosphorus oil and Stannum, but we also had to give Levico Water injections to enhance the effect. The boy was at a very acute inflammatory stage of arthritis in the hip, and in his case, too, all symptoms regressed and he was completely free of pain. The damage to the joints and cartilage was, of course, already so severe that there was no question of restoring joint mobility.

That is altogether the problem, of course. Let us now consider the two cases, for this can teach us a great deal. How old was our patient Mrs X?

Dr Palmer. Perhaps in her late twenties, and the boy will have been 12 or 13; it was the American boy.

Dr Kaçer states that her patient is 27, and has had the condition from her twelfth year; a second patient is 45, sick for three years, and one patient was about 70 years old.

The question, is, however, if you achieved a cure. Did you give the same treatment?

Dr Kaçer *states that she had only now started to use it.*

The matter is extraordinarily important because with this condition enormously much depends on the kind of person we are dealing with. And we can indeed say that with arthritis deformans it truly is the case that in a certain respect we really have to individualize treatment in all cases, for the genesis of the condition relates greatly to the whole development of the person. In a condition which develops in the middle years, as in the case I first asked Dr Palmer to interpret, you sometimes have to ask: Does the cause lie far back in childhood, or did the causes only develop in later years?

The peculiar thing is exactly that with the relevant bodily disposition, especially if there is a constitutional weakness of the etheric body, the cause of arthritis deformans lies in mental processes, especially in people who bring their astral body down into a weak etheric body on waking, so that because of the weakness in the etheric body the astral body comes to be stronger than it really should be, is not sufficiently toned down as it enters into the etheric body. Pain, care, shocks and consuming sorrow then truly act as the cause for the disease.

The peculiar thing is this, however. If you have a child, let's take an ideal case, a child in his tenth year, and somehow, let us say due to having had measles or the like, his etheric body is weakened, even if only for a time; the astral body is too powerful. At this time of life—I won't say 10, but 12 years, you'll see why in a minute—if the child has a grouchy teacher who gets him into states of all kinds so that he is at odds with himself, such a child's worries will be predominantly active at first. As the fourteenth year approaches, approximately of course, two years will have passed from his twelfth to fourteenth year, another two years take him to his sixteenth year, and in that sixteenth year—just as long after the end of the period following sexual maturity as the insult came before sexual maturity—there is a possibility of the business repeating itself rhythmically. Then it will not be new worry coming from outside, but the organic counter-image of those worries. Now the question is: How long does this process need after the periods which develop there to be thoroughly peripheral? At another period, in the twenty-first year, that is, in the nineteenth, two years before, and again two years later, at age 23, the possibility for this child will again exist for the matter progressing.

It just is a question as to how long this process needs to be thoroughly peripheral, to appear as a deformation. Depending on circumstance, this may extend from the twelfth year, where the first causes are, to the 30s, or indeed the early 40s. This is a very different picture than if someone, say, only comes up against the psychic cause after his fiftieth year or in the late 40s, when the experience may also come. In that case these deformations come from a completely different depth in the organism. We are therefore able to say—let as assume we have a patient who is in his late 30s or early 40s, if you like, and suffers from severe arthritis deformans, an indication that the causes are really a long way back. On the basis of these facts one might suggest the following treatment. I have construed an ideal case in response to your question, and it would now be a matter of provoking what has been the subject of our discussion here by means of arsenic injection and Stannum and so on, by giving hydrogen sulphide baths, thus acting first of all on the neurosensory system, which always responds to such baths, thus taking hold of the peripheral human being from outside. If you then give high potencies of Arnica, Arnica tincture or Equisetum by mouth—both the same in this case—you are acting in the same direction from inside out, and you will probably get a cure even with a long-established arthritis deformans.

We can certainly say that this would be a case which might be treated in this way. Cases like the first one given by Dr Palmer, where the cause definitely did not go back such a long way, might be treated with Stannum and with phosphorus oil. I was pleased to mention this case because it is instructive to see from a condition just like this, though it does go very deep, how we must individualize.

A case is described where a woman had gone through something like this in her youth. In her 20s she then had a gonorrhoeal infection and immediately after this developed a very severe chronic arthritis. She is now about 45 and in a truly desolate state.

It is almost as if I had construed this case as an ideal one just now! Hydrogen sulphide baths and Equisetum or Arnica by mouth—or perhaps, if there is no immediate response, by injection.

Dr Kaçer. *The case to which you were referring is exactly that of the woman aged 27 who is my patient. You gave an accurate outline without knowing the case.*

Here again an interesting question arises—diseases of the gastro-intestinal tract due to shock. They may develop due to shock, but I think also due to other psychic influences such as long-lasting worries or the like, constantly provided with more food; this will be the case especially with females. Very painful colicky states may develop. Lethargy of the whole gastrointestinal tract may also occur, or even complete failure, but a failure frequently also involving sensations of pain. Isn't that more or less the picture one gets? (*Answer: yes.*)

This is a very common condition and it is highly interesting to observe what has really happened. In every one of these cases the following has happened. The human astral body is a highly differentiated organism, and when you get to know this human astral body you find it greatly adapts itself to the ether body for all organs that lie behind the sexual organs in the direction of the renal tract, their upper limits defined by the lung and heart tract—in this area, therefore. We may say, therefore, that the ether body sets the tone in this tract. The astral body adopts what the ether body does in its movements, its forms. It is very different in the sexual tract. The astral body is strongly active in the sexual tract, in some respect suppressing ether body activity. If a shock of this kind occurs here, the activity which the astral body develops in the sexual tract forces its way into the digestive tract, and we have a displacement of astral activity, with all the symptoms I mentioned. We need to initiate the process which will take the astral body to its proper place again in such a case.

We must truly understand this situation which really takes place wholly among the higher levels of existence in the human organism. Anything taking place in the physical body is merely a sequel, an outer symptom. The process is between ether body and astral body, partially so in that particular region of the body.

You will always get a result with compresses or *einreibungen* [special medicated rubs] with oxalic acid, simply oxalic acid which is most easily obtained by expressing clover. You express clover and thus obtain oxalic acid. It is most effective, and best used in *einreibungen*. It is extraordinarily powerful in energizing the etheric system in the digestive tract. The system develops especially powerful activity with this. And you must then try and get this astral sexual system which has gone in there to go back again. You get it to go back either with a silver preparation, given in suitable dosage by mouth, or with a silver injection, using the fifth or sixth decimal. Silver introduced into the circulatory and the digestive systems always tends to restore deformation in the higher levels of the human organization.

You see, if you use these two processes one after the other you will get very good results especially with the effects of shock. Shocks are extraordinarily interesting. And if you have brought about a cure for shock effects, when the kind of typical shock effect we have been describing is evident, you will be able to note the following as you continue to observe the patient. If you know how to put the right questions the answers given by the patient will be more or less: 'It is very odd indeed. From the time when I got well at that time, my heart seems completely different; when I hear something that gives a shock, cannon shot or the like, my heart feels as if it wanted to calm me, as if it was an entity which seeks to calm me down.'

You see from this that polar opposite processes are indeed present with any regulatory intervention, not only those intended to heal, in the human organism. This action of the heart of which the patient was speaking, an action essentially in the etheric and the astral, is the polar opposite effect to what you were actually doing to restore the right relationship between sexual and digestive tract. This is what can be said with regard to this shock effect.

Tomorrow I will go more into an interesting question concerning nervous disorders, especially spinal cord disorders, the first of the written questions, as it were. We'll meet again at half past eight in the morning. Now I'd just like to say one more thing, as it really is highly topical—or at least I think so—and also noted in this list, about incontinence in children, bed-wetting. It does indeed appear to occur in a greatly increased form.

With bed-wetting in childhood we are dealing with a typical weakness of the astral body. The astral body simply does not have the strength it should have. But if you use arsenic, also in the healthy form of Levico Water or Roncegno Water, especially to treat bed-wetting, you will as a rule get powerful but extraordinarily short-term activity especially in bed-wetters, through their total organization a short movement of the astral body as appropriate for that body. The children will continue to wet their beds. But you will quite definitely get good results if you use the substance you obtain by expressing the leaves and flowers of St John's wort, *Hypericum perforatum*.[40] I don't know if you know that it is the only plant with stamens in three bundles. It is a member of Linnaeus' 18th class, has yellow petals and leaves that appear to have holes in them when seen against the light. Expressing this plant you get a juice. Essentially it is this bitter extracted principle found in the plant which matters, a substance which also acts powerfully and lastingly on the inner mobility of the astral body, making it strong.

Recovery will be achieved in the right circumstances if one then also exerts a moral influence on the children simply by telling them that they are obliged to pay attention to their functions. This moral influence should really be brought to bear exactly with things which, you know, are on the border between bad behaviour and sickness. Please do not misunderstand me, I do of course know that it is a disease, but it is on the borderline between bad behaviour and sickness. And we should not fail to pay attention to the moral will which does indeed have considerable influence. If you cure such a thing in children—you can, of course, cure it with Hypericum—you weaken the children's will if you do not at the same time encourage them, giving them an impulse on the moral side. This would be what can be said about bed-wetting.

Tomorrow we'll talk about children with neuropathies, especially dementia praecox[41] in various forms. Also some other issues, and I'll try and cover all these questions.

Dr ... *Question as to the age of the plant juice.*

You should not let it to be too old, but if you give it more or less by expressing it well, using a specific quantity, let us say a gram of leaf and flower, half and half, you will be able to add this to a glass of water, and you can then divide it into portions and use for half a year in this way.

LECTURE 12

Today I would like to deal with some of the questions put to me, some of which I deem to be particularly important.

One concerns gonorrhoea, the clap. To see what needs to be done we must study the nature of the matter. It seems to me that people are too easily satisfied, particularly in this area, simply saying it is infection, infection and once more infection. This is what people really say. The possibility of infection is of course extraordinarily great with this and similar conditions; but knowing about the infection is least likely to lead to knowledge of the medicinal agents. It does not help much to know that the condition is infectious. The only thing is that you do, of course, ensure that the risk of infection is reduced. That is a matter of course, really. But it will be good to go into things like this more deeply.

Well, we have to understand that the human organism truly is a system complete in itself and that everything outside it is to a greater or lesser degree poison to it. Everything outside the human organism really is poison to it. But there are certain adaptations where an otherwise toxic effect is isolated. This isolation of what is otherwise the action of a poison brings about the realization of etheric impulses and astral impulses when female and male seed unite. It also comes into play in numerous other cases, but especially when female and male seed unite. The action is eminently toxic when the two substances which are polar opposites come together. It is isolated, however, and in that isolation exposed to the powers of the cosmos, powers that can actually be described in detail. These are the concentrated powers of sun and moon, and the outcome of the unification is exposed to them.

Such exposure is only possible when male and female seed actually interact. With every substance that is outside the female seed, i.e. produced in organs that are not the female sexual organs, the male seed produces a poison which has no use anywhere in the human organism, nor anywhere in the world outside. Conversely, the female seed produces a poison with every substance, except the one secreted by the male sexual organ, a poison that cannot be processed. This poison essentially but in metamorphosed form is chancre poison on the one occasion, clap poison on the other. We are therefore dealing with diseases that are something greatly different from the syphilitic conditions we have been considering. We are dealing with the production of toxins that do not stand up to exposure in the human organism nor beyond the human organism.

Such substances are essentially also tremendously powerful infectious agents. They are altogether vehicles for parasites of the smallest kind, hypermicroscopic organisms. This is the kind of effect we are dealing with, with the astral and etheric organization in the male and female interacting, and producing these toxins by acting down into the physical. That is the essence of it. The risk of infection is secondary. It always exists, particularly because this is the way in which the altogether most powerful toxins that exist for the organ are produced.

I think it is extraordinarily important to gain insight into such things, so that we won't always really, I'd say, consider the relevant phenomena in the way in which the whole of human reproduction was regarded at one time—by tracing the whole human race back to Eve's ovaries for all of earth's future. That is, of course, an easy way of looking at it. And people also take the easy way when they say: This disease is due to infection; infection in its turn due to infection. And they get back, of course, into something indefinite, gaining no real insight. But when we gain the kind of insight I have just been referring to, we will of course ask ourselves the following. We will say: How can we deal with the activity which arises in the human organism under the influence of this poison?

We have to produce something to which this poison may be exposed, just as one can expose the fertilized female seed to the universe, for instance. We have to create an atmosphere, as it were, in the astral and etheric organism that has some capacity for absorption—not of the poison, however, for this will be eliminated when the poison-producing powers in the astral and etheric are absorbed.

With things like this in particular it is often the case that you get healing powers to come in from two sides. You will really be able to bring about something good in such a case if you give a preparation such as an alkali carbonate by mouth and apply compresses locally, strong oily eucalyptus compresses, letting the two things act together. This will definitely lead to a cure, slowly but all the more thoroughly. For essentially the action of alkali carbonates is that they produce a special ether body, as it were, from the whole human ether body; the eucalyptus extract then flows through this manufactured ether tract in an astral-like way. You literally create an atmosphere around the genital tract which absorbs the poison-producing powers. This is what one may consider in such a case.

Are there any comments, perhaps? All these things are not really for discussion; they have to be tried out and will prove their value. I'd now like to consider a question I found here. It is this.

Can a patient who has become addicted to morphine because of severe asthma be got off the drugs, including morphine, by treating him with the agents used at the Institute of Clinical Medicine in Stuttgart—citric acid, Prunus spinosa *and* Nicotiana tabacum?

Asthma is a problem because essentially it is due to the fact that exhalation, the stream of exhalation, meets with resistance in the respiratory tract. It catches there, as it were. It is something which one can see very strongly in the astral organism.

It is, of course, always somewhat problematical to put these things on record, but you are all of you anthroposophists and will, of course, take these things as they are meant to be taken. You actually see something like hooks facing the outgoing air flow and it runs into them [Plate 6]. That is the status. It shows that asthma is quite specifically the condition which is right on the border to purely mental conditions. I do not mean the so-called mental diseases, but conditions connected with the life of the psyche. Mental diseases need not at all be connected with the life of the psyche but may merely be physical conditions, with the mental aspect merely a symptom. In most cases they should not be called mental diseases for it is almost always an organic disease with its mental counter-image, a shadow image which is merely a symptom. The best way of curing the so-called mental diseases is to consider the physical status as a syndrome which may be renal disease, liver disease or a truly organic disease of the brain. For me, real mental diseases are those where you have truly mental causes, such as shock or anxiety and the like. With asthma the situation is that we must often go a very long way back for the mental causes.

When you have reached my age you have come across all kinds of different types of asthma. I have to say that in cases of asthma, looking for the cause and origin—leaving aside the karmic aspects—you often have to go back as far as embryonic life. The external causes truly do often lie in embryonic life. The mother will have suffered shocks or worries that would have come up again and again at irregular intervals during the pregnancy. Such things have an extraordinarily powerful effect on the whole system of mucous membranes in the respiratory tract, and this establishes the causes for something which will later show itself in the phenomena of asthma.

The following is particularly important with those phenomena. Asthma takes very different forms, depending on the person's individual nature, and much depends on our ability truly to combat the other sequels of asthma in the organism. This makes the organism strong enough so that it can do something itself to combat the asthma later on. Let me now refer to the possibilities for dealing with the situation, which truly is an irregular movement of the astral body in the region of bronchi and lungs.

There is something behind it which I'd say is really cunning, just as asthma is a really cunning disease. If you examine someone suffering from asthma using occult vision, if I may be permitted to say so, you will find that something which I'd like to call the organism's inner appetite has been cut out.

Let us first of all consider the concept of the 'inner appetite of the organism'. You really only arrive at this when you observe very young children. They taste things not only with their tongue. I have always said so to teachers; young children taste things not only with their tongue, they taste things with the whole of their organism. The whole organism is something like a subtle taste organ. Later this becomes localized around the palate, tongue and so on. This differentiation, which comes relatively early, is only partial, however. In subconscious spheres human beings taste things and thus generate this inner experience of appetite throughout the whole organism. The whole organism simply has that power to strive which we call appetite.

Well, you know, just as there is such a thing as lack of appetite in the separate head region, so there is also lack of appetite in the organism, and that is very much the case with asthma. There the whole organism lacks appetite; it does not at all feel like taking up the ingested nutrients, especially the parts that end up in the circulation as a whole. It even has a distaste—though it is not aware of this, since it is inwardly unconscious—especially for cooked food. It is fairly easy to observe this in the outer symptoms in the asthmatic's life. This needs to be dealt with first of all. We have to make the organism able to have an appetite again.

It is altogether a good thing for you to know how to deal with an organism where you think you notice lack of appetite, with the proper connection between ether organism and astral organism disrupted, for that is what it means to be without appetite. It is a good thing to know quite generally what will benefit in that case. And it is always good to introduce into the organism in the right dosage the tannic acid to be gained from sage leaves, for example, from nut leaves, from oak or willow bark, in short, if you present the human organism with tannic acid in perhaps the first decimal, that is, just a percentage.

This is particularly important for the astral body in such a case. It is stimulated to extend its activity to the ether body when given tannic acid. The ether body on its part does not react to this. We merely create chaos if we give only tannic acid. We therefore have to help the ether body as well. This is done by making an extract of the leaves of *Veronica officinalis*, heath speedwell, and obtaining above all the bitter principles from this. The bitter principles found in such plants—they can also be obtained from other plants, any that contain such bitter principles—are given in alternation, let us say the one in the morning, the other at night. With this we can regulate the rhythm between astral and etheric body and so initiate healing. If you then instruct the patient to be truly patient and not lie in bed for weeks but sleep in a chair, and to try and meditate on his breathing when going to sleep, that is, mentally to see or feel—inhalation, spread the breath out, then exhalation (breathing very consciously on going to sleep)—and on waking up immediately start again to breathe consciously for some minutes; if you strengthen his moral powers, applying them to his own organism, his breathing, but so that he is able to use them undeterred (it will be quite impossible for the patient to do this consistently in any other position except for sleeping in a chair, that is, especially not lying down) and you make this the third act in the treatment, there is hope of dealing with asthma even at very late stages of its development. Addiction to morphine is merely a sequel and we must then deal with it. You must then try and combat the addiction.

Now to another interesting case put before me. I would stress, however, that one tends to produce things that are more or less problematical when one does not actually see the patient. We can only construe the case in theory, but let us briefly consider the situation of a post office secretary who has had a nervous breakdown from some cause or other. At first, it seems, he was sleepless, and got himself into a situation where he lost control of himself, thinking only with the head, which means automatically. That was probably the first stage. It seems that it then turned into something else, with a tremor developing in the limbs after two years, and spasms, probably also in the limbs.

In such a case we must above all know that the whole condition is not located in organs other than those which out of the I organization[42] and the astral organization give direction to the human will system. The will system must be considered. The irregular and abnormal element in the will system is indeed involved in this strange way of being given up to cerebral automatism. It has nothing to do with the thoughts; it has to do with the will that lies behind the development of a thought. Everything goes in the direction of being active deep down in the subconscious mind, to generate the will really only in the organism of metabolism and limbs, withdrawing it from the rhythmic organism, withdrawing it from the neurosensory organism. The tendency is really to shift all physical and etheric organs of will down towards the lower organism.

I am sure you could have seen this very well also in external symptoms if you'd had opportunity, let us say, to observe the post office secretary from some point in time and then again two years later. You would notice that the mutual relationship between lower and upper lip had changed in those two years. Two years earlier, it would have seemed to you that there may have been a particular, not entirely harmonious relationship in moving the upper lip relative to the lower lip; you'd have the feeling that it does not fit together as in normal people, and this would have been more so after two years. The lower lip would have continued its unruly movements more than the upper lip. You will be able to observe such things. You will also be able to observe the relationship between leg and arm movements that are not in tune.

In a case like this we need to combine medical treatment, meaning physical treatment, and treatment of the psyche in eurythmy therapy. These two things must be combined, and the case is indeed typical for this.

Give Equisetum baths in such a case, using relatively much Equisetum, which means that you are counting on the silica. Equisetum contains a very high percentage of silica. Give Equisetum baths, therefore, and you'll be able to strengthen the I organization quite considerably. But it needs the influence of the bath. There is always the risk of the effect being lost again after a short time. It is encouraged towards a tendency to be lasting if you now have vowels done in eurythmy therapy, simply vowels, for one hour after the bath. You are then stimulating something for which the Equisetum bath has provided the basis. You may thus hope to combat the matter, doing so mainly from the periphery. We must always try and find the point from which we can combat things.

Here is another case I have been finding most interesting; it is just that it is not very clearly presented. It says here:

Lupus-type proliferation of mucosa in the palate spreading progressively, causes problems swallowing for a woman aged 37. She had pulmonary tuberculosis seven years ago, second or third degree, but there are largely adhesions now. Surgery for non-existent gallstones.

I would like to know what happened immediately after the operation for non-existent gallstones.

Suffers from disorders of the digestive tract, flatulence responding to the S exercise in eurythmy therapy and now minimal. Has had serious worries for years. Might a successful I exercise have causes the lupus? What would need to be done?

Do you think that it really is something like lupus?

It might be scurvy; but it does look like it.

We need not assume that. In reality it can really only be that the form-giving power of the etheric organism is simply not acting sufficiently strongly in the peripheral parts. It cannot be anything else. And we'd have to deal with it simply by injecting bee venom in perhaps the sixth decimal, making the process a total one which happens because the bee venom stimulates the etheric body most powerfully to take up the astral powers truly into the whole human organism.

Bee venom is a most interesting substance. At the base of it is a system of forces that truly is also the basis of the whole form of the human organism. The influence at work in the hive between production of bee venom and the bee food and everything the bee gathers—what will then be the wax cells in the honeycomb—is not for the individual bee but for the whole hive and marvellously similar to the organic processes in the human organism. For if we study bees from the point where they land on the flowers to the point where they return to the hive, secrete the products they have gathered and then build the cells, we have an activity of the hive which truly is inwardly, in terms of the I, the astral and the etheric, highly similar to what happens between the processes that occur inwardly in the brain when human beings have sensory perceptions, then take substances into their powers of perception, and all the way to the process of configuration—that strange configuration—of bone cells. In the honeycombs we see something that has stayed soft, different, from the activity that has led to bone cells, and we see human sensory perception in the way the bee sits on the flower. The whole human organism is indeed encompassed in what comes between the sucking process when bees are on the flower and the process of producing the wax cells.

Bee venom is the organizing principle behind it all, coming in from the spiritual sphere. So if you are able to see that the organic activity breaks off, as it were, in the periphery, does not want to enter into the periphery, then you can do much good with bee or wasp venom, and also support the action of the injection from within by making a thin paste of honey and milk which you give daily as a dietary supplement.

This is something where we can really see how the organism, which had contracted in spasm and showed such abnormal phenomena in different areas in the periphery, is spreading its activity out again on the one hand under the influence of the insect venom which enters into the circulatory system and on the other under the influence of something which is related to milk and honey as a substance in the organization, developing and spreading. I think this is what one may recommend in such a case.

I would now like to talk about the issue which, it seems, is also close to your hearts. It is the matter of neuropathies, spinal cord disorders and so on.

Among neurological disorders those of the spinal cord are of course hardest to reach. Others can be dealt with more easily. But we would be able to deal with so-called neurological disorders much more easily if we considered that the nerve, the nerve strand, the nerve altogether, contains a substance which always tends to crumble and break up. Unlike other parts of the organism, nerves contain no up-building, sprouting powers of growth. Nerves everywhere contain matter tending towards the I organization in always really wanting to separate off and crumble. The moment the I organization is not strong enough to prevent the nerve from crumbling, all kinds of phenomena develop. Depending on whether it is the I organization or the astral organization which is not strong enough, you get either the neurological disorders as such, where the astral organization is not strong enough, or the different conditions with half-mental symptoms and so on where the I organization is not strong enough.

You have to understand that it is possible to influence the nervous system so that a kind of phantom of the astral and the I organism arises in it. This really happens if you attempt to get powers of silica action into the whole nervous system— for a severe neurological disorder, not a partial one. This is like a postulate, as it were, to get silica into the nerve organization.

Unless there are special obstacles and inhibitions we get silica into the nervous system because there truly is an extraordinarily great affinity of the form of the human nervous system to the Arnica substance. It truly is very great. And if you give injections of Arnica in a high potency—the 15th, 25th or even 30th potency—you will find that in most cases the effect of Arnica injections is that patients feel themselves the urge and drive to do something for their nervous disorder. For this must always be our aim, to have the patient suddenly realize: A medicine is relieving me of the problem in the nerves and I am now able to use my I organization, my astral organization. It is the taking over, relieving, which matters in this case. In neurological patients, I organism and astral organism are intensely involved in the nerve process. We have to introduce something into the nerve process which imitates I organization and astral organization. The remarkable configuration which exists in Arnica does exactly that; it is a compound mixture of all kinds of things, truly also a kind of microcosmic imitation of all kinds of macrocosmic elements. Arnica substance does this to a particularly great degree.

Just consider everything that is going on. First we have the silica contained in *Arnica montana*. It is the base material. It is tremendously sensitive, a deeply significant reagent for all kinds of cosmic influences. Silica is an uncommonly subtle reagent to everything that influences the earth. *Arnica montana* always has a tendency to transmit these subtle silica 'perceptions', as we might call them, of the cosmos and give them form in the potassium salts and the calcium salts which are likewise distributed in a marvellous way in the plant.

Think of the whole action of tannic acid as I described it; this action on the astral organism is also present in the arnica plant. We thus take something brought in from the cosmos, configurations imprinted, as it were, in the potassium and calcium salts, directly into the organism with the tannin contained in arnica. At the same time arnica substance miraculously develops a sedative action so that the human being does not feel disquiet as foreign matter enters into the physical correlate of the astral body. Arnica substance has something camphor-like in it and thus its own sedative. It also contains protein, marvellously embedded in latex and similar material, which means affinity to the ether body. We also have phosphorus-like principles in its volatile oils. The whole is constructed in such a way that it turns directly into a phantom of the human I organism.

If you therefore introduce *Arnica montana* substance into the organism in the right dosage—by injection, the other things will not act as powerfully given by injection—you will as a rule find that at least initially there is a powerful effect on the nervous system. Things will be going the right way when you are able to note that the patient feels stronger now, and believes he can now cope with the situation himself. This is the feeling we must evoke. If it does not develop, alternate something with the *Arnica montana* that will help to support him by getting the arnica action going also from the respiratory side. Alternate arnica with formic acid injections in relatively high percentage. You will see that the matter will then arise.

If you do not achieve this, it will of course be necessary to make an extract of the corresponding part of an animal's nervous system, depending on whether the origin of the disease is in the brain or the spinal cord, and inject a high potency of this rather than formic acid in alternation with arnica. If you suspect, for instance, that the neurological disorder originates in the visual region, take the secretion from the quadrigeminal substance or some such substance from an animal, extract it, and inject it in a fairly high potency to support the *Arnica montana*. Let the support go to the place where it is needed. These things must always be observed.

A mildly toxic effect will develop, especially if the *Arnica montana* treatment proves successful. We do indeed want it to develop. It may be evident from something or other. But you'll always find that this mildly toxic effect can be cancelled out with alkali compounds of some kind taken by mouth.[43]

I think that what I have been saying tells us something of great importance about what needs to be done with neurological disorders, including those of the spinal cord. These can only be diagnosed at the right stage, and we should get out of the bad medical habit, so common especially in western Europe, of ascribing almost all forms of tabes dorsalis to some form of syphilitic causes. That is utter nonsense. And if you blinker yourself from the beginning you will, of course, not see things as they are. The majority of spinal cord disorders do not have any kind of syphilitic origin but arise from chills in the gastric and pelvic tracts, which people generally consider harmless, or from the spine being exposed to cold on some occasion. The situation is, of course, that due to social conditions over the last decades the purely external complication would very frequently arise with both syphilis and spinal cord disorder, which distracts attention and people did not do the right thing, which is to combat the sequels of syphilis on their own and the sequels of spinal cord disorders with something of the kind I have just described.

The interesting thing is that when you have located the neurological disorders as being still in the digestive tract or indeed the gastric tract, not going beyond the digestive organs, you can achieve the same result—and that is so extraordinarily interesting—by using *Chamomilla* instead of *Arnica montana*, again by injection, and apart from this do the same. It is interesting because you can see from this—chamomile having practically no silica—that silica is only needed when you get beyond the digestive tract with the nerves. Silica is absent. On the other hand the tract contains sulphur, and essentially this is particularly beneficial when you need to stimulate the ether body in the digestive system.

Some more questions have come up, but we don't have the time to go into them in detail. 'What is the nature of far-sightedness and short-sightedness?'

I know you mean to ask if these things can be treated. The origins are perfectly evident and one doesn't enquire into them with things like this. You mean how one might influence them medically? It is possible to cure short-sightedness and far-sightedness, and also take preventive action, for you are quite right, glaucoma is very much connected with far-sightedness. People who are not far-sighted do not easily develop glaucoma. Medical treatment, which is certainly possible, will, however, only be successful if you initiate it perhaps even before the third year of life. So we have to notice the potential for short-sightedness or far-sightedness very early in children. You can do much then with Belladonna in high potency. But you really have to spot it before the child has fully learned to talk and walk. Once the organism is physically established as far as it is when the child has learned to walk, stand and talk, the whole tendency is there to give form to the crystalline lens and the vitreous body which is the basis for far- and short-sightedness. And then it is difficult to do anything, for it is something purely mechanical and formal. On the other hand, for as long as the unformed principle in the infant's undirected movements, when arm movements and so on have as yet no orientation, influences the infant eye, high potencies of Belladonna induce a very inward sensing experience, a certain sentience, and so one might well think that something can be done at that point. But it probably won't be easy to make one's observations then. This is what can be said on the subject.

I am sorry but we now have to come to a conclusion. I hope that we will be able to continue at a suitable time. It will always give us very particular satisfaction to be able to add something, as it were, to the medical programme of the School, to be able to give something to the physicians when they come to such gatherings. I hope that this can happen again in the future, in one way of another. Essentially it will also be possible for friends who keep in touch with the School in Dornach to be given information on various things from time to time—we'll see to it that this is done in the right way. So if you send questions to Dr Wegman we will answer them together, not of course in the supplement to *Das Goetheanum*[44] but in a form in which it will go to physicians only. I think we should arrange things so that if someone asks a question the answer will reach all our anthroposophical physicians, for it is really always of interest to everyone, and this will be the best way forward for us. We'll try and also initiate communication with the physicians from here, in Dornach, in a suitable way.

Dr Palmer. *Esteemed Dr Steiner, please permit me on behalf of my colleagues to express our heartfelt thanks that in spite of all the work you have to do you have found the time to devote a few hours to us. Those of us who are working at the Institute for Clinical Medicine in Stuttgart are well aware of our great need for these sessions, and we would ask that you continue to give your support and advice, give us your help.*

The only thing I would have liked to see would have been a greater number of sessions. Thinking about it as much as we might, Dr Wegman and myself, no more than these three sessions proved possible. As I said, I wish there could have been more sessions. Let us hope for another time!

IV
HYGIENE AS A SOCIAL ISSUE

LECTURE 13
HYGIENE AS A SOCIAL ISSUE

PUBLIC LECTURE, DORNACH, 7 APRIL 1920 *

T H E social question must be one of the most important issues today, beyond doubt so for many people. Wherever people have just a bit of a heart for present developments in human history, impulses that pose a threat or need to be given serious consideration for the future—all this comes together under the social issue heading. We have to say to ourselves, however, that the consideration, the treatment, of this social issue does at the present time suffer from a basic evil, one that sticks to so many elements in our life of the mind, our moral life, and indeed the whole of our civilization. This is the intellectualism of our time, with problems so often merely considered in a highly intellectual way. The social question is dealt with by one individual or another who is leaning more to the right or to the left. The intellectual nature is evident in that people start with particular theories that things ought to be one way or another, that one thing or another should be abolished. Little heed is paid to the human being as such in all of this. People treat the human being as if there were a general thing, 'the human being', as if there were something which is not in a particular respect developed individually in every single human being. Attention is not given to the particular nature of every individual. This makes the whole way in which we look at the social issue into something abstract, something which enters so

---

* Please note. Hygiene here refers to the set of practices perceived by a community to be associated with the preservation of health and healthy living. Translator.

little today into social awareness, into the attitudes that come into play between one person and another. We are probably most aware of the deficit which exists in social studies when we focus our attention on a specific area, one which is perhaps more suited than another to being subjected to social scrutiny, an example being the field of hygiene, in so far as hygiene is a public issue concerning not the individual person but the human community.

There is no shortage of rules, treatises and articles about health care also in the public domain. We have to ask, however: These rules, these reflections on hygiene, how do they relate to social life? And we have to say: They relate in such a way that some talks on proper health care are published as the outcome of medical and physiological studies. Trust in a subject area the inner nature of which one is unable to test for oneself is meant to be the basis for our acceptance of such rules. Purely on authority the populace at large is supposed to accept things about hygiene coming from the desks and examination rooms, the laboratories of the medical profession. Yet if you are convinced that in more recent history, over the last four centuries, a longing has arisen among people for a democratic order in all affairs, then, however grotesque it may seem to many people today, you will come up against the undemocratic nature of the pure belief in authority demanded of us in the field of hygiene. The undemocratic nature of this belief in authority goes against the longing for democracy which at the present time, we might say, has come to a culmination, albeit often in a highly paradoxical way.

I know very well that the words I have just spoken will be felt to be paradoxical by many, for people simply do not put together the way in which someone accepts things relating to health care with the democratic urge to form one's own opinion concerning public affairs that concern all who are of age, and the community of these people who are of age, be it directly or be it through their representatives. We do of course have to say that something like views on hygiene, hygienic measures in public life, cannot completely go their own way because it depends on the judgement of someone who is seeking insight in a field such as this. On the other hand there does have to be the question: Should it not be possible to be more democratic in such a field than is possible under present conditions, a field such as public health which intimately concerns every individual and hence the human community?

We are certainly told much today about the way in which people should live their lives with regard to air and light, with regard to diet, disposing of waste material produced by the individual himself or his environment, and so on and so forth. But most of the rules let loose on humanity cannot be tested by those to whom they are intended to apply.

Let there be no misunderstanding. Please do not think that I represent any particular view in this lecture, which is meant to be on the subject of hygiene as a social issue. My intention is to be unbiased on a subject that tends to be presented from a party point of view or on the basis of a particular scientific conviction. Please permit me to drop out of my role, seemingly, in the introduction. I do not want to take sides in any way for the old superstition that devils and demons go about as diseases, entering into people and departing again, nor for the modern superstition that bacilli and bacteria enter into people and leave them again, causing disease. It shall not matter so much to us today if we are dealing with spiritualist, spiritual superstition from the past or a materialistic superstition. I would, however, wish to touch on something that is to be found everywhere in modern education, especially in so far as it derives from the basic scientific convictions of our time. We are assured from many different sides today that with science the materialism of the middle and the last third of the nineteenth century has been overcome. This cannot be true, however, for someone who truly understands the nature of materialism and its opposite, for this materialism has at most been overcome by some who see that modern scientific facts no longer permit the wholesale declaration that everything which exists is only some kind of mechanical, physical or chemical process taking place in the material world. It is not enough that, compelled by the weight of facts, some have come to be convinced of this.

On the other hand there is also the fact that in spite of their conviction those people, and others just as much, take up the materialistic trend in their thinking when there is need to explain something in concrete terms, to have a view concerning something real and concrete.

People say that atoms and molecules are harmless coinage of account, and that no one would say that they are anything but elements of thought. Yet their view has nevertheless remained atomistic, molecularistic. We explain the phenomena in the world from the behaviour and mutual relationship of atoms or of molecular processes, and in that case it is irrelevant if we have the idea that some thought, feeling or any other kind of process is wholly due to material processes among atoms and molecules. What matters and has relevance is the direction taken in our whole state of mind, the direction in which the mind goes when the only basis accepted for its explanations are things seen in atomistic terms, arising from the smallest, from something that is pure invention. It is not that one is convinced, literally or in one's thoughts, that there is something else apart from atomistic effects, from material atomic activities. What matters is if it is possible for us to make other explanations of the world the guiding principle for the mind rather than to derive phenomena from atomistic processes. It is not *what* we believe that matters but *how* we explain things, our inner attitude. And here, in this place, we have to represent the conviction that only a genuine, real science of the spirit can help us to overcome the evil which may be characterized in this way.

Let me give you a real example where this is truly the case. I think there is hardly anything causing more confusion than the frequently addressed differences between the living human body and the human soul principle or the human mind and spirit, between physical diseases and so-called mental diseases. Objective distinction and the establishment of objective relationships between such facts of human life as a sick body or a seemingly sick mind suffer from the materialistic and atomistic way of thinking when insight is sought. For what is the essential nature of the materialism which has gradually developed as a more recent philosophy of life for many people and which has not been overcome but is in fact in full flower today? What is the nature of it? It is not that people look to the material processes, look to material processes also in the living human body, and devotedly study the marvellous composition and activities of the human nervous system and the other human organs or the nervous system of animals or the organs of other life forms. You do not turn into a materialist when you study these things. What makes you into a materialist is that the spirit is not with you when you study material processes, that you look into the world of matter and see nothing but matter and material processes.

This is what the science of the spirit must show—I can only speak of this in summary form today—that wherever material processes become evident to the senses (the only processes which are accepted as observable and exact in modern science), they are always mere external signs, the external revelation of spiritual forces and powers at work behind them and within them. It is not a characteristic of spiritual science that one looks at someone and says: 'Ah, there he has his body; this body is a sum of material processes. But that cannot be all there is to the human being; independent of this he has his immortal soul.' And one then begins to develop all kinds of abstract theories, all kinds of abstract views of this immortal soul which is independent of the living body. That does not characterize a spiritual philosophy of life. We can certainly say that apart from a body consisting in material processes human beings also have an immortal soul which is taken to some spiritual realm after death. In terms of anthroposophical spiritual science this does not make you a spiritual scientist. You will only be that if you realize that this material body with its material processes has been created by the soul principle.

To be a spiritual scientist you need to know how to enter in detail into the way in which the soul principle, which existed before birth or let us say before conception, acts to configure, to shape the composition and indeed the material nature of the human body; you must be able to perceive everywhere the immediate oneness of this living body and soul, and to understand how with mind and spirit active in it this body as such is used up, worn out, partly dying every minute, and how the moment of death means the radical deconfiguration, as I'd put it, of the processes happening at every moment in the body under the influence of mind and soul; you have to understand this living interplay, with the soul always active in the living body, understand this in every detail, and you must endeavour to say: The soul differentiates itself into absolutely concrete processes, entering *thus* into the processes of liver function, *thus* into breathing function, *thus* into heart function, *thus* into brain function—in short, in describing the material aspect of the human being you must know how to present the physical human being as the outcome of a spiritual principle. In spiritual science we come to genuinely appreciate the material world because we see an individual, concrete material process not merely the way it is seen in modern science, as something visible to the eye, or something established as outcome in abstract terms, having observed its outer form. Spiritual science is spiritual science because it always shows how the spirit works in matter, and one looks with devotion at the material effects of the spirit. This is what matters on the one hand.

On the other hand it matters that exactly because of this we are shielded from all the abstract nonsense talked about a soul independent of the human being, something one can really only fantasize about in so far as life between birth and death is concerned. For between birth and death, mind and soul are, except in sleep, given up so much to the bodily functions that they live in them, come to expression in them. We must learn to study spirit and soul outside the course of human life, and accept that human life between birth and death is an outcome of spirit and soul activity. We then see the true, concrete oneness of mind and soul with the living body. This is anthroposophical spiritual science, for we then have hope of having the human being with all individual differentiations before us as an outcome of soul and spirit activity also for the gaining of knowledge. The mystical theosophical view, where beautiful theories are developed of all kinds of spirits free of the body, cannot serve us for gaining real knowledge of life; it cannot serve life at all but only be intellectualistic, mental indulgence, wanting to put life, outward life, aside as quickly as possible and then, for inner satisfaction, to give oneself up to an inner self-indulgence, spinning out all kinds of fantasies concerning spirit and soul.

Here, in this spiritual movement with anthroposophical orientation, we are concerned to do serious work, to cultivate a science of the spirit that will truly enliven physics, mathematics, chemistry, physiology, biology and anthropology. It is not a matter of pronouncing in a religious or philosophical way: Human beings bear an immortal soul in them, and then to pursue anthropology, biology, physics and chemistry as if one was dealing with material processes only. No, it is a matter of applying the insights we can gain into soul and spirit to the individual aspects of life, of looking into the wondrous composition of the body itself. We may certainly say, though it will sound paradoxical in some respects: Some people deem themselves to be good mystics or good theosophists and hold forth in all kinds of ways about the human being consisting of physical body, ether body, astral body, I and so on, but they have not the least notion of how the soul comes to expression when you blow your nose. The point is that we must see matter not as matter but as revelation of the spirit. We will then also have sound views, rich in content, of the spirit. And this will give us a science of the spirit that can be fruitful for the life sciences.

Something else is also achieved with this. It is that we can overcome the element which in more recent times, when scientific insights grew materialistic, has moved towards specialization. I certainly do not wish to enter into a diatribe against specialization, being well aware of its justification. I know that today some things have to be done by specialists, simply because you need specialized technology for them. But someone who is wholly attached to the sphere of matter when he becomes a specialist will never have a philosophy of life that is relevant to life. For the field of material processes is infinite. You only have to study the human nervous system, taking note of everything known so far, and you will need a long time for this, at least as much time as specialists usually want to devote to their specialist studies. However, if you have only the knowledge of material processes in the nervous system, things presented in abstract terms in modern science, you will have nothing to guide you to anything that is universal and can be the basis for a philosophy of life. The moment you start to take a spiritual-scientific view, let us say of the human nervous system, you will not be able to do so unless the spirit you find at work in it immediately takes you to the element of spirit and soul which is behind the muscle system, the bone system, the senses. The spiritual is not something which divides into separate parts. It is something—and this is just the most basic explanation—which spreads like a differentiated form, an organism. Just as I cannot study a human being by just looking at his five fingers, covering up the rest of him, so I cannot study anything in spiritual science without the things which I perceive in this one thing taking me to a whole. When I am thus taken to such a whole—

admittedly it may perhaps be just for a specialist in brain and neurological research—it will nevertheless be possible for me to get an idea of
the whole human being from my study of this individual member of
humanity as an organism. I will then be in a position where I truly have
something universal for a philosophy of life. And the strange thing is
that I can then begin also to speak of something relating to the human
being which will be understood by anyone of sound mind and sound
common sense. That is the big difference between the way we may
speak about the human being on the basis of spiritual science and how
people must do so who are specialists in materialistic science.

Let us take the simple case of the kind of handbooks published in the
field of specialist science. As an ordinary person who has not been taught
a great deal about the nervous system, picking up such a handbook
about the nervous system—well, you'll probably soon put it down again.
At least you will not find much there that can give you a basis for looking
at the human being as truly human in his value, his dignity. However,
when you hear what can be said about the human nervous system from
the fund of spiritual-scientific knowledge, it always takes you to the
whole human being, things that give a clear picture of the whole human
being, and the idea that arises has in it something of the value, essential
nature and dignity of the human being you are dealing with.

There is nothing where this is not more evident than if we consider
not only the human being with regard to the state of health of one of his
members but also the sick individual, someone deviating from the norm
in many ways, and especially if we are able to consider the whole human
being under the influence of one disease or another. Nature shows us
something in the sick individual that can take us deep into the nature of
the world, show us how this human being is organized and how because
of his organization the atmospheric influences and those from beyond
this earth can affect him, how this human organization is connected
with different substances in nature which then prove to be medicinal,
and so on. We are taken into far-reaching relationships and it is fair to
say that if we add the things we can get to know through the sick
human being to all that may be known about the healthy human being
in this way profound insight arises into the whole situation and the
deeper significance of life. Everything which comes to you in this way is

the basis for knowledge of human nature, is the basis for something which can then be put into words that can be spoken to all people. We have not yet reached that point because spiritual science in this sense has only been working for a short time. The lectures given here, as Dr Boos[45] said just now in his introduction, are in many ways only a beginning. But this science of the spirit tends to develop the subject matter of the individual sciences into a form where the things everyone should know about the human being can indeed be conveyed to everyone.

Now, once spiritual science brings such a change to conventional science, and if it then proves possible to develop forms of insight into the human being in sickness and in health that can be made accessible to general human understanding—just think how people will relate to one another in social life, how individuals see others with a different kind of insight than is the case today when we go past one another without having insight into the special individual nature of a person! The social question will only be freed from its intellectualism when it is based on objective knowledge and on real life experiences. This is particularly evident in the field of health care. Consider the social effect if people learn to see what is healthy in another person and what is not; consider what it will mean if the whole of humanity takes health care in hand with understanding. To be sure, the intention is not to encourage scientific or medical amateurism—that must be so—but think what it will mean if sympathetic understanding rather than just feeling for health and sickness in others develops, understanding based on insight into human nature. Think of the social effect of such a thing and you'll have to say to yourselves: There we see that objective knowledge in specific areas must lead to social reform, to new developments in the social sphere, not on the basis of general theories, be they Marxist, Oppenheimer's[46] or whatever, theories that disregard the human being and are intended to shape the world on abstract ideas. Salvation will not come from this but from dedicated insight into the individual spheres. Health care, hygiene, is one such specific area, for I think it takes us closest to the pleasure others gain from a normal, healthy way of life, or to the pain and suffering, the limitations, due to the more or less pathological changes in them.

Something like this immediately makes us aware of the special social style which spiritual science can create in the field of hygiene. For when those who cultivate anthroposophy, knowledge of human beings in sickness and health, and also those who specialize in being physicians are members of human society who have that kind of insight, they will be able to bring enlightenment to human society and will be met with understanding. The relationship between physician and society will then not be such that unless you happen to be a friend or relative you do not pass by his or her house, and only ask the physician to come when you suffer pain or have broken your leg. The relationship to the physician will then be such that the physician is your constant teacher and instructor on health care; the physician will intervene all the time, not merely to cure someone sick enough to notice it but to maintain people's health as much as possible. Lively social activity will take place between physicians and the whole rest of society. And then the soundness of such insight will shine out on medicine itself. For with materialism extending also to the medical view of life, we have indeed come to have strange views today.

On the one hand there are the physical diseases. They are studied by looking for abnormalities in organs or whatever physically perceptible or physically envisaged processes are thought to exist within the human integument, and aiming to correct the damage which has been found. Here the bodily principle in its normal and abnormal states is considered in a wholly materialistic way. Then there are the 'mental' diseases. On the one hand, thinking in materialistic terms, these were considered to be mere diseases of the brain or of other parts of the nervous system, and people were no doubt also looking for causes elsewhere in the system of human organs. As no idea at all has been developed on the way in which mind and soul are indeed active in the living human body, no view has been gained as to how mental illness, so-called, relates to the rest of the human being. The result, I'd say, is that we have the mental diseases on the one hand, even partly understood in a strangely hermaphrodite science, psychoanalysis, where the thinking is materialistic though the nature of matter is not at all understood. So there they are, these mental conditions, and people are unable to connect them in a rational way with the things that really go on in the human organism.

In spiritual science it is possible to show—and I have drawn attention to this—that what I am now saying is not mere agenda, but is studied in detail, especially on occasions such as have just now been available when giving a course for physicians[47] here in these weeks. With spiritual science we can certainly show in detail how everything by way of mental illness is due to changes in the organs, degeneration of organs, enlargement of organs, reduction in the size of organs in the human organism. Something is not in order somewhere in the heart, in the liver, in the lungs when 'mental' disease develops at the same time or later. If spiritual science enables us to perceive the spirit at work in a normal heart, it is also possible—and perfectly reasonable—to look for the causes of such sickness of the mind or soul in degeneration of the heart, defects in the heart.

The main problem with materialism is not the denial of the spirit. Religion might see to it that the spirit is nevertheless acknowledged. The main problem with materialism is that one gains no insight into matter, for example with purely psychoanalytic therapy, or by merely observing something or other that happened in the psyche, referring to it as an island in the psyche, which is an abstract idea. Instead we must study how certain impressions gained at some time or other in life, impressions normally bound to the normal organism, come up against faulty organs, a sick liver rather than a healthy one, for instance, and this may become evident at a time which differs from the time when the defect in the organ can be identified.

We need not be afraid in spiritual science to show how 'mental' disease is always connected with something in the living body. In fact we must insist that one gets at best a one-sided diagnosis if one studies only the psyche and where it deviates from 'normal' life in the psyche. Psychoanalysis can thus never be anything but at best diagnostic; it will never lead to genuine therapy in this field. Because of this, with therapy for mental conditions in particular having to start with treatment for the living body we must know all the ramifications of the spiritual aspect if we want to know where to start, treating the material body, which is however filled with the spirit—where to start in treating something where the abnormal conditions in the psyche are merely symptomatic. It really must be stressed in spiritual science that the 'mental' diseases need to be traced all the way to the human being's organology. We will, however, only be able to see into the abnormal human organology if we are able to trace the spirit down to the smallest particle of matter.

Conversely, the temperaments and people's life in the temperaments, evident in the whole way in which the individual plays when a young child, the way they walk, the things they do, all the things considered to be mind and soul as phenomena of life that appear to be influencing the psyche or be active within it, these also have their bodily side. Things not done in many ways when bringing up children may at a later time show themselves in an absolutely common type of disease. There are cases of mental illness where we are literally guided to consider the living body in order to establish the real cause, whilst with physical diseases we must look to mind and spirit to do so.

It is the very essence of spiritual science that one does not talk about some nebulous spiritual element in abstract terms, as mystics and one-sided theosophists do, but trace the spirit's actions in the sphere of matter. In spiritual science we do not ever see matter the way it is seen in modern science, but always penetrate to the spirit when considering matter and thus are also able to observe how an abnormal life in the psyche must come to expression in an abnormal life in the body though this may not be outwardly in evidence. Very many people have entirely the wrong idea about serious anthroposophical spiritual science, perhaps justifiably so on occasion, when one hears people talk who do not in truth want to consider the reality of it but only to present abstract theories. The human being is made up of such and such, and there are repeated lives on earth, and so on. These things are of course most important and very good. But when it is a matter of working in all seriousness in this spiritual-scientific movement, it is a question of giving full consideration to the individual chapters, the individual spheres of this life.

In the widest sense this will in turn take us to a social spirit in human togetherness. For when you see how the seemingly sick mind lets its impulses shine into the organism, when you can feel this connection between the organism and the seemingly sick mind—feel it with understanding—and when on the other hand you know that the ways in which life is lived also influence the physical health of people, that the spiritual principle, seemingly only superficial in social institutions, also influences physical health care, then you are part of human society in a very different way. You begin to gain a real understanding of human nature, and you treat others in a very different way. You study their character in a very different way. You know that certain characteristics are connected with one thing or another, you know the attitude to take in relation to these characteristics, you know, especially if tasks have to be performed in relation to this, how to place people's temperaments in society in the right way and above all develop them in the right way. One social sphere will need to be influenced with particular intensity with regard to hygiene by the insight into human nature you have gained and that is the sphere of education, of teaching. Unless you have truly comprehensive insight into the human being you cannot really judge what it means when children sit in class, their backs bent, so that their breathing is always impeded, or when they are not taught to speak loudly and clearly, enunciating vowels and consonants clearly. All their later life essentially depends on whether they breathe properly in school and are taught to speak loudly and clearly, articulating well.

With things like this—I am merely taking the odd example, for much the same would apply in other fields—we see specialization for hygiene as a whole in schools, which shows the whole social significance of hygiene, but also how life demands that we do not specialize further but take an overall view of everything specialized. We must know not only what enables a teacher to know that there have to be educational standards for teaching children in this way or that way, but also what enables a teacher to form an opinion as to what it means when he makes a child articulate clearly in saying a sentence or lets the child gasp for air after half a sentence, and so on, not making sure that the air is used up in saying the sentence. Yes, there are also many reference points and rules. But we only come to recognize and apply these things rightly once we are aware of the whole significance of this for human life and social health. This alone makes the matter into a social impulse.

This was the background to my thinking when I gave the course on education and didactics[48] for the teachers in Stuttgart when we started the Waldorf School there.[49] It was that to educate and teach the children we need teachers who are able to work out of the whole depth of a philosophy of life based on understanding the human being. Everything said there as art of education and didactics was said with the aim of making the children into people who have been taught as children to perform the functions of life in the right way and would therefore have sound lungs and livers and hearts and stomachs, because their minds and souls would have worked on them in the right way. In this philosophy of life one would never use the old phrase 'a sound mind in a sound body'. In materialistic terms this would mean that if the body is sound, with all kinds of physical means used to make it so, it will of its own accord be the vehicle for a sound mind. That is nonsense. It makes sense to say 'a sound mind in a sound body' only if we proceed as follows. I mean by saying: There I have a sound body before me, and it shows that the powers of a sound mind, or soul, have put it together, shaped it and made it sound. I perceive as I consider this body that an autonomous, sound mind has been working on it. That is the meaning of the phrase. And it is the only way in which those words can also be the basis for a sound hygiene.

In other words, with teachers who do not base their work on an abstract science of education we do not need a school doctor who at best walks through the school every two weeks and also cannot think of anything sensible to do. We must create a living link between medical knowledge and the art of education. We need an art of education where the children are taught and educated in the right hygienic way in all respects. It is this which makes hygiene a social issue, for the social issue is essentially one of education, and the issue of education is essentially medical, though it needs a medicine fructified by spiritual science, a hygiene fructified by spiritual science.

This points to something which is of extraordinary significance especially with regard to hygiene as a social issue. If the science of the spirit is cultivated and if it is indeed real to you, you will know that there is something in the things you gain from spiritual science that is different from anything you get in mere intellectualism—present-day natural science, too, is mere intellectualism—or in only intellectually trained natural science or in only intellectually trained history or law. All sciences are intellectualistic today; any claims made that they are empirical merely mean that they give sensory experiences an intellectualistic interpretation. The knowledge provided in spiritual science differs greatly from this. It would be sad indeed if the fruits of our intellectualistic culture were not mere image but a real power with deeper influence on human beings. Everything intellectualistic actually remains on the surface for people. This statement is made as a comprehensive one. People who work with spiritual science in an intellectualistic way, merely making notes—physical body, ether body, astral body, I, repeated earth lives, karma and so on—noting this down the way one notes things down in natural science or modern social science are not serious about that work, for they are applying their usual way of thinking to the things they meet with in spiritual science. The very essence of spiritual science is that it must be thought, felt and live in one's mind in a very different way from the intellectualistic approach. This is how we gain a living relationship to people in health and sickness with spiritual science, but in a somewhat different way than people would often imagine. I think people will fully realize how powerless we are with what is given as a warning or as encouragement to those believed to be mentally ill in a purely intellectualistic culture. The mentally sick individual says he hears voices. You tell him all kinds of things that come to you from intellectual rational thinking—in vain, for he knows all possible objections and so on. This in itself might tell us that we are neither dealing with a disorder of the conscious mind nor of the subconscious, but with a disorder in the organism.

In spiritual science we come to realize that one also cannot cope with 'mental' diseases in a way said to be 'spiritual', where you use hypnosis and suggestion, for instance. No, they have to be dealt with by 'physical' means, that is, by treating organs, but this does indeed need spiritual insight into the human being. With spiritual insight one knows that one really should not intervene in the field of 'mental' diseases with procedures in mind and spirit only, for mental illness means that the spiritual part of the human being has been forced out, which normally happens only in sleep, and is weak when it has been forced out. We have to treat the organ so that it will receive soul and spirit in a healthy way on their return. The fruits of spiritual science, which do not arise from the intellect, the head, but from the whole human being when they arise

as Imagination, Inspiration and Intuition will influence the whole
human being, the whole organism, when taken up by a person. Spiritual
science in the true sense does indeed intervene in the human physical
organization to heal it.

The fact that some dreamers feel sick within spiritual science or
demonstrate the opposite of what I have just said does not prove anything. There are infinitely many people who are not spiritual scientists
but intellectualistic gatherers of notes on spiritual-scientific findings. To
make the substance of spiritual science genuinely known is in itself
preventive social care, for it acts on the whole human being, normalizing
his organology when this threatens to go in the direction of dreams or
on the other hand shows a tendency to deviate to the abnormal. That is
the tremendous difference between anything given in the field of
spiritual science and anything arising in purely intellectualistic science.
The concepts arising in the field of intellectualism are only pictorial,
two-dimensional, and much too weak to influence human beings and
bring health. Spiritual-scientific concepts on the other hand have been
taken from the whole human being. Truly, not only the brain but lungs
and liver and heart and the whole human being were involved in
developing them, and anything gained from the strength of the whole
human being 'is glued to them', penetrates them, if I may say so, in a
three-dimensional form. If you make them your own, take them in with
sound common sense in gaining insight, they will in turn be beneficial
for the whole human being. Spiritual science can thus provide something that points the way to hygiene as a social principle.

Spiritual science can also have an influence on the whole health
situation of humanity in many other ways—I can only pick a few
examples—if it is ever taken up in a truly serious way.

Let me refer to just one thing. The relationship of the waking to the
sleeping human being is a chapter that has to be studied again and
again; it covers the tremendous difference in the human organization
when awake or asleep. Great attention is given to the relationship
between mind and soul in waking hours, when they interpenetrate in
the human body, soul and spirit, and in sleep, when they are temporarily separated.

I can only refer in passing to a statement which, however, is a fully substantiated finding in spiritual science. We see epidemic diseases, as they are called, affect large numbers of people, which definitely also makes these diseases a matter of social concern. In ordinary materialistic science investigations are done on the human physical organism. People do not know how tremendously significant an abnormal attitude to waking and sleeping is particularly with regard to epidemics and a disposition to catch epidemic diseases. Developments in the human organism seriously predispose people for epidemic diseases if sleep is excessive. People who create processes in the human organism that should not be there by sleeping too long—for sleep should not interrupt waking life for too long—have a very different predisposition to epidemic diseases and also relate to epidemics in a completely different way.

You can judge for yourselves what it means to enlighten people about the proper relative amounts of sleep and waking. You cannot make rules about this. At best you can instruct people not to send their children to school when they have scarlet fever, and you can't give lectures during an influenza epidemic. In that case people will obey; they tend towards 'freedom' today and belief in authority is no longer what it was. In a case like this they'll obey. I am not saying that it is right for them to toe the line; I am not saying anything against such rules and regulations, but you cannot possibly tell people in the same way: 'You must have seven hours' sleep.' Yet it is more important than those other rules that people who need it sleep for seven hours, whilst others who do not need it may sleep much less, and so on. Things like this, which are so intimately bound up with the most personal aspects of human life, have a magnificent social effect. The form which the social effects take does indeed depend on the most intimate element in us— whether a greater or lesser number are not able to take up one vocation or another, which may have an effect perhaps in quite a different area or not. Here hygiene does indeed influence social life quite tremendously. Quite apart from any ideas we may have about infection or non-infection, this element influences social life during epidemics. You cannot make rules from outside; you can only influence things by bringing a lay population into human society who meet the physicians' endeavours to enlighten us about hygiene with human understanding, and by constant, lively collaboration between the experts and lay people who understand the human being, so that health may be maintained.

Considering all these things we'll say to ourselves that we have spoken of one aspect of hygiene as a social issue which in the most eminent sense depends on our having an independent cultural life, truly a cultural life where those concerned with the nurture of cultural life, also where it extends to individual practical fields such as hygiene, are completely independent of anything not coming from pure insight, from the nurture of cultural life itself. Anything an individual can do for the benefit of others must come wholly from his own abilities, there can be no government standards, nor dependence on economic powers; it must be within the personal dependency sphere of the individual and also within the trust and understanding which others who depend on his skills have for that capable individual. We need a cultural life independent of all authorities, government and economic life, a cultural life with its own expertise gained solely from the powers of the mind.

It is particularly when you give full consideration to the element which will truly make hygiene into something which is closely bound up with genuine insight into the human being and social behaviour, when you objectively consider the individual branch—hygiene, for instance—that you will realize (whatever abstract theories may have to say against the independent position of cultural life) that the individual field, this one or any other, specifically demands that the spirit in the field must be under the management of the people who are involved in its cultivation. Not experts at the ministries, but people actively involved in cultural life must also be managing this cultural life and are indeed the only ones to manage it. Once hygiene based on social insight has truly become a social institution it will be possible to work for it in a very different way financially. It will then be possible to serve the idea of a threefold social organism I described in my *Threefold Social Order/Towards Social Renewal*[50] and it has been repeatedly discussed in journals[51] such as the Swiss *Soziale Zukunft* published by Dr Boos.

Once the latent potential for hygiene that rests in the womb of society is accepted with understanding of the human being and becomes the established order, it will be possible to bring everything that can come into effect out of this into economic life, into an independent economic life, independent of any considerations as to gain or of government impulses, but purely out of this independent economic life. This needs to be cultivated with the resources of economic life to serve genuine, true hygiene. Then, and only then, the greatness of mind will enter into economic life which is needed if we are to cultivate hygiene in human life. If mere business acumen from economic life prevails, with its growing tendency to be incorporated into a centralized state, and it is generally believed that one must produce whatever brings greatest profit, the independent impulses of cultural life, also in this field of hygiene, cannot be brought to bear. Economics will then gain mastery over cultural life. Economic life must not govern cultural life. This is most clearly evident when we are required to bring about the things demanded by culture, by the spirit, in economic life and we are meant to serve a genuine hygiene, true hygiene. The forces of economic life, a free economy, will join insight in the threefold social organism, insight that becomes a public concern, and it will join the understanding of the human being that will be a public concern in that organism.

People need to have an independent cultural life where a truly objective hygiene can flourish. On the other hand they need to develop that greatness of mind where everyone meets production processes with an understanding that arises not only from business sense but also from the insights gained in the independent cultural application of hygiene. Once people have this social understanding of the human being, full of insight, and that greatness of mind where one wants to work in the economic sphere simply so that humanity is provided with that hygiene in the social sense, people will be able to come together democratically in parliaments or otherwise. Then insight into the need for hygiene as a social phenomenon will arise in that independent cultural life to culti-vate what is needed for hygiene as a social issue, an economic life that is objective and expert, thanks to the great-mindedness developed in it. Humanity will then have come of age and be able to negotiate in the sphere of economics on the one hand from insight and their under-standing of the human being, and on the other hand from their con-nection with the economic life which serves hygiene. People will then be able to deal as equals in the sphere of government, rights or economic life concerning measures to be taken with regard to hygiene and public health. It will not be lay people or amateurs who restore health then, but people who have come of age will meet the medical expert who tells one thing or another to them as equals and with understanding. Insight into the nature of the human being will make it possible for lay people to use their understanding of the human being, cultivated together with medical people in social life, and relate to expert knowledge to such effect that they are able to agree with medical opinion in a parliament meant to be democratic not merely because they believe in authority but because they have a degree of understanding.

If we are objective in considering how the three elements in the threefold social organism work together in a specific field such as this, we will find that the idea of the social organism being threefold by nature is fully justified. One may fight this idea of a threefold social organism if initially one has only an abstract idea of it.

Today I have again only been able to give you brief indications of the necessity for a threefold social organism becoming evident if we think in the right way about a specific field such as hygiene. I have been able to indicate first steps in this direction; if they are followed and taken further you will find that someone who approaches the impulse for a threefold social organism with certain abstract notions may well fight it in a way. The reasons that he will usually give are those one has oneself produced long ago as possible objections. But to anyone who enters into the individual spheres of life with full inner understanding, considering how they come into their own, with all the individual aspects they bring into human life (these are what social life is about), someone who truly knows his way about in a particular sphere of life, endeavouring to understand something of true life practice in some field or other, will be guided more and more in the direction indicated with the idea of the threefold social organism.

The idea truly did not spring from a dream state, nor from abstract idealism; it arose as a social need for the present day and immediate future, from genuine, objective study of the individual spheres of life. And if you then penetrate these individual spheres of life with what lives in you out of the impulse for a threefold social organism you will find exactly what these spheres need today, as it seems to me. I just wanted to give you some indications this evening as to how with something like the idea of the threefold social organism, which spiritual science can give for social life, the things which today can only be accepted by believing in authority, blindly subjugating oneself to this, can instead arise from a genuine understanding of the human being which is cultivated in the social sphere and can be a social concern and element in human society. Because of this I am able to say here: Hygiene can indeed be a social, a truly social affair if fructified in the way this particular field can be by a medicine made fruitful by spiritual science. In the truest sense and to a high degree it can become a general issue, democratically cultivated, for the whole nation.

In the discussion which followed, Rudolf Steiner said the following:

Ladies and gentlemen, with the kind of things we have been discussing today it matters above all that one is first of all able to enter into the whole spirit of what has been said. Because of this it is sometimes difficult to answer questions formulated out of present-day thinking and attitudes, to answer them objectively without rephrasing them or at least going into explanation. The question that you, or many of you, may consider to be terribly simple, requiring only a few sentences or a single one, is the following: 'How does one get out of the habit of sleeping too long?'

To answer this question it would be necessary for me to give a lecture that is almost longer than the one I have just given; for I would first have to present the different elements that are needed to answer the question properly. However, the following may perhaps be said. Today almost the whole of humanity lives in an intellectualistic state of mind. People who think they are forming opinions or live according to their feelings, or think they are not intellectualistic for some other reason, are in fact highly intellectualistic. The basic character of intellectualistic life in mind and organs is that it ruins our instincts. It is actually the case that if you want to refer to instincts today that are not completely ruined you have to refer to early humanity or perhaps even the animal world. I had occasion these days to speak of an instance that tells us a great deal. There are greedy birds who'll eat insects such as garden spiders. Garden spiders are poison to them, however, and so the birds develop convulsions, twitches, and have to die a miserable death soon after swallowing the garden spider. But if there's any henbane growing nearby the bird will fly to it, suck the healing juice from it and save its life. Just consider how the instinctive life has developed there, whilst in us human beings it has shrunk to the few instinctive reflexes we still have, so that if a fly settles on one's nose one does instinctively brush it off. A defensive instinct comes up in response to the insult. In a bird which has eaten a garden spider, the response to the effect which this has on the organism is such a defensive instinct driving the bird to do something really sensible. Such instincts can still be found in people who lived in the dim distant past if we know how to interpret their history correctly. Today we live differently. I have always found it tremendously painful to see people at their midday meal—where I used to see knife and fork and similar implements lying beside the plate—and see scales beside their plate, literally a set of scales. This is a genuine experience. They would weigh out this small piece of meat, for only then would they know how much meat to eat, doing right by their organism—by weighing it! Just think how much human beings who need to have things prescribed for them are lacking in all genuine original instincts. It is therefore necessary not to stop at intellectualism but rise to spiritual-scientific insight.

You may think I am speaking *pro domo* [for the house], albeit this great house,[52] but I am not doing so. In fact I am speaking of things which I believe I have perceived to be the truth, quite apart from the fact that I represent that truth. You will find that if you do penetrate not merely the intellectualistic thinking but also the things that need to be grasped in spiritual science, so that they come to one more in the form of images, that if we grasp such insights, which are not accessible to the mere intellect, we are guided back to healthy instincts, perhaps not in the individual life but more in the things that lie in the deeper foundations of life. Someone who seeks, at least for a time—however little time it may be—to develop the very different state of mind that has to be developed if one truly wishes to understand aspects of spiritual science, is taken back to sound instincts again in things such as the need for sleep, for instance. Animals do not sleep too much under normal conditions of life, nor did early man. You have to train yourself to gain sound instincts again, instincts we lose the habit of in today's intellectualistic civilization. We may say, therefore, that a truly effective way of getting out of the habit of sleeping for too long is to be able to take in spiritual-scientific truths without going to sleep in the process. If you immediately go to sleep on hearing spiritual-scientific truths you will indeed not get out of the habit of sleeping too long. But if you manage to be present with a true inner human interest when spiritual-scientific truths are gone through, this inner human quality will be activated to the effect of actually discovering what length of sleep is exactly right for your organism.

It is again enormously difficult to give intellectualistic rules, saying for instance that an individual person with one problem or other in the liver or kidney, something that does not make him sick in the usual sense but is nevertheless there, should sleep for such and such a length of time. In general this will not get us anywhere. And again it is not the same when we induce sleep artificially or if the body in its need for sleep refuses entry to the spirit for as long as it needs. We may say, therefore, that the right kind of hygiene based on the science of the spirit will enable people to find the right measure for their sleep.

This is also why the other question that has been asked cannot be easily answered. 'How do we know how much sleep we need?' I'd say that this is something we need not know in discursive thinking, no need for that, but we will no doubt need to acquire the kind of instincts one acquires not by simply taking in sets of notes relating to spiritual science but by the way in which one understands things in that science—being really involved in it. We gain this instinct and will then individually find the right measure of sleep. This, then, is what can be said about this in general terms. As I said, I can merely point the way in answering this question and not give what may perhaps be expected. However, the things people expect are not always the right things.

Is it healthy to sleep with the window open?

Questions like this also cannot always be answered in completely general terms. It is perfectly conceivable that sleeping with the window open is very healthy for a person, but this depends on the particular nature of his respiratory organs. For someone else it may be better to air the room well and then close the windows before going to sleep. We really need to understand how human beings relate to their environment and base our opinion on this in the individual case.

How do you explain, on the basis of spiritual science, mental disorders developing because a crime has been committed? I mean where do you look for the physical condition that is behind the mental problems?

Well, to answer this properly and fully we would also have to go into the whole criminal and essentially also psychiatric anthropology. Let me just say the following. In the first place we have to assume, when considering such things, that there is something abnormal in the disposition of the organs of someone who becomes a criminal even before he does so. You really only have to consider the truly objective studies of any more significant criminal anthropologist and you will see that the pathological study of the forms of individual human organs can indeed be connected with a disposition to criminality. But the abnormality does already exist. Materialistic thinkers like Moritz Benedikt[53] may, of course, draw the wrong conclusions, for not everyone showing these particular signs is a born criminal. The point is that we can indeed influence defects in the organism—as I just said organ defects, not the existing mental conditions, but organ defects—especially through education and later with appropriate cultural elements, that is, through mind and spirit, providing the factual situation is spiritual-scientifically investigated. The conclusions drawn by Benedikt are not correct, therefore. But we can refer to defects in organs. We have to be clear, however, that above all the things that are not intellectualistic, but are related to feelings and emotions in everyday human life, have an influence in turn. Initially they act on glandular functions or the like, secretory functions, and in the process also on the organs.

Here I'd advise you, for instance, to read an interesting small volume written by a Danish neurologist about the mechanics of emotions.[54] It says all kinds of things you will find useful. And now consider the bodily disposition, which you can study with anyone who truly may be considered a criminal, add all the consequences for the caught criminal by way of emotional shocks, which will in turn influence the organs, and this gives you later on the way of looking for the defective organs for the evident sequels of a committed crime that brought about mental illness. This is the way in which we can look for enlightenment in situations like this.

How does theosophy relate to anthroposophy? Is the theosophy that used to be represented here no longer considered tenable to its full extent?

All I want to say is that nothing but spiritual science with anthroposophical orientation has ever been presented here. What is presented here today has always been presented, and if it was taken to be the 'theosophy' which is presented in other places, then that was a misunderstanding. This misunderstanding will persist also because, within limits, anthroposophical spiritual science was for a time active within the Theosophical Society.[55] Even within that Society the representatives of spiritual science with anthroposophical orientation presented nothing but what is said here today. This was accepted within the Theosophical Society for as long as it did not seem too heretical. But when people realized that anthroposophy was something very different from the abstract mysticism which tends to be widely considered to be theosophy, they threw out the anthroposophists. That procedure was definitely the work of the other side. The approach presented here has never had any other form than it has today. People who take a superficial view of things and listen only to people who have come to such a superficial approach as members of the Society—one does not always need to be on the outside to take a superficial view of anthroposophy or confuse anthroposophy with theosophy, one may actually be a member—people therefore who merely gain knowledge by such a superficial approach will arrive at such confusion. What is represented here, and today I have characterized it for a specific area, and nothing else has ever been presented here, though work is, of course, continuing all the time and certain things can be characterized more precisely, more fully and intensively today than was possible 15, 10 or 5 years ago. It is in the very nature of the work that we progress, especially in formulation to make ourselves understood about a subject as difficult as spiritual science. We really do not have to listen to people who from ill will have made a noose for our necks of the fact that things said in a less perfect way before are later said in a more perfect way, making this into all kinds of changes in philosophies of life; we need not pay heed to such ill-intentioned people and the things they say. The spiritual science we represent is alive; it is not something dead. Someone who thinks that it cannot progress, who wants to nail it down at a point where it once was, which does happen now and then, does not believe in the life in it but wants to make it into something dead.

Would you please tell us how an epidemic such as influenza or scarlet fever has come about if not by transmission of bacilli. Pathological organisms have been established for many diseases. What is your view on this?

Well, I did say earlier on that I do not want to take sides particularly when it comes to this question, and it would need a whole lecture to discuss it. But let me draw your attention to the following. Someone who has insights that compel him to point out that the causes for conditions where bacilli or bacteria make their appearance are deeper than primary, deeper than the appearance of bacilli, certainly is not denying their existence. It is quite a different matter to say the bacilli are there and appear in the course of the disease than to consider them to be the primary cause. I have just developed the theme fully in the course which is currently in progress.[56] But it does need time to do so. The same applies to certain elements that need to be considered first. It is not something to be dealt with quickly in a question-and-answer session.

Let me say this, however. This human constitution is not such a simple matter as people tend to think. The human being is highly complex. I initially wrote of this in my book *Von Seelenrätseln.** Human beings are threefold by nature, and we may speak of the human being of senses and nerves, secondly the rhythmic human being, and thirdly the metabolic human being. That simply is the way they are. And these three parts of human nature interact, and if the individual is to be in good health they must not interact in any other way but so that in a way the spheres are also separate. Thus the human being of nerves and senses, who is more than people imagine in modern physiology, must not simply transmit its influences to the metabolic human being without the mediation of the rhythmic movements of circulatory and respiratory processes which do, of course, extend to the outermost periphery of the organism. This interaction may be interrupted in a particular way. But the combined activities have a quite specific effect.

When questions like this are put, you must forgive me but they have to be properly answered. I intend to be as objective as possible, but some

---

* Extracts in *The Case for Anthroposophy.*[57]

things will have to be said and must be objectively received. It is definitely the case, for instance, that processes in the human pelvis are part and parcel of the whole organism. They function properly if integrated into the whole organism. If something or other causes them to be either made stronger directly in the pelvis so that they are more active there, or if the corresponding processes—there always are such corresponding processes—in the human head or in the human lung lose some of their intensity, are reduced, something quite specific will occur. It will then be evident that for a normal life the human organism must develop inner processes that must only develop up to a certain point if they are to lay claim to the whole human being. If the process increases it becomes local and a process may develop in the pelvis, for example, which causes the processes in the head or in the lung that correspond to particular processes in the pelvis not to be properly separate. Processes always correspond so that they run parallel. This means, however, that something which should only exist up to a certain level in the human being in order to maintain his vitality, the vitality sustained by spirit and soul, is taken beyond a specific level. It then becomes the atmosphere, as I'd like to put it, for all kinds of lower organisms, all kinds of small organisms; these are then able to unfold there. The element in which the small organisms are able to be active is always there in the human being, but it extends over the whole organism. If it becomes concentrated it provides the soil for small organisms, microbes; they find there the soil they need. The reason why they are able to flourish there must be sought in extremely subtle processes in the organism which then prove to be the primary cause.

Truly, I am not saying this from antipathy to the bacillus theory. I do fully understand the reason why people pay homage to that belief in bacilli. You may believe me, if I did not have to say this for objective reasons I would acknowledge these reasons, but in this case insight is of necessity leading to the acknowledgement of something different, forcing one to say: 'I see a particular landscape with great numbers of extraordinarily beautiful, well cared for cattle. My question is: Why do particular conditions of life apply in this region? They come from the beautiful cattle. I explain the conditions of life in the region by saying that beautiful cattle have come into it from somewhere and have spread there.' I am not going to do so, of course, but investigate the primary causes, the local people's diligence and insight, and this will tell me why these beautiful cattle thrive on this soil. It would be superficial merely to say that it's nice here, life is good, for beautiful cattle have come here.

Essentially the same logic applies when I find typhoid fever bacilli and think that people have the condition because typhoid fever bacilli have entered. Very different things are needed to explain typhoid fever, not just reliance on typhoid fever bacilli.

We are led astray in quite a different way if we adopt that kind of false logic. Yes, the primary processes provide the soil on which the typhoid fever bacilli can live, but they also cause all kinds of other things that are not primary. It is very easy to confuse secondary elements with the actual, original syndrome completely, or to confound them. These are the things which take us to the right view or show how something which in a sense has its justification must be placed within its limits.

Perhaps you see from the way in which I have answered this question—only briefly, in outline, so that there is a risk of it being misunderstood—that it really is not a matter of taking the popular line and condemning the bacillus theory. No, it is a matter of investigating things in all seriousness.

Request for some examples of physical and organic disorders possibly causing mental problems.

Well, answered in detail this, too, would go much too far. But let me say just one thing. You see, medical thinking has not developed in the way in which it is presented in the history of medicine today—of Hippocrates establishing the beginnings of medicine, and Hippocratic views then developing further. As far as one is able to trace this we know that very peculiar things were taught by Hippocrates, and we have the last remnants of an ancient medicine of instinct rather than just the beginning of today's intellectual medicine. And we also find something else.

You see, when this ancient medicine of instinct still applied people would not speak of depression of a particular kind, which is a very abstract way of putting it, but of hypochondria, indurations developing in the abdomen. They knew that disorders developed in the abdomen, hardening, when hypochondria arose. We cannot say that the ancients were more materialistic than we are.

It is also very easy to show that certain chronic lung conditions are clearly connected with something we may call a false mystical attitude. We might refer to all kinds of things, quite apart from the fact that—and this again is connected with a good instinct—the ancients certainly related the temperaments to organic aspects. They let the choleric temperament arise from the bile, the white bile, the melancholic temperament from the black bile and everything the black bile brings about in the abdomen. They then had the sanguine temperament arising from the blood and the phlegmatic temperament from phlegm, from what they called phlegm. Any degeneration of the temperaments was clearly something to them which pointed to degeneration in the relevant organic aspect. The way this was done in the medicine of instinct and hygiene of instinct can certainly be taken up again in a strictly scientific way and cultivated from the point of view of present-day insight.

Now comes the question where one may be even more seriously misunderstood.

Do you have knowledge of eye diagnosis? Do you recognize it as scientific?

Well, it is generally correct that with an organism, and especially the complex human organism, all kinds of individual things, seen in the right way, may permit conclusions as to the whole. Equally, the relationship of the individual part to the organism is of great importance. In a way, the iris in the eye studied by someone practising iris diagnosis is too isolated from the rest of the human organism, and on the other hand it is part of the rest of the organism in such a peculiar way that we do indeed have an organ that can tell us a great deal. However, we must not be schematic, especially with things like this. The problem with things like this is that people are schematic about it. It is certainly the case that people of a different constitution in soul and body show different characteristics in the iris compared to others. It needs such intimate knowledge of what goes on in the human organism that if you have that knowledge there is really no longer any need to base the investigation on a single organ. And if you are instructed to follow particular intellectualistic rules and do things schematically, nothing of much value will result.

How do diseases relate to the progress of world history, especially those appearing now?

One chapter in a whole history of civilization! Well, let me just say the following. Students of history must have a feel for doing symptomatology, that is, to see many of the things which are today considered to be history as mere symptoms of something much deeper down lying behind them. This is the spiritual current, and it merely bears these symptoms. Developments in the depths of human evolution thus appear symptomatically as the diseases of a particular age. It is interesting to study the connections between developments in the depths of human evolution and the symptoms of one disease or another. Conclusions may also be drawn from the presence of certain diseases as to impulses in historical evolution which go unrecognized with a symptomatology that is not of this nature.

The question may also refer to something else, something not without significance for the study of the evolution of human history. It is this. Irrespective of whether they affect individuals or occur in epidemic form in society, diseases are often also reactions to other kinds of degeneration which are perhaps considered to be less serious from a health point of view but seen as very serious indeed from the moral or spiritual point of view. We must not apply what I am saying to medicine or hygiene. That would be quite wrong. Diseases need to be cured. In hygiene we must support humanity. You cannot say anything like: 'I'll check first if it is not perhaps your karma to have this disease, in which case I must let you keep it, and if it is not I may treat it.' That is not the way you proceed in the work of healing. But something which does not apply to human intervention in nature does objectively apply in the outside world. There it has to be said that many things that arise as a disposition for moral excesses enter so deeply into the human organization that reactions develop, taking the form of specific diseases, and in that case the disease suppresses a moral excess. It is not so important to consider this in the case of an individual; we should leave it to his individual destiny and essentially not interfere, just as we should not concern ourselves with someone's personal correspondence—unless it is from the particular standpoint we meet with at the present time, 'Opened officially under martial law'—we should not interfere with someone's personal correspondence and certainly also not in their personal karma. It is different with world history. The individual person has merely a statistical role in the laws of world history. We always have to point out that the statistics of life insurance companies provide a good basis for estimating mortality. They do, of course, base their rates on this. It is fairly accurate and the calculations are correct, everything is wholly scientific—but, well, you don't have to die exactly at the time established in life insurance statistics, nor do you have to live for as long as they say. Other elements come in where the individual person is concerned. But when it comes to groups of people or the whole of human evolution, it may well be that you are not superstitious but properly scientific if you investigate in how far pathological symptoms, diseases that make their appearance, provide correction for other excesses. We may indeed look there for a certain repercussion also of the disease or at least the fact of the disease being brought about, on something which would have taken a very different form had it not been for the disease.

These are a few aspects in considering the matter touched on in this question.

The time is advanced, and we will now follow the others, so many of them, who have left already.

V

Aspects of Psychiatry

QUESTIONS AND ANSWERS

DORNACH, 26 MARCH 1920

THIS subject would need to be considered exhaustively if we wanted to tackle it at all. Today we can only make some brief references, for the study of psychiatry undoubtedly needs the most thorough revision especially in our day. Just consider the way it is really impossible today to know what issues need to be addressed in psychiatry and you'll soon realize the great need for reform. This will not be possible—or so it seems to me after hearing Dr Husemann[58] speak—unless spiritual science truly renders the individual specialized subject areas fruitful first. The development of science so beautifully described by Dr Husemann today, a development which began and reached its height in the nineteenth century, has really driven the whole of human thinking apart in two directions that are extreme opposites. On the one hand there are the ideas people have of the material world and its processes, and on the other hand we have the life of thought as such, which, I'd say, has become progressively more abstract in character. Abstractions have no power in the world, nor have they any power in human beings, and offer no possibility for human beings to grasp matter—the physical world—out of the psyche, to build a bridge somehow between the psyche and the material world.

Today people have at best an idea of a sum of abstractions or abstract sentiments and the like when they speak of the psyche. This sum of abstractions clearly cannot set an organism in motion, nor build some kind of bridge to the organism. It therefore also cannot be said that we can somehow influence the outer, physical, real organism through the psyche, doing so with something which is but a sum of abstractions. On the other hand knowledge has been gained in science of the physical organism; it is pure fiction to say the phenomena of the psyche are but parallels to or indeed due to activities of the physical organism. None of the actual ideas developed concerning this physical organism are such that one might squeeze anything out of them by way of ideas concerning the psyche.

As a result we have a view of the inner life—irrespective of whether one is more or less of a materialist—where one looks only on abstractions, and side by side with it a view of physical life, organic life, that will not in any way yield anything relating to mind and spirit.

It is only natural, really, that a method that would serve psychiatry is not easy to find. This is also why people have most recently ceased to talk in any way about the connection between the physical, organic aspect of the human being on the one hand and the psyche as a process in the conscious mind on the other.

As we are truly in constant danger of sitting between the two chairs, the physical and material and the abstract and psychic, it has been necessary to invent a wholly unconscious world, a world that is both strange and unconscious. This has been done in psychoanalysis, analytical psychology, a scientific subject that is really extraordinarily interesting. Once psychiatry has been reformed so that we shall again have a proper psychiatry, this scientific subject will have to be thoroughly tested from the new psychiatric standpoint, for it is really an object for psychiatry.

To avoid ending up on the floor between these two chairs, attempts have thus been made to discern an unconscious world. I am not against the unconscious world, of course, but it has to be investigated, truly recognized, using the vision introduced in spiritual science; one cannot fantasize, dream it up in the way Freudians or others like them do.

Spiritual science will contribute to a reform of psychiatry in taking us from merely abstract concepts that have no life in them to concepts that are in accord with reality, concepts which already live in the world as concepts and are gained by entering wholly into reality with our methods. Rising to such spiritual methods, which on their part provide concepts that are in accord with reality, we will be able to make the transition to actual reality. It means that we will be able to build a bridge between psyche and physical body. The psyche and the physical body must look different in our mind to what they look like today if we seriously want to have a psychiatry.

Today's sum of abstractions, including all the abstract laws of nature—they are filtered more and more, these laws of nature—cannot enter fully into a process that is real.

Just imagine how, with the abstractions that figure in science today, one might actually find something like the two important facts, as I am right to call them—for they are facts—of which I spoke in the first lecture in this series: the thesis, grounded in spiritual science, of cardiac function and the basic biogenetic law being reversed for the historical development of events on earth.

Examples like this show that the methods used in spiritual science truly allow one to find one's way into the world of facts, doing so out of the inner life of the psyche, to build a bridge from the 'mental' to the 'physical', as they are called.

This is particularly necessary in psychiatry, for we will only get somewhere once we are able to observe the relevant facts in the right way. And the facts of psychiatry are essentially even harder to observe because they call for greater freedom from bias than the facts relating to the effects of physical laws. Essentially there is practically no way of isolating the human being completely as soon as we come from health, relative health, to relative sickness. The human being does indeed develop into a single individual, an isolated life. He does this exactly through his soul element, but it is through something which in the psyche deviates from linear development. Anything which deviates from the linear development which we call 'normal' in the physical aspect (I can, of course, only make brief reference, otherwise one would have to go on for hours, going into detail) is not something which we can consider in isolation. Human beings are much more social creatures, also in the deeper sense, than we tend to think. And actual mental diseases can only in the rarest instances be assessed according to, let us say, the biography of the individual in isolation. This is practically impossible.

I'd like to use a hypothetical example to indicate what I really mean. You see, it is possible, for example, that two people live side by side in a community, be it a family or some other kind of community. One of them has the misfortune after some time to suffer an episode, something classified as belonging to the field of psychiatry. Now it is, of course, possible to treat that individual in isolation. But if you do this, especially if you base your view on a study of this individual in isolation, you will in many cases really just fall victim to a thought mask. For the situation may well be, and this is so in many cases, that someone else who lives in the family or other kind of community with the sick individual really has the complex of powers, as we may call it, in him which has led to the mental condition of the other person. Considering these two people initially we have this: A has the episode, from the psychiatric point of view; B has a complex of powers in him that is psychic and organic by nature. If we were to consider him on his own he might probably show the element which in the case of A we call the cause of the illness to a much greater degree. It means that B, who has no evident mental problem, has much more of the cause of this mental condition in him than A, who had to be taken to a clinic.

This is something which is wholly in the sphere of reality and not just conjecture. It is based on the fact that apart from the complex of powers considered to be the cause of his mental condition, A has a weak constitution and does not tolerate this complex of powers. The other person, B, who also has that complex of powers in him, has a much stronger constitution than the other; it does not harm him. B tolerates it, A does not. A would not have developed the condition if he had not been constantly influenced mentally by B, who lives next to him. B's influence would be extraordinarily great because he is more robust than A.

Here you have an example which is a reality in a great many cases. You see how important the psychiatric way of looking at things is if the aim is to consider things that are real, rather than playing around, which is often done in this field today. It really is a matter of not looking at a person in isolation, but in the whole of his social environment.

What I mean to say here must, however, be put on a very broad basis. For it also applies in all other pathology that there is a great difference between a weak individual affected by some complex or other and a strong, robust individual. Let us assume two people live side by side from a certain age onwards. One still has the robust country person's nature due to his young years and his origins, the other comes from three generations of nothing but town people. The one with the healthy countryman's nature, who is well able to cope with inner damage, may perhaps bear much more of a complex in him but he tolerates it and does not fall ill. The other, who only has the complex because of psychic infection, by imitation, due to the things that always exist between people, is not able to cope with its influence.

Here you see everything that needs to be considered if you want to talk about psychiatry not in theory and in terms of programmes, but on the basis of reality. Now is the time to be serious, realizing that essentially our scientists have grown so one-sided, especially from the time of Galileo, and there is need to take in new things that will make science fruitful in all fields. Otherwise human insight must fall into utter decadence, especially so in the areas that are to take us into practical life.

I might thus say that basically the same holds true for psychiatry as for the things we say when talking about the Waldorf school and speaking of the art of education—that one should not just come up with some new formulations of a theoretical nature, but take the living science of the spirit itself into this field. What may be said about the field of education must also be said about the field of psychiatry. We will certainly never be able to say in a biased way: This or that needs to be improved in psychiatry. No, we must come to accept the idea that either we accept the spiritual-scientific basis altogether in the search for insight—and it will certainly change psychiatry, making something particularly of psychiatry which so many people are truly longing for today, though it cannot be found with the latest natural-scientific methods of which you have heard a great deal both yesterday and today.

You see, what must above all result when spiritual science becomes popular—to use a commonplace term—is a much, much better insight into the nature of the human being than any found today. People relate to one another in such a way today that one simply cannot speak of insight. They pass each other by, everyone lives for himself. Spiritual science will make people open to one another. And much which today is perhaps still thought to be in the field of mental pathology will with this be driven across into the field of mental hygiene. For the situation is, I'd say, that straight currents may be traced everywhere from the syndromes of disrupted mental life to the ideas, often accepted as a matter of course in public life, which are not considered pathological at all but are indeed generally accepted. If we were to follow up some of the concepts which are so generally accepted, we would find that more slowly, perhaps, but nevertheless the same route has been followed as that used to trace an abnormal mental syndrome, though it then progresses speedily in someone whom people consider mentally abnormal today.

It is evident from all this that ultimately all the talk about details in reforming individual sciences does not give us much, but if one decided—sadly souls, many souls, are too sleepy today—to look for scientific life to be made fruitful in terms of spiritual science, then all kinds of different fields in science, and especially the field where various deviations from normal mental life are considered, psychiatry, would suffer an automatic reform, as I'd like to put it. Even if such cases go in the direction of the most extreme rebellion, raving madness, feeblemindedness and so on—we will only discover what these mental aberrations from normal life signify within the whole of normal development. And we shall in many respects find that if our philosophy of life grows progressively more sound, many of the unhealthy public errors that cast their light into the pathological aberrations of the mentally ill will grow sound.

For it is absolutely remarkable how difficult it is to draw a clear boundary between 'normal life' as it is called and abnormal mental life. It is difficult to say, for instance, if a normal mental state pertained in a case that happened not far from here, in Basel, not that long ago. A man bequeathed a large sum in his will to anyone who would shut himself up, in complete isolation, until he succeeded in establishing that the soul is truly immortal. Someone in Basel wrote that will, and I do not know what happened after that. I think his heirs raised objections and sought to get a decision—not psychiatric but legal—as to how far this goes towards the psychiatric or not. However if you, every single one of you, set out to investigate if this is a matter for psychiatry or a whim or indeed excessive religiosity or whatever, you'll hardly arrive at anything that is wholly accurate.

It is very much the case that our concepts have grown feeble as compared to reality; they need to grow strong again. But they will only gain strength with spiritual science. And psychiatry will be one field among many where people will grow aware of this.

VI

ADDRESS (FOLLOWED BY DISCUSSION) AT A MEETING WITH MEDICAL PRACTITIONERS

ADDRESS

DORNACH, 21 APRIL 1924

I think the main subject we need to discuss should be in response to definite questions put by you. I merely have a few things to say first, matters of principle.

Real values have been lost in the course of human evolution because people have lost insight into the spiritual element, which truly is present in all things physical. Medicine is undoubtedly a field where most has been lost, the reason being that limiting oneself entirely to knowledge of the natural world must inevitably lead to all insight into the essential human being and human life being lost. Again and again we have to stress that the nature of all processes in the natural world is such that they cannot take place in the same way within the human organism.

Let us leave aside the animal and plant organisms. The prevalent idea today is that a process that can be observed in the natural world outside can also exist in some way within the human organism. People talk of combustion and all kinds of other physical processes within the human organism. In fact there is no such thing. Compared to something in the natural world outside we have a self-contained human organism which seen from the outside is different from any object in the natural world, and every single process in the human organism is something thoroughly different. All processes in the natural world, outside the human being, have an effect on human beings, being constructive or destructive. To understand the essential human being we have to accept three different kinds of degradation or destruction.

The first kind of destruction happens from inside, in a way, due to all the influences which earth has on human beings. The powers of earth destroy human beings from the inside. The powers acting from the air, mainly through respiration and transferred to the human being, bring in destruction from the earth's surroundings. And the powers of light act destructively on man from the cosmos. Thus the powers of the cosmos, powers outside the human body, bring destruction in three ways, and destruction starts as soon as the I organization and the astral body are not acting on the human organization as well. Astral body and I organization counteract the destructive principles in human beings. Destruction due to extra-human powers must therefore begin the very moment when I and astral body are no longer active in human beings. This also tells us that we cannot in the least manage to understand essential human nature unless we gain more and more genuine insight into the higher levels of human existence also when considering the medical aspects.

Medicine has come to be mere experimentation, trying things out, merely because in more recent times people no longer dared to count on the higher levels of essential human nature, on the supersensible. It is, however, impossible to understand the disease process unless we see it as being connected with those higher levels. Nor can we understand the process of getting well, of healing, unless we see it in relationship to them. Let us consider the following. Destructive processes of the physical body and the ether body are mainly active in the human head. They actually make it possible for the astral principle and the I to be independently active in the head. In the organization of metabolism and limbs, in everything connected with motor function and metabolism, we have the constructive, anabolic, processes in the human organism of both ether body and physical body. I and astral body are most eminently active in these anabolic processes solely for metabolism and motor system. Astral body and I are active in everything that happens in metabolism. The I organization is active in all movement. We thus have I and astral body engaged in the system of metabolism and limbs; in the human head they are exposed, as it were; I and astral organization are absolutely free there.

To draw a diagram [Plate 7] we might have the physical head, etheric head, but astral body and I free, not engaged in the physical and etheric

[head]. If on the other hand—leaving aside for the moment the middle human being, the rhythmic, blood human being—we consider the human being of metabolism and limbs, the etheric body is fully involved in the first place. It is so also in the head, but here astral body and I organization are also active—not left free inwardly but bringing the processes about.

Looking at a child we have a complete connection between everything by way of astral body and I organization that is free in the head, and the principles bound to the physical organization as they are in the body, whilst in adults we do not have such inner cohesion, so that the whole body is not dependent on anything that happens in the head to the same degree as in a child. In children the whole body is still wholly dependent on anything happening in the whole head.

It is quite impossible to gain knowledge of essential human nature unless one really takes the higher levels of it into account. No one can really understand what goes on in the motor system, the metabolic system, unless they take recourse also to the mind and spirit. At best one can draw on the head organization; it is inwardly very much taking its physical form from the way laws outside the human being apply. The head organization has an etheric body present within it and differs from organizations that are not human, but it is still most similar to the organization outside man.

What does it really mean to understand a disease? Let us assume you are dealing with some organ in metabolism, and have to assume a quite specific connection between the physical and etheric and the way in which astral body and I organization intervene in this organ, let's say the liver. Astral body and I organization must intervene in a quite specific way. The moment they withdraw a little from this organ it will grow similar to the head organ, and one must always keep in mind that when any metabolic organ and also anything connected with metabolism shows an irregularity, astral body and I organization are not sufficiently involved in the organization of the organ concerned. It is the other way round in the head. If astral body and I intervene too much, a morbid state develops in the human head. The head is really the part of the human being that is inwardly most strongly vegetable and mineral in disposition, whilst motor and metabolic organs are most strongly animal and human. People really only see the opposite of this. They think the head organization is most spiritual in organization. Yet when the head organization becomes the most spiritual the conscious mind gets clouded. Now the moment processes coming from I or astral body do not intervene sufficiently in the organism of metabolism and limbs, the moment the system of metabolism and limbs grows similar to the head system, this system will be morbid.

The physician's approach must therefore be to ask: 'When I see that a disease involves clouding of the mind, how do I prevent this? I have to prevent the I and astral body from intervening too strongly.' Or: 'How do I manage to get the astral body to intervene more strongly where its intervention is not strong enough?' Now you see, these things show the extraordinarily great role which the way of thinking, the method of thinking, plays especially in medicine. Yes, we must indeed know the medicinal substances, the medicinal agents. But you will be perfectly right in asking how one will get to know the medicinal agents. We cannot get to know them unless we first gain living experience in mind and spirit of what is truly going on in the human being. To do so we need a particular way of thinking. This is what I really wanted to say by way of introduction, that the physician must be wholly given to a particular way of thinking. Initially, for instance, I'd say one has to start with things that are more outside, in nature. The physician must first of all understand that everything we may call heat, light and so on really exists in two ways. You see, initially, if it's summer, light and warmth come down to the earth from the sun. Sunlight and the heat of the sun take hold of everything on earth that is sprouting, shooting, about to flower and bear fruit. And things that flower and fruit are essentially interesting for us because they are vehicles for the sun's light and heat.

But how are things in winter? In summer, the sun's light and heat enter into the soil; staying in the earth, the sun's light and heat continue to be active through the winter. Light and sun thus have to be considered from two angles.

But when we look at the sun's and altogether the cosmic surroundings' effect on earth we realize that all of it has an effect on the human system of metabolism and limbs. The whole system of metabolism and limbs is already affected by influences from the cosmos.

Everything in the head is influenced by cosmic powers that have been preserved in the earth. In this respect the human being is upside down on earth. The system of metabolism and limbs is affected by influences from outside the earth, cosmic influences. But you can extend this to every single substance. Take lead, for instance, lead being a definite medicinal agent for certain things. We find lead in nature outside the human being to be as it has arisen through the totality of cosmic powers; when it exists because of the cosmic powers, it will most eminently act through the system of limbs and metabolism up into the head. If we melt the lead, using an earthly process and subjecting the lead to it, it will act directly on the head system. This is why there is such a great difference.

Antimony, grey antimony glance, is an important medicine we have. If we take the fibrous ore existing in the world outside—the spearlike habit comes from the cosmos—we have a medicament which acts on metabolism. If we subject the antimony to an earthly process, making it into a black mirror deposit, we get a specific action on the human head.

Now you see, with this way of thinking it is a matter of entering not only into the substance, but into the processes, into what is going on. It is not right to say that lead is a medicine for this or that. It is a matter of knowing how the process went, if we have a raw material or if the substance has been subjected to some process or other. The way substances are treated—that is essentially what matters. And we ought to stop looking for the medicinal property in the substance as such. We should more and more say to ourselves, if there's a disease, it is a process that is not embraced by the human organism as a whole. If we want a medicine, we must strengthen the organism; we must subject the human being to processes that we fully understand. This is what matters.

I now want to tell you something that is the aim and purpose of the whole of this introduction. It may seem paradoxical at first, but it needs to be fully grasped in the whole of medical life. It is this. You have to study all the processes that need to be studied in the universe to establish if they are cosmic or telluric or processes where both come into it. We have no way of really getting to these processes unless we are able to understand how the soul element is also differentiated into three different regions in the threefold human being. It is really not possible to get to the human being in any real way unless we understand the soul principle.

And you see, for this we have to consider the following. The soul principle really has much greater unity in adults than the physical organism does. The latter is clearly differentiated into three—neurosensory system, rhythmic system and system of metabolism and limbs. These must be distinguished. The soul principle fills the head system, the neurosensory system, as much as it does the rhythmic system and also metabolism and limbs. In the lower system it is very sleepy, dreaming, but it does fill the whole human being in his three aspects. Now if someone is meant to develop one system especially, that is, if the soul principle is to pour its activity especially into one system, what happens in that case? I think you'll agree that a person can be busy thinking, he can walk, occupy himself using his hands, his legs—we'll have to consider the middle system separately. But what happens with the soul principle when a person is busy with an activity, or is walking? When a person walks or works with his hands, it truly is the case that the same power comes to expression in everything in the world we call love; this remains in arms and hands, in legs and feet [missing text]. Human beings have to go to the limits of their skin when they stir into activity, and when this flows out beyond them it unfolds as love.

What does it mean to say 'Someone is walking'? It means he lives and loves the human organism within his skin; it means he makes the necessary effort with his astral or I organization. And in walking he works his I organization in such a way that he draws it out to some degree of his physical and etheric organization. Human beings withdraw their astral limbs and I limbs when they walk; stretching their legs as they walk they are withdrawing astral body and I. Thinking, they shine them in, only as far as the skin of course. If we take this into account we can say that in getting the organism going we simply have the beginning of morbidity. You get morbid states when astral body and I organization withdraw from the system of metabolism and limbs without the individual lovingly filling his organism. When etheric body and physical body are filled completely in the head and it is not from arbitrary choice, you'll again have morbid states. Anything a person does arbitrarily will immediately afterwards correct itself. Daily life in thought and motion—it is a continuous process of making ourselves ill. But the human organism is immediately able to restore health to itself.

To understand these things depends on being truly able to have enough love for what is going on in a case of sickness, so that we can look at it as something which really shows us the spiritual in the human being in a physical way. You see, when someone develops liver disease, does in some way develop abnormalities in the liver, let us say, his astral body is not sufficiently active in the liver. What kind of mental activity involves a similar process? It is when I take a particularly great inner interest in something external. The moment someone looks at something with great attention, that person really has liver disease. The astral body is withdrawing from the liver in that case, but the situation is immediately corrected. Going through the different disease processes in the human organism we can always see what happens in a healthy individual through arbitrariness, through arbitrary life. If the arbitrary processes were not always balanced out again, people would make themselves sick all the time with those processes. It is therefore possible to learn how the soul principle, the spiritual principle, is if we *like* disease processes as study processes—truly love them.

This love for the diseases must of course be combined with something else. We don't just want to study the disease; this is of lesser significance. But if we are able to cure, what do we have then? We have insight into the way in which the divine world has come into existence, the world has been created, out of all kinds of different spiritual activities and entities. And that is the first step in the physician's work, to say to oneself that disease processes take one to insight into essential human nature. They are genuine insight processes. The healing processes can only be grasped, however, in a religious mood. Everything a physician does must be filled with a religious attitude to the world. Without this, insight will never be ours in the individual case.

Of course, you can always say to yourselves: Well, here we have the medicines, and anthroposophy comes along to tell us which to use, but one can't really understand the whole of it. You can understand it if you consider things like those I have just been characterizing, if you can penetrate a genuine process of gaining insight for diagnosis and a genuine process for treatment. These things must be taken very seriously. This must be our attitude if we want to understand everything said from the anthroposophical point of view in medicine. For application in practice we have to go into detail. But it is necessary to let this attitude prevail in everything one does in medicine.

I'd now like you to ask further questions so that we may move on and consider actual situations tomorrow. It has been my intention merely to bring in the qualitative aspect.

First question. As a physician one is sometimes forced today to use medicines which one does not like to use, and some of those medicines are surely such that they should not be used. Would it not be possible to say something about medicines which we should not be using?

[Rudolf Steiner.] I'd like to say the following in response to this question, wholly in principle. There is a great difference between saying 'I see how this medicine works in the human organism' and 'I do not understand it'. Initially the difference is of course relative when it comes to practice, so long as we do not have medical faculties where one has courses of the kind it is possible to teach in anthroposophy. Until then it will happen again and again that practitioners make notes also of recommendations made on the basis of anthroposophy: This is a medicine for this or that. We who are here would, of course, like nothing better than to start presenting insight into essential human nature, so that looking at an onion we know how the onion process acts in the human organism, the antecedents being such and such. We'd certainly like this better than anything. But initially it is relative, and for the time being it is only possible to speak of a medicine for this or that. We are, however, most unlikely to speak of a medicine where we do not know how its action continues on within essential human nature. It will not be said, for instance, that silica from Equisetum should be taken unless we know exactly that it evokes a kidney process. The hyper-excitability of an irritable kidney is reduced by it. Hyper-excitability of the kidney is thus reduced if you provide the kidney with silica from Equisetum. That is understood, therefore, and one would need to know [text missing].

But let me ask you, confidentially: How are investigations done out there? They are done very superficially, using statistics; they are done by giving the medicament to so and so many patients. People do not really know what is going on, and above all the big difference between a genuine medicinal agent and one of this kind is that one fully understands the process and knows how it influences the whole of human life. If you successfully treat something with some medicament or other today, you will not know what this will lead to in five years' time. But if you fully understand the process, you will above all need no statistics.

Statistics never come into it with our medicines. The book which is due to appear soon will tell you that it does not depend on statistics if a medicament proves effective or not but on study of the individual case. If you have a box of matches and test the matches you'll not light all the matches, knowing that once you have lit one of them they can all be lit. You also know that every process has to go the way you know it does. So it is not a matter of statistics but of fully understanding the individual case. Because of this we'll always have great problems when people say: Hand over your medicines for testing. This will not get us anywhere, it will not create confidence in our medicines. Yes, statistics will give extraordinarily good results with our medicines, but the usual cases either have not been diagnosed correctly or they are cases where other things are needed as well. In my opinion, the real point with medicines that heal is to understand, above all truly to understand, how things go.

You see, strangely enough even to test things leads to all kinds of interesting things. There are all kinds of medicines for syphilis today. And arsenic is always involved. Why? We say that arsenic is something which stimulates the astral body when it is not greatly inclined to intervene in the physical body, so that it will intervene more. This astral body is stirred to action by giving a person arsenic. The medicines investigated in tests are really based on this. Now you can also see how people are deceived, how illusions come in. You rely on the intense action of arsenic in cases where the astral body truly can gain such strength with arsenic. And only arsenic will really cure syphilis. We really must always fully understand how such medicines act. It should be our aim always to do so. Our way of thinking must become more and more widely known and our aim in producing the book is indeed to introduce the way of thinking we seek to cultivate here, and not so much to suggest medicines. It will also be important to refer to this way of thinking when it comes to medicines that are not suggested by us. There are good medicines also outside our sphere, and one will give the one or other as need arises.

Second question. We talked about asthma here the last time. You said that one should meditate on breathing. Are we entitled to give a meditation in such cases? I could not think of anything else. I found a verse by Goethe:

> *In every breath lies twofold benison—*
> *Drawing air in, letting it go again,*
> *Oppression first, and then refreshment comes;*
> *Life wondrously combines the two.*
> *Give thanks to God when he oppresses*
> *And thanks again when he releases you.*[59]

I was not sure if that was the right thing.

[Rudolf Steiner.] You see, with things like that it does have to be accepted that because they are halfway, if you like, or three-quarters psychological, your response must also have soul quality if your attitude is such as I have spoken of today. The way human beings are in the earthly world and through their head in the cosmic world—when physicians have learned to think and feel spiritually, and also approach their patients in that way, then it is reasonable to do so. But if you approach patients with the attitude which is so common with the materialistic view today, not really caring about them at all, you will generally achieve the opposite of what you really want to achieve. You see, many people turn up again and again today—and physicians also do not completely exclude it—who work with things of this kind. They will sometimes ameliorate conditions but not cure them. If the patient is made strong by it, the amelioration may actually lead to a cure. But when people ask if you can really achieve this, I have to say that it will be possible if you truly love the patient. But it will not help if you are indifferent to the patient.

We should really have the courage to heal. This is why I have always referred to the courage to heal at our institute here, where that is the case. The worst thing you can do if you want to heal is to think of death when you have a patient before you, however sick he may be. As a physician one should really forbid oneself to think of a patient's death as any kind of possibility. The imponderables are indeed most powerful. You have the power to strengthen someone enormously if, come what may, you put aside the thought of death—to the very last moment!—and think only of what you may do to save whatever can be saved of the power of life. Many more people are saved when this attitude is developed than when the other attitude develops where the prognosis based on one thing or another somehow is death. This is something you should never do. And things like this must indeed be properly taken into account. You are then justified in having the will to heal.

Question. Working as an assistant at a hospital where you have to prescribe morphine and other drugs—is there anything else that can perhaps stop the action, exactly because of one's attitude to the patient?

[Rudolf Steiner.] You can achieve much just by your attitude. But if intervention is necessary, using physical substances, these should as far as possible be taken from the plant world and not be derivatives, depending on what you feel is needed, using the actual poppy juice, for instance. And this not in thinking of the inner processes; quite the contrary, but turning to the outer form of the plant, that which delights us in it. It is difficult to give rules for such things, for even if you are forced to give the medicament, your attitude plays a great role—if you capture what shows itself in the patient. You need to take note of the mood which shows itself in the patient with the medicament, and then you can intervene. The medicine has made the patient more transparent with regard to the help needed. We'll continue tomorrow, and I'd ask you to put all the questions that cause you concern.

DISCUSSIONS WITH MEDICAL PRACTITIONERS (FRAGMENTARY NOTES) I

DORNACH, 22 APRIL 1924[60]

A member of the group asks about the significance of the latex in spurge and dandelion for treating leukaemia. This had come to him during a meditation.

It is, of course, also a matter of giving some consideration to the secondary phenomena, for leukaemia can have all kinds of causes. If there is definite awareness that one is dealing with a disorder somehow in the rhythmic human being, then you'll be right; you'll get results. It's like this: whenever you use products of the plant world that still have remnants of the ether body in them—and that is the case with resinous, with these latex-type juices both of dandelion and spurge; it is also the case with wax, plant wax for instance—with all these substances you get a powerful action in the human rhythmic system. If on the other hand the primary cause is something which does not have its basis in the human rhythmic system but in metabolism—these things merge one into the other, but one has to make the essential distinction—you are unlikely to get results. Everything that still has the ether body in it acts most powerfully on the inner mobility of the astral body, stimulating all activity in the organism from the astral body. And one can get results this way. It is due to the fact that the astral body is greatly influenced by these substances and by acting on the ether body establishes a balance in the ether body.

What are the conditions in which a smallpox epidemic develops? It seems that the disease has lost its malignancy. I have observed such cases.

What view is taken of vaccination in spiritual science?

With a condition such as smallpox, the situation for the individual person is that the I organization withdraws to a great degree from all three other human bodies, from physical, ether and astral body. This powerful withdrawal, this weakening of the I organization, may be due to the fact that the individual slips very much into the Is of earlier lives on earth with his present I; because of this the I organization shows marked affinity to the spiritual world altogether. With smallpox, it is worth noting that there is some similarity with the things a person goes through with certain forms of initiation. Strange though it may seem, that is how it is.

When someone gets to know the actions of the figures in the zodiac on human beings, really gets to know them inwardly, such states of insight involve powerful inner shocks. This the individual can at least go through in that it acts in a more controlled way, this situation with smallpox, more at the soul level, because human beings live very powerfully in the spiritual sphere with smallpox, though in a different way.

We may say that with smallpox the danger of infection is extraordinarily great. We should not carelessly plump straight for physical means of transmitting the disease, however. With smallpox the mental disposition plays a particularly great role. One proof of this would be that one is able to protect oneself extremely well if one is able to contain oneself in the right way. I am entitled to say this because at the age of 22—I need not go into the circumstances—I tutored a youngster whose mother, suffering from Variola major, was right next to us, with only a screen between her and the room where I was teaching. I did not do anything about it, continuing my teaching until the mother was well again. But I was quite pleased to do it, so that I might see how one can protect oneself if one absolutely treats the sick person objectively, like any object, a stone or a shrub, with no feelings of fear or other emotions, but treats them as an objective fact. With this you counter the risk of infection to a high degree. The mental factor can thus play a considerable role also when it comes to catching things.

I have actually never shied away from exposing myself to any danger of infection and have really never caught anything, have never got myself infected. This did show that mere awareness, powerful awareness of the existence of a disease, can bring about the disease through the astral body. Powerful awareness of a disease can be the cause of that disease arising from the astral body.

And smallpox vaccination? There we find ourselves in a peculiar position. You see, when you vaccinate someone and you are an anthroposophist, bringing him up in the anthroposophical way, it will do no harm. It will harm only those who grow up with mainly materialistic ideas. Then vaccination becomes a kind of ahrimanic power; the individual can no longer rise above a certain materialistic way of feeling. And that is really why vaccination causes us concern, because people are 'garbed through' with a phantom. The individual has a phantom which prevents him from freeing the psychic entities as far from the physical organism as in a normal state of consciousness. He grows constitutionally materialistic, is no longer able to rise to the spiritual sphere. This is what causes concern with vaccination. Statistics will of course be quoted, and we must ask ourselves if we really must rate statistics so highly exactly in this respect. Smallpox vaccination has very much to do with the psyche. It is certainly possible that belief that the vaccination is effective plays an incalculably great role in this. If we were to replace this belief with something else, if we were to educate people in a way that is in accord with nature, so that they would be impressed by something other than that we are vaccinating them, let us say by taking them closer to the spirit again, then it would certainly be possible for us to be as effective against the unconscious imposition of 'there's a smallpox epidemic here' with fully conscious awareness that 'there's a spiritual element here, unjustifiable, yes, but I must stand up to it' which is just as effective, and we must altogether make the person strong in the face of such influences.

How should one handle this under the kind of difficult conditions in our area, with education and so on having such a negative influence?

Then you simply have to vaccinate. There's no other choice. I would be absolutely against opposing these things in a fanatical way, not for medical but for generally anthroposophical reasons. Fanatical opposition to these things is not something we aim for, wanting instead to provide insight so that things might change on the greater scale. I have always seen this as something I had to combat when with medical friends such as Dr Asch,[61] for instance, who absolutely did not vaccinate. I would always fight against this. For if he does not vaccinate, someone else will. It is utterly absurd to be fanatical in particular situations.

Dr Kolisko. As a school doctor I have to say that children starting school show a colossal inner restlessness, evident particularly in their sleep. The parents of these children, who are in their 6th or 7th year, complain that the children are plagued with nightmares and motor unrest at night, and have difficulties in going to sleep. What would this be due to?

The states in which the children are when they now start school—in Germany, that is—are due not to conditions in general but to conditions relating to diet. These conditions, persisting for years now, seriously upset the powers of taking nourishment, an inner ability—not what happens initially in the stomach, but the inner ability to take the chyme further there where it matters, out of the intestine. The situation is that these children are really unable to get their astral body to interact in the right way with the ether body. Because of this they are not able, as a rule, truly to take the food they eat, even if provided by charities, into their organism. As you know, every food has its own inherent laws and must become inorganic at a particular stage in the digestive process. It is not known in external science that the protein we eat, vegetable or animal protein, is taken into the mineral state and then changed back into human protein. The whole process takes place in the nascent state, but it does take place. This conversion must happen, otherwise the process is not human but foreign. We may say, therefore, that within the human skin, roughly speaking, there must not be anything, except for direct salts, which occurs outside the human organism. Nothing within the human skin is external, except for salt. Everything else is metamorphosed. These children lose the ability to fully and properly organize their ether body via the astral body at the very time when this ether body comes free. It comes free at the time when they enter primary school. This is the cause of their digestive disorder. They have processes belonging outside the human being inside them, and things like this must be quite rationally combated physically. We have the medicament we produced at the time when we had some particularly serious instances of such children. I think you'll always get excellent results in this direction. You'll remember the small, pale boy in class 2? How is he?

He's a lot better.

He is pretty good now, relatively speaking.

We have also used it for many other children.

That was the next occasion which arose. A pale boy, already given up by the medical profession, he was said to be close to death. We gave him the medicament, calcium carbonate and phosphate. It turned out that this takes digestion forward in a quite outstanding way; internal conditions improve with it. Dyspnoea and breathing difficulties will always appear if the astral body is not able to work properly. Dyspnoea develops when it is held back, and may also be the cause of hidden anxiety states. All this can improve with the medicament. It is of a kind where we can say that it is an extraordinarily good medicine when someone is no longer able to benefit from his food, though he is eating it.

What do you do for a spinal (paralysis)?

What are the symptoms?

Only sensitivity to pressure over the affected vertebra. X-rays show that it may have fused slightly on one side, and the vertebra now is this {shown or drawn, Plate 8, left}[62] rather than its normal shape.

It is of course difficult to get to the heart of things when the condition is so highly localized, unless we go back to the primary cause. Which vertebra is it?

The sixth thoracic vertebra.

Has there been any demonstrable mechanical insult?

No, but the condition derives from pulmonary tuberculosis.

But changes in the hilar lymph nodes.

The X-ray shows largish shadows in this site which enter into lung tissue in a scattered way.

How old is the patient?

35 years.

Has the problem persisted for a long time?

For about three months. I have four such patients, all of them women. Two had a trauma by falling down the stairs onto their back. For the other two the X-ray might lead one to conclude that the problem comes from the lung.

Is there no evidence of other vertebrae being affected?

Not a single one. In one case it is the tenth, in others the sixth. These are adults, about 36 to 39 years of age. In the case of a child, the origin is traumatic, and it is also traumatic for a young woman of 20.

In such a case one will have to try and see if the lung—the cause does not lie there, of course—somehow does not have enough room at some point or other, perhaps because it has expanded. And you will indeed find something or other in this case that concerns the unfolding of the lung. And it will then be highly probable that you find expansion in some part of the lung, widening out, reciprocal to this shrinkage—it is a shrinkage process. It may perhaps not be in the region of the lung; it could even be in the bone or one of the ribs. You'll have to look for it. It will then be a matter of using something which can even out the formation of the human body. We do have one substance which is absolutely perfect in making up for trauma. This is tobacco. Injected in dilute form it proves to be the principle which corrects deformation. If you want the medicament to be freely active in the organism you'll need phosphorus. In this way you can be sure of achieving healing processes. It may be said absolutely that healing processes will be achieved if the individual concerned is less than 28 years of age. But it is not impossible that they will also be achieved at a later age, especially with women. And if you get very stubborn situations, with marked resistance, you would need to get the people concerned artificially brightened up, lightening their powers of growth, their vital energies a bit and so helping the medicine to act. This, I think, is what one might do in such a case.

Going back to what was said about syphilis I'd like to ask how one can relieve a patient who has been given mercury and Salvarsan of the damage done by those drugs.

Extraordinarily much of the damage caused by mercury can be removed. Give the patient a very hot bath daily or every second day, letting him sweat it out completely, thoroughly, in the steam. This stimulates the organism to an extraordinary degree to defend itself against the mercury. It is necessary to fight the mercury even in the bones when one has been treated with it. I expect you'll all have heard that tiny droplets of mercury are demonstrable even in the bones when someone has been treated with mercury. You'll realize that the effect is adequate because the bathwater will turn black with the mercury that is released. Did you not notice this? You can't fail to notice! For one can't understand why the bathwater is getting so dark. If that does not happen, one would have to have an arsenic bath, adding about 5% of water containing arsenic to the bath; again let the patient take a hot bath and above all see to it that the peculiar smell of ink is actually smelt by the patient, giving him a sensory impression. [Text missing.]

You will need a follow-up treatment in such a case. The mercury may have been almost completely removed; but the destructive tendency it brought with it will remain in the organism. You have to consider that mercury has an extraordinarily powerful action on the human organism. You have to consider: What is mercury to the human organism? If you study embryonic development you'll have an ascending embryonic development, that is, rising from the ovum to the developing human being, and you have a descending development, something which drops away, is destroyed in stages. The regulator of this destructive process is the human being's mercurial inner nature. If it were to happen that there are too many vital energies, you can throttle them back with mercury, which constitutionally works to destroy the human being. This destructive tendency must be combated in the psyche. If you can induce someone to study a wholly abstract science, regularly so, for instance half an hour's geometry dutifully every day, this would be the follow-up treatment. Clear thoughts, logically combining and separating, challenging the mind and helping to develop inner activity rather than giving oneself up passively to the world. This lively inner activity really needs to be applied for a long period. You will then be able to cure someone of the mercury powers.

Women sometimes have nodular indurations in the mammary gland. Would it be safe to use Viscum prophylactically in that case, even if the diagnosis of cancer is in doubt?

Did you find that prophylaxis caused any kind of damage in such a case?

You once said that with this medicament, which may be suitable in a case of illness, there is also the danger of provoking something in the wrong case.

We use Viscum injections in quite a specific way. Let us assume the wrong diagnosis has been made. This can happen. Of course you won't use prophylaxis when a diagnosis of cancer in its early stages has been made. As soon as the tendency is there, prophylaxis can no longer do harm. But let us assume there has been an error. We give seven injections in succession; then there's a pause. If there really had been an error, we would immediately see this, because a kind of carcinomatous inclination will have developed that would disappear as soon as we give the second sequence of seven injections. We would then go no further. Any inclination which developed would regress again when a process of a similar nature is applied. If you are careful, there is absolutely no way in which you might cause any harm with Viscum treatment.

Dr Koeller. I talked with a lay practitioner about the treatment of cancer. I told him that I believed Viscum to be a medicine for it. He replied that this was indeed the case but one would have to add something else, wild thyme. Without this it would not be possible to get to the problem with Viscum. Wild or shepherd's thyme provided the opportunity to do so.

Did the man know this from personal experience?

Dr Koeller. I got to know him because he had achieved a remarkable cure. A girl who was almost blind came to see him. He does iris diagnosis. It is not clear how he does this. He has 750 kinds of tea. It is really difficult to talk with these people. One characteristic is that they are enormously optimistic. He said one can cure everything, including cancer. He did not ask how we do it but said 'with mistletoe'. He told me he had once walked in the country with some friends and come across a cherry tree with mistletoe. The tree was stunted, cancerous. And the man said to himself that mistletoe had great healing powers.

Viscum certainly is the specific for carcinoma. Nothing one can do about it. But of course, since every illness turns into something different because every organism is in a particular condition, the medicinal agents are in given cases helped by adding something else. It is possible that he got a cure with mistletoe. He did not give it by injection, and so he probably needed to add something. But given by injection Viscum is the specific agent. You have to consider the differences, however, as to whether the mistletoe comes from an oak, a cherry tree or some other tree, perhaps an apple tree. The important thing is, of course, also that the use of mistletoe extract truly depends on actually enhancing the medicinal action. I do not know if you've seen that we are not seeking to use Viscum in such a simple way but need an apparatus for it. We first set the extracts in motion vertically, and then have a horizontal rotation enter into this [Plate 8, centre]. What we must achieve is that the mistletoe extract comes in drops and as it drops meets the rotation and in the horizontal rotation combines again with mistletoe extract, so that a special structure is produced even in the smallest cycles. The actual healing principle for the mistletoe arises in this process. Yes, it is an effective medicament in itself; but it only becomes the absolutely specific medicament in this complicated process.

It can only be a matter of a complicated case of the disease calling for the addition of wild thyme. For a pure carcinoma, which is complete in itself, is not like influenza, for example, where there are all kinds of other things as well. It is a condition complete in itself, and a medicament which is complete in itself will deal with it.

It is interesting to note that someone discovers this simply because the things he told you and the things you said are but a mask—not a mask he knew of, for knowledge can only be gained in sleep by such individuals. 'It came to him in his sleep', as the saying goes. He went to sleep in the expectation of finding a mistletoe. He would then recall this unconscious prophetic experience just as he came to mistletoe. A conversation came later that was quite irrelevant to the business. We have to understand that a degree of foreknowledge is possible especially in a case of sickness. Let me remind you of the case given by Schleich where the individual concerned knew that he would die the next night.[63]

Dr Koeller. Basically it became clear that he also heals people by another method. He said it had given him no peace; he did not think that I would get any further.

He does not give injections. You cannot touch cancer if you give mistletoe by mouth. This will rather touch the psyche. But you do come upon a malformation in the etheric body that is reflected in damage to the sensory functions. You cannot cure internally by giving mistletoe by mouth, only by injection. I understand what he is telling you; he does not dare tackle it.

Is the cause of cancer the same for women and men? Is the cause different in the upper and the lower human being? I think I noted that the medicament gave satisfaction with cancer of the stomach but not with cancer of the uterus. Success was evident with cancer of the stomach in men. With cancer of the uterus the business drags on. In some cases we cannot get at it, we have always injected in the periphery, also with cancer of the uterus.

The situation is, of course, that we do have to make a distinction if we give the injection further away from the tumour site or get very close to it. If you get very close to the focus you will get a more rapid result than when the cancer is in a location where you cannot get close.

You can get much closer if it is cancer of the uterus. With cancer of the stomach you are much further away.

Yes, that's right. But on the other hand communication between surface and stomach is much greater than between surface and uterus. The uterus is more of an internal organ. The difference in results is, however, not due to any difference between men and women. There must be other circumstances. We have to exclude all sources of error. It is definitely the case that some of our medicines have got a reputation of being less effective; the way in which they were formerly produced made them less stable. I think this is no longer the case now; they will no longer be less effective when they have grown old.

With some of the medicines we are still at the experimental stage.

It has rather become evident to me that the cancer medicine, the way is has so far been manufactured, loses a great deal when it is a year old, but is absolutely effective if it is not so old. This matter would also have to be excluded, taken up and excluded as a source of error. Perhaps one also needs to use a considerably larger dose with cancer of the uterus.

A member of the audience wanted ask a question concerning a young woman who is now 29 and went insane when 18 or 19. As a child she'd always been recalcitrant and disobedient; now she had grown quite dull. She would be wild particularly during her periods. In the time when she grew duller and duller she also grew bigger and bigger; she now weighs 97 kg. So she was a naughty child, as we might call it, and then between the ages of 18 and 19 her waywardness, dullness and nonsense grew very much worse, not reacting, raving during her periods, so that she had to be put in a straitjacket; then she grew duller and duller, less and less lively, bigger and bigger, her periods being regular. She was treated with thyroid extract with the result that the dullness and weight gain grew less.

These symptoms all indicate that her I organization was greatly weakened. And it is highly probable that in such a case the I organization is strengthened by giving a course of silica, a course of silicon. One should advise to make it a double treatment—silica by mouth and above all silica baths. Also Equisetum, which is a good thing. It is probable that this will achieve something with her.

She was given silica for a time, no baths, two years ago; but there was no change.

I would consider silica action by baths of value, above all because it would be specific in its action if brought into play. The peculiar rhythmic states that arise with silica would restrain the weight gain and they would also combat the dullness, making her easier to deal with. It is also possible that she may be in a state where she does not take up silica. In that case one would have to try a phosphate in very high potency, potassium phosphate. One would need to get the things active again.

In response to a further question:

The silica in about the 6th decimal. But use actual quartz by mouth, Equisetum for the bath.

Question concerning a neurasthenic patient. The problem went away very well with formic acid injections, but recurred this year and would not go away again with formic acid injections. I finally lost my way and removed an ingrown toenail. Things got even worse after this. I tried formic acid once again, enhanced with silicon. But I did not succeed. The pain grew intolerable, from the foot up into the calf. The type of pain varied, rhythmic on one occasion. I had to give morphine injections, increasing the dose greatly; I would hardly touch him, to keep the pain at a tolerable level. He was no longer able to sleep. He sat there, holding his foot, complaining of horrendous pain; I tried alternating foot baths. The foot had to be amputated at mid-calf height. I am asking because the process is unfortunately about to develop on the other leg now. What can one do?

With something like this we must look for the primary cause.

He says it happened when he was in the army and usually did not have decent shoes. He is 47 now and often had to lie on wet ground.

But in that case the pain surely did first appear not in the leg but perhaps in the abdomen? It is perfectly possible that the whole situation is due to a deformation at some point in the intestine, that he got hit by shrapnel, fell of his horse, bumped into something, and that the deformation in the intestine comes from this. This intestinal deformation characteristically migrates downwards and provokes conditions like those you have described in the legs, first in one but then also shifting to the other. This will usually end in tuberculosis of the bone. But we can do something in that situation with the agent which acts against deformation—tobacco (in a case like this with tobacco enemas).[64]

He does smoke quite a lot.

That has nothing to do with it. Tobacco smoke does not make an impression on the organism similar to the one you get if you give tobacco by injection or enema. It is an altogether different action on the organism. With smoking the tobacco does not have opportunity to exert its re-deforming action.

A boy, now 11 years old, learned to walk at one year, was also able to talk a little. When two years old he was rather close to an exercise shooting with cannon. They say he's been deaf and dumb from that time. His speech is an incomprehensible babble, and he hears absolutely nothing at all. Is it still possible to do something for him? He can walk, and actually looks very intelligent.

Otherwise there are no problems, except for being unable to hear and talk? How is it if some impression or other is made on the eye?

In that case, he reacts like any normal person; only the ear and his talking are subject to change.

What about his second dentition?

Quite normal, at seven and a half years.

So one would have to assume that the vitality of the auditory nerve was destroyed in some way. We do at least have quite considerable successes with edelweiss, especially in the 10th decimal, or first in the 6th, then in the 10th, to re-enliven the auditory nerve. Failures have also been known, but essentially these were observed with relatively old people, not really with younger people. I do think that you may try this. It is indeed extraordinarily difficult to do something about these devitalized nerves; but with edelweiss one may certainly get results on occasion.

A woman suffered some kind of shock during the war. She thought her fiancé was dead. She was alone at home and had no one to whom she could talk about it. Since then she's been epileptic. The seizures always come just before she has her period. They involve biting her tongue and so on, quite typical. It is over as soon as her period starts. She is in an institution for epileptics, although her seizures come only before her periods.

What treatment does she have?

{Answer missing}

You start with Belladonna in such a case. If it does not help, move on to reindeer moss or lichen in the 6th decimal, and finally inoculate fly agaric. It is most difficult to say anything definite particularly in such a case, unless one sees the patient. There may be all kinds of causes.

A 50-year-old man had a hard time in earlier years. He suffered from rheumatoid arthritis for 11 years, and one of his brothers died of it. Now a change is still evident in the left knee. Until two years ago he would have states where the blood rose to his head. A definite change came two years ago. He has put on weight, and then this rush of blood to the head disappeared. Instead something he would refer to in short as asthma developed. He has breathing problems, has to gasp for air when talking. It is my impression that the business is now located in the bronchi.

At age 48. Before the rush was to the head, now it is to the chest. Is it the case that the man changes colour a bit now and then, only slightly so, turning a bit blue, perhaps?

It's possible.

It is highly probable that the man has been too much in a position to change the oxygen he took in into carbon dioxide and therefore would always have too much carbon dioxide in his blood. You can check if he does not feel relieved if given air containing more oxygen. If that proves to be the case, the situation will be quite clear. The man is producing too much carbon dioxide, and we need to give him—what does he do?—

—An engineer—

silicon in the first decimal, i.e. 5%, and ask him to make some mental effort for about half an hour after taking the silicon. He may then improve. He will put a brake on his overweening capacity for producing carbon dioxide.

We have to come to a conclusion now. More of the same kind tomorrow.

I do not find it helpful to have this way of asking questions. The individual gains much, but the others do not. The questions should be more general, something more interesting. So we should do things a bit differently tomorrow. Would you not agree, Dr Steiner?

I am prepared to consider any question put to me. Every question could be answered by giving a whole lecture. When the first person put a question I could have gone on to discuss the matter until now, but in that case only one person would have had a turn. I think it was quite a good thing to hear a variety of things. It is not, after all, a matter of our satisfaction, but of the audience's.

I think that this is something like having a clinic at the university, because the way of asking questions does not allow the other question to come about, as to how we can develop powers of understanding.

It would come about if a question to this effect were to be put. Tomorrow then let us have a question to this effect right away, and then it can be that way. I do not think that it is entirely useless to consider this question. But other answers do also arise. We merely put such a value on them that the audience may be satisfied.

Would you say something about deepening the diagnosis? We can have many different thoughts about one patient. Many questions then arise, and one often has the problem of deciding what is to be done. It cannot be done intellectually; the will must be there to make a decision. My question is: Would it not be possible to hold this intellectual will impulse back at that moment, so that it may come to one what needs to be done? Would you be able to say something about this?

You mean how the diagnosis may be made more transparent?

There are a number of possibilities when it comes to treatment. You can't decide if you should use vegetable or mineral medicines; you have to come to a decision. It should be possible to approach the patient on a deeper basis and let all these ideas come together, so that you will then know: That is the right thing.

We will make something up tomorrow and then develop an idea for diagnosis.

DISCUSSIONS WITH MEDICAL PRACTITIONERS (FRAGMENTARY NOTES) II

DORNACH, 23 APRIL 1924

In connection with the question put by Dr Husemann yesterday we have decided to read out two case records from the book which thanks to Dr Wegman[65] is due to appear shortly. This may be followed by things you would wish to know, in the spirit of your question.

I would ask you, of course, to be very discreet about these cases for the time being, as they will be integral parts of the book due to appear shortly.

The cases are meant to show how you arrive at treatment specifically from the diagnosis. This is to be demonstrated, doing so on the basis of anthroposophy. We will not shy away from speaking in wholly anthroposophical terms in this book.

Dr Wegman read out Case 4 on pages 95 ff. of Extending Practical Medicine: *'A child who had been brought to the Clinic twice, first at age 4, then at 5½. Also the child's mother and the mother's sister.'*

It is important that the mother and sister were there. You'll see why in a minute.

'The process of diagnosis led from the child's illness to the mother's and also that of her sister. With the child, we found the following. It was a twin, born six weeks prematurely. The other child had died in the final embryonic stage. At the age of six weeks the child fell ill, crying a great deal, and was taken to hospital. Pylorospasm was diagnosed. The child was fed partly by a wet nurse, partly

artificially. It was discharged from hospital at eight months. Arrived at home it had a seizure the first day, and this recurred daily for the first two months. The child would stiffen in an attack, turning up its eyes. Attacks were preceded by timidity and crying. The child also had a squint in the right eye and would vomit before an attack. At age 2½ another attack occurred, lasting five hours. The child went stiff again and lay there as if dead. At age 4 it had an attack lasting 30 minutes. This was the first attack reported to be accompanied by pyrexia. The parents noted that the convulsions that happened after the child came back from hospital were followed by paralysis of the right arm and leg. The child made its first attempts at walking at age 2½. It was only able to step out with the left leg, dragging the right leg after it. The right arm also remained without will impulses. The condition still persisted when the child was brought to see us. What we had to do was establish the situation with regard to the aspects of the child's organization. This was done independent of the syndrome. We found the ether body to be greatly atrophied, in some parts only accepting a very low level of astral body influence.'

Those essentially were the findings. The ether body was atrophied in many different locations and did not accept the influence of the astral body in those places. You got such lacunae in the ether body [Plate 9]. The astral body did not enter the sites where the ether body was atrophied. This was the case in a number of sites in the organism.

'The region of the right chest was as if paralysed in the ether body. On the other hand we noted something like a hypertrophy of the astral body in the stomach region.'

One has to use unusual terminology. Just as the term 'hypertrophy' is used for areas that are too active, too lively.

'Then the syndrome had to be considered in relation to this. The astral body was clearly putting a considerable strain on the stomach in the digestive process, which, however, was static at the transition from intestine to lymph vessels because of paralysis of the ether body. This resulted in malnutrition of the blood. The symptoms of nausea and retching thus had to be taken very seriously. Seizures always result if the etheric body grows atrophic and the astral body comes to have a direct influence on the physical body, without mediation from the ether body.'

This is important on principle. The seizures developed because astral body, ether body and physical body were no longer in their regular relationship. The way you have to think of this is of the astral body only acting on the physical body with the help of the ether body. When there are such areas of atrophy the astral body influences the physical body, leaving the ether body aside. Spasms will occur wherever this is the case. We know that in a site where spasms develop the ether body is not mediating properly between astral body and physical body.

'This applied very much in the case of this child. If the condition becomes permanent during the growth period, which was the case here, processes that make the motor system ready to receive the will in the normal way do not occur. This took the form of the child not being able to use the right side. We then had to connect the child's condition with that of the mother. She was 37 years of age when she came to us. She stated that she had been as tall as she was now at age 13. Her teeth were bad at an early age.'

Please take special note of this. She did not grow any further from her thirteenth year until now, meaning that growth was complete by the time she reached sexual maturity.

'Her teeth were bad at an early age, she had rheumatic fever as a child and maintained that she had had rickets. Menarche was relatively early. The patient said she had had a kidney disease at age 16, and also referred to some kind of seizures she had had. At age 15 she had chronic constipation because of spasms in the anal sphincter, which had to be stretched. She still had spasms with every stool. Diagnosis of her condition, based on direct observation, with no conclusions drawn from her syndrome, showed remarkable similarity with that of the child. Only everything was much milder in form. It had to be considered that the human ether body develops especially between the changing of the teeth and puberty. In the patient this was evident from the fact that the available forces of the ether body, which were not very strong, made growth possible only until she reached puberty. This is the point where the special development of the astral body began which, being hypertrophic, overwhelmed the ether body and intervened too strongly in the physical organization.'

Both were of the same type. Mother and child showed excessive intervention of the astral body in the physical body.

'This came to expression in cessation of growth at age 13. The patient was anything but dwarf size, however, and in fact very tall, which was due to the fact that the ether body's growth forces, uninhibited by the astral body, caused a tremendous increase in the volume of her physical body. These forces were not yet able at the time to intervene in the functions of the physical body in a regular *way. This was evident in the development of rheumatic fever and later on of seizures.'*

The rheumatic fever as such was also connected with the fact that the astral body intervenes directly in the physical body at the joints. This also leads to inflammatory changes where such are possible. So one has either seizures or inflammatory conditions.

'Because of weakness of the ether body, the action of the astral body on the physical body was particularly powerful. This was a destructive effect. In a normally developing life it is balanced out by constructive forces during sleep, when the astral body has separated from the physical and ether body. If the ether body is too weak, as in the case of our patient, excessive destruction occurs, and in her case this could be seen from the fact that she needed her first filling in her teeth in her twelfth year.'

There is too much destruction due to excessive intervention from the astral body. Physical body and ether body build up; astral body and I organization deteriorate. If there is excessive destructive activity this is evident in a phenomenon such as having to have fillings at age 12. Her teeth got worse with every pregnancy.

'If the ether body has extra demands made on it, as in pregnancy, this will always cause dental deterioration. The weakness of the ether body as far as its connection with the astral body was concerned was also particularly evident in the frequency of dreams and in the fact that the patient slept soundly, despite all the irregularities.'

If the relationship between astral body, ether body and physical body is completely regular, there will be no excess of dreams. The moment the astral body is able to be overweening because the ether body has weakened, dreams will be frequent and lively. Also, the astral body, being strong, can easily go out and sleep nevertheless remains sound.

'The weakness of the ether body was also apparent from the fact that foreign processes not controlled by the ether body occurred in the physical body, presenting as proteins, occasional hyaline casts and salts in her urine.'

These products of degradation develop due to astral body hypertrophy. One must always look for them when it is a case of astral body hypertrophy.

'It is interesting to note the way these pathological processes relate to those of the mother's sister. The diagnosis concerning the composition of the aspects of the

human being is almost entirely the same. Weak ether body activity, therefore dominance of the astral body. Only in her case the astral body itself is weaker than her sister's. Menarche was therefore early, too, but instead of inflammation she merely had pain due to irritation of the organs, e.g. the joints.'

That is really most interesting. You have almost the same morbid constitution in mother and child. The sister, parallel to this, only gets as far as milder symptoms; everything is to a lesser degree with her, in miniature we might say, in hints.

'The ether body has to be especially active in the joints if vitality is to go normally. If ether body activity is weak the activity of the physical body becomes dominant, which showed in swellings and chronic arthritis in this case. The weakness of the astral body, which is not acting sufficiently on subjective feelings, is evident from a preference for sweet foods, which increase sensation for the astral body.'

That is most interesting. If you want to cope with these things you do actually have to ask what the individual concerned likes to eat—sweet or bitter things, preference for sensory impressions of one kind or another. Some have a peculiar weakness when it comes to smells. It all shows that the astral body must get involved in some way. This preference shown by the astral body indicates that it is not involved; it gets involved as soon as it is given sweets.

'If in addition daily life has worn out a weak astral body, the pain will be more significant if the weakness persists. The patient complained of pain getting worse in the evenings. The connection between the disease states of the three patients pointed to the generation ascendant to the two sisters, and especially the child's grandmother. The cause must lie with her. The upset balance between astral and ether body in all three patients can only have arisen from an equal imbalance in the child's grandmother. This irregularity must go back to the grandmother's astral and ether body not achieving adequate nutrition of the foetal membranes which feed the embryo, especially the allantois.'

This case is particularly interesting because one discovers that the cause truly lies in inadequate development of the grandmother's allantois. The whole condition of the astral body, which of course presents vehemently in one of them, the mother, and less in the other, takes us back to the grandmother. It is not bound up with one part but goes constitutionally through the whole astral body and can only go back to that peculiar development, to the allantois, to the embryonic period.

This is an occult finding that must be taken in. But once one has found it, the individual phenomena are perfectly in line for verification. You must definitely get in the habit of verifying causes from causes. The composition of symptoms really only gives one an unclear picture.

'The inadequate development of the allantois has to be looked for in all three patients. The physical allantois is metamorphosed, becoming non-physical, into the capability of the astral body's forces.'

This comes in as well (we were only able to suggest it as a principle) in the physical allantois, which also can only be embryonic; all the organs which are abandoned in the embryo exist as the higher aspects of the human being once born. Physical as an accessory organ, it is spiritual in the adult state, so that we only have to see the physical correlate of the embryonic period in the allantois.

'A degenerated allantois results in reduced capability of the astral body, which shows itself especially in all motor organs. All this held true for all three patients. It is indeed possible to perceive the quality of the allantois by considering that of the astral body.'

The point is that we have to know: The amnion is the physical correlate of the adult person's ether body, the allantois that of the astral body, the chorion of the I organization.

'It will be evident from this that our reference to the ascendance does not derive from hazardous conclusions based on fantasy but from genuine observations using the methods developed in the science of the spirit. To anyone who feels irritated by this truth we would say that the above has nothing to do with a love for going against accepted views but a desire not to withhold insights, which after all have been gained, from anyone. The mystical concepts of heredity will remain for ever obscure if we shy away from accepting the idea of metamorphosis from physical to non-physical and the reverse in successive generations. As regards treatment, an insight like the above must inevitably give us an idea as to where the healing process should be initiated.'

We now come to the treatment aspect.

'If we had not been pointed in the direction of the hereditary aspect but had merely noted the irregularity in the relationship between ether body and astral body, we would have used medicines that act on these two aspects of the human

being. In the present case this would have proved ineffective, however, for the damage going through generations lies too deep to be balanced out in these aspects of the human organizations themselves.'

It is particularly important that we consider this case. We have a situation which relates to the question asked yesterday. If the findings were merely that astral body and ether body are not in close accord and therefore one must take this or that medicine, we would be unlikely to get any kind of result. If we strictly go on to the cause, treatment too will be more definite. The focus of attention moved from direct observation and we considered the sequence of generations, and this pointed the way to strict exactitude.

'In a case like this we have to influence the I organization, bringing every-thing into play that has to do with harmonizing and strengthening the ether and astral body. We achieve this by addressing the I organization in enhanced sensory stimuli, as it were (sensory stimuli act on the I organization). We attempted to do so in the following way for the child. A 5% pyrites ointment dressing was applied to the right hand and at the same time golden agaric ointment (Amanita caesarea) *was massaged into the left half of the head.'*

So here you have the treatment. We have a direct action on the hand with pyrites, FeS. This puts us in a position where it stimulates the I organization to make the astral body more lively and at the same time influence the ether body and so bring about harmonization. We must endeavour to bring ether body and astral body more closely together. The cure depends on this. It means we must use agents that go beyond the immediate, for it was a matter of generations.

'Externally applied, pyrites, an iron sulphide, stimulates the I organization to make the astral body more lively and increase its affinity to the ether body. The action of golden agaric substance, with organized nitrogen a special constituent, is to let an action going via the I organization evolve from the head, which makes the ether body more lively and increases its affinity to the astral body. The healing process was supported by eurythmy therapy, which makes the I organization as such lively and active. This results in externally applied principles being taken to the depths of the organization. The healing process thus initiated was further enhanced by measures designed to make astral and ether body particularly sensitive to the influence of the I organization. Using a rhythmic diurnal sequence, baths were given with a decoction of Solidago, back rubs with a

decoction of Stellaria media, *and both a tea made of willow bark (acts speci-*
fically on the astral body's receptivity) and Stannum 0.001 (specifically makes
the ether body receptive) by mouth. We also gave poppy juice in weak doses to
induce the individual's damaged inherent organization to make room for the
medicinal actions.

　'*The mother had more of the last of the above treatments, since she was one*
generation earlier so that hereditary forces were less involved. The same applied to
the mother's sister. We were able to note that whilst still at the Clinic the child
was more biddable and the general psychological condition had improved. It was
more obedient, for instance, and movements that had been very clumsy were done
in a more skilful way. Later the aunt reported that the child had gone through a
big change. It had grown quieter, the excess of involuntary movements was
reduced; it has gained sufficient skills to be able to play on its own; and, with
reference to the psychology, the former obstinacy had disappeared.'

　Now perhaps you'd like to say something? This is the way of taking
diagnosis forward to treatment. It then comes about that we get the
higher aspects of the human being, the higher levels of human existence,
to help us. We have the syndrome as our starting point. In this case it is
that the sick organism was subject to a process that took a particular
course. We have to follow it back to its beginning. If we have a clear
view of the evolution we are able to trace it back, seeing how not just an
organ but the whole inner human being is connected with the things
that happen out in the world.

　Let us say you want to learn how some kind of lesion, perhaps in the
gall bladder, may be treated. For this you must study it in its opposite
process out there—at least getting this opposite process to aid you. If
you perceive one process to be going one way, let us say, you perceive
the other to be coming the other way, which gives you the complete
cycle. Would someone still have a question, perhaps?

　One can sometimes get to the diagnosis in adults, sometimes in people who are
alive in their souls. I have tried this also with children, but gained the impression
that I went too far there with this method of diagnosis.

　That you did not achieve what you intended by entering into the
psyche? This is something that may be true and may also be incorrect. It
entirely depends on how far one is able to worm the things one wants to
know out of the child; also on whether the child is chatty or not; and on

the memory function; also on whether one is getting the right things from the soul. In principle a child can truly provide magnificent things, especially when there are condensed soul phenomena. When you take account of child nature and the child speaks of things seen in terms of condensed soul phenomena, you can look deeply into irregularities; these are always the correlate. You have to consider the case in a completely individual way.

With adults it is, of course, fairly easy to enter into the mind and soul if you know the soul organism as such, if you know how people are apt to tell one any old thing. You then move on. The things they tell are mostly untrue. It starts with the patient not saying how it is. You then have to pick it up at some point. You get to something which is the most true. Having grasped this you can move on. You have to make out if the one goes with the other. A creature with an eagle's beak cannot at the same time have an ostrich's feet. In the soul, too, things go together or not. You have to guide the patient towards this. Until you pick it up at some point you believe everything, that is, you don't believe anything, but you make it clear to him that you believe everything he says. Once you have picked it up at a point where it has to be true, you make very clear to him what cannot be. This creates a kind of soul organism for you which strongly points to the bodily organism. And so it is indeed useful to base yourself on a diagnostic process at the level of mind and soul.

A member of the audience said something.

The direction in which you pointed yesterday is like this: I make a diagnosis, have the diagnosis before me. I know that when I have this, such and such medicines are available to me. I am able to choose among them. You wanted to know how one can actually make a choice. The answer can only be that one says: If I am able to choose between a number of medicines I have to assume that my diagnosis is not yet complete. I must go further in making the diagnosis until I arrive at one definite medicine. In principle there is no arbitrary choice. This was really a fortunate case, and it amazed me. Going from the condition of the child to the grandmother's allantois is something which does not generally come up in making a diagnosis. It did greatly amaze me that this was the motif. On the other hand the results show that one must aim to penetrate to the very last cause.

Dr Wegman then read out Case 5 in the book.

'A woman aged 26 came to the Clinic suffering from serious consequences of an attack of influenza in 1918 in conjunction with pulmonary catarrh that had followed a pleurisy she had had in 1917. The patient had never been really well since she had the influenza. In 1920 she was greatly emaciated, weak, with a slight temperature and night sweats. Soon after the attack of influenza she developed low back pain, which got worse until late in 1920, then the pain was extremely severe and a curvature was noted in the sacral region. Her right index finger became swollen. Bed rest was stated to improve the back pain. When the patient came to us she had a gravitation abscess in the right thigh, bloated abdomen with slight ascites, and catarrhal sounds over the apices of both the left and the right lung. Digestion and appetite were good. The urine was concentrated, with traces of protein. Investigation using the science of the spirit showed hypersensitivity of the astral body and the I organization; this kind of abnormality initially comes to expression in the ether body in that it does not develop proper ether functions but an etheric offprint of the astral functions.'

It is most interesting when in such a case as this the ether body is so weak that it does not perform its own functions but is like a matrix, like wax, with the astral body imprinting its own functions on it. We have here an ether body functioning like a disguised astral body. That is the situation here.

'Astral functions are destructive. Vitality and the normal process in the physical organs therefore had to show atrophy. This is always connected with processes that are normally outside the human being, as it were, taking place within the human organism.'

This we must firmly hold on to. When something enters into the human organism, be it from some state of aggregation or other or be it warm air and so on, it must go through a change within the human organism, or roughly speaking within the human skin. Nothing is the same outside of and within the human organism. The human organization has to transform everything coming into it from outside. No temperature process may run in the human organism the way it does in a stone where a temperature simply passes through, warming the whole stone. When warmth comes to us from outside, the way it does to an inorganic body, we transform the warmth which comes to us in this way so profoundly that it is wholly filled with life. If a chill develops, even if it is a chill in the internal organs, it does not come from inside but from a temperature condition imposed from outside.

This extends down to the conditions existing in metabolism. Any substance that comes in must be transformed right down to its most subtle processes in the human organism. Anything we take in—let's say a carbohydrate—must go through a further process in the organism. The carbon-hydrogen-oxygen process in the world outside the human being must not exist in there in the same way. In that case a process foreign to human nature would exist in the human being. All pathological conditions based on metabolic deposits are essentially due to this. Basically they are due to warmth processes not coming from the human being but arising as processes inherent in the foreign matter, because the human organization is not strong enough in some area. If the I organization is too weak, for example, you'll find that ingested fats are not properly processed. If the astral organization is too weak you'll find that carbohydrates are not properly processed. If the ether organization is too weak, you'll find that the ingested proteinic states are not properly processed. This is something you must take note of.

'*The gravitation abscess, the back pain, the bloated abdomen, the catarrhal symptoms in the lung, and inadequate processing of protein were due to this. Treatment had to consist in reducing the sensitivity of the astral body and the I organization. This is done by giving silica, which always increases the inherent powers to counter sensitivity.*'

Silica always strengthens the inherent powers to counter sensitivity.

'*In this case we added powdered silica to the food and gave it in enemas. We also derived the sensitivity by putting mustard plasters on the lower back. The action of this is to generate sensitivity on its own accord, which relieves the astral body and I organization of sensitivity.*'

You see how one can help oneself—you apply mustard plasters and this produces an artificial sensitivity which relieves the astral body of its inner sensitivity, creating a stimulus[*] in this way. It is often the case,

---

[*] Following consultation with Dr Hans Broder von Laue, I have put 'creating a stimulus'; or one might think of 'giving a hint'. If the word appearing in the transcript was heard correctly, Rudolf Steiner said 'Intimation', using the term three times. Translator.

when something is not right in the human levels of existence, that one creates a stimulus—in this case, a powerful downward stimulus of the astral body. If this grows sufficiently powerful the sensitivity will have gone. The sensitivity of the astral body decreases in a downward direction. Sensitivity is increased when it moves upwards.

'*A process to reduce astral body sensitivity in the digestive tract was used to channel this astral activity to the ether body, which is where it normally should be. This was achieved with copper and Carbo animalis in low doses. The possibility of the ether body refusing to take up normal digestive activity, having got out of the habit, was countered by giving pancreatic juice.*'

That is merely an aid, a final aid.

'*The gravitation abscess was aspirated a number of times, removing large quantities of pus. The abscess was reduced and the abdominal swelling decreased, with pus formation decreasing steadily and finally ceasing. When pus was still being discharged, a further elevation of temperature took us by surprise one day. It did not seem inexplicable; the constitution of the astral body being as described, even minor mental upsets could cause such a fever. Distinction must be made, however, between the explicable nature of such a fever and the severe damage it can cause. Under the given conditions, such a fever actually mediates profound intervention of destructive processes in the organism. Care must be taken immediately to strengthen the ether body, so that it will inhibit the damaging effect of the astral body. We used silver injections in high potency and this resulted in the temperature being reduced. The patient had gained 10 kg in weight when she left the Clinic and was much stronger. We are perfectly aware that in this case follow-up treatment will be needed to reinforce the cure.*'

The case is meant to show how one can really find a way of making practical use in treatment of aspects otherwise considered in a more theoretical way concerning astral body and ether body. We may now come up against the question always put by 'well-meaning' people: Should we use the terms we have been using here, making them the naked truth and reality, or should we paraphrase? 'Well-meaning' people have said that we should not say 'ether body' but 'functional processes' or something like that. In that case we cannot get as far as the astral body. Now the situation is that we do not get to the essence of most diseases unless we go up as far as the astral body. The damage caused by the I organization, that is, the serious damage due to metabolic deposits—here the situation is that it is evidently there, this damage. The destructive damage due to the astral body is more insidious. And it is simply the case that we must speak of the astral body.

Well, the case will be that we can simply say—yes, many people will say this—that one should not talk straight away about astral body and ether body. But if you do not talk about them there will simply be no reason for anyone to think that this is something new. People think that one thing or another has just been changed a little; the approach is the same as everywhere else, at best it is just a tiny step forward. But that is not the case. And this must be made radically clear to people. If we show that these are not abstract things but point out the nature of the individual case in these many, wholly concrete individual cases, and then show how diagnosis leads to treatment and how healing comes as soon as the treatment is applied—the point is that this must be understood, otherwise we would have to despair altogether when it comes to human ability to understand. I am fully convinced that this is the only way for us—say things boldly, with courage.

A question is asked as to how the scientific picture appears if a close study is made of carcinoma.

With cancer it is altogether a matter of a sense organ being called into existence at a point in the organization where there is no reason for this. Take the most radical sensory organization, as I'd call it; take the eye. What makes the eye develop? You know that it is really half created from outside; it is integrated into the organism. The organism on its part leaves room for the eye socket, to put it crudely. The eye is then placed in this [Plate 9]. This indicates that processes from outside the human being are mainly involved in creating the eye. The eye is merely embraced by the human being. With a sense organ as striking as the eye we are able to say: A foreign body is integrated into the human organism. This is putting it in radical terms, in a truly unfamiliar way. Something like the lens or the vitreous body or the material composition in lens and vitreous body could never arise from the human organism. And everything placed there, being partly still etheric and not merely physical deposits in the case of the eye, is enveloped by the astral body and I organization, which are really as far as possible emancipated from the physical and etheric in the case of the eye. The relationship between

I, astral body, ether body and physical body is very different in the eye than it is, say, in a piece of muscle. In a piece of calf muscle you see I, astral body, ether body and physical body brought very close together. If I were to put this in the style of a chemical formula it is that in the eye [Plate 9], I and astral body (I and A in the drawing) are closely bound up with each other, and the other two are also intensely bound up with one another. The affinity between ether body and astral body is a loose one. This situation pertains only to the eye.

It is not the same for other sense organs such as the ear, for example. There it cannot be said to be like this. There the affinity between I organization and astral body and also between physical body and ether body is a loose one. It is slightly different for each of the senses.

If the tendency to develop a sensory organization arises somewhere in the human organism where there should not be any sensory organization—the tendency may develop in every part of the human organism; something due to happen elsewhere may come up as a tendency in any other place—we can see how physical body and ether body on the one hand and astral body and I on the other fall apart.

Take a concrete case. If there is a strong physical impact on, let us say, the mammary gland, the impact continues on inside, showing the evolution of an effect within the skin—roughly speaking—which had its origin outside. A mechanical insult, therefore, continuing on inside. This will in most cases be the true origin of breast cancer. Otherwise it could only be a protracted overheating or combustion process. It will always—speaking in external terms, as I put it here—be an insult which brings it about. What happens in such a case is that the astral body comes up very strongly in the site, where it is normally absorbed by the ether body. When the astral body comes up suddenly in the site, it appears in gleaming form; it looks as if it was afire. If it shows itself like this, we have a tendency to develop sensory effects in the site, a carcinoma develops. It is beyond question that we may at the least start with the first seven inoculations.

The situation there gets particularly interesting if we see how one thing relates to another. Imagine you have someone who is no longer all that young. You need to remove the carcinoma. But the principle you have with a fairly well-developed carcinoma is a tendency to let processes from outside the human being take place really in the whole body, for the organism is a whole. The carcinoma changes in a quite peculiar way as it progresses. After a time the local carcinoma becomes a valve for concentrating carcinomatous development. If you cut it out, the valve will suddenly be gone. But if you are dealing with an older person you get this ability now to have valves for that existing tendency to have outside principles in the human being in the organ which takes in the inorganic outside world most in the human being, which is the lung. With a carcinoma existing in an older person you will therefore dissolve the process into pneumonia. If the organism is sclerotic, the process concludes with pneumonia in old age. The reason is that an old organism takes in more of the outside world, doing so more easily than a younger organism does. The lung is the organ which takes in external processes most easily and suffers damage in the process. The liver is an organ which easily takes up external processes without suffering damage. It is quite thick-skinned when it comes to external processes. The lung takes them in and is damaged by them. This is the crux of the matter, that the lung takes them in easily and suffers damage.

Question about heredity relating to the tendency to develop cancer.

That is connected with ideas people pick up. Essentially people are not inclined to fear cancer. This is evident from the fact that the fear exists more among educated people in more highly civilized countries. Country people do not have that fear. They have cancer, die of it, never knew anything about carcinoma. It is something that comes with education and must be combated.

How far is supersensible vision necessary in these two cases, and how is it applied?

The procedure must be like this. Initially, in order to make any kind of start, you have to master spiritual vision fully—something which comes in the course of time—see how something you are able to establish in spiritual science relates to symptoms evident to the outside. If nothing else is given, the purely spiritual-scientific findings are always evident.

How is it perceived from outside?

Well, one may just as well say again that it should, of course, be meditative. You can meditate on rheumarthritis, you can meditate on diabetes. This will, however, drive you back again. A good way of arriving at spiritual-scientific observation is to meditate on a disease process in its symptoms. Only it is not easy to go in the opposite direction. You may even do what homoeopaths do—collect all the symptoms and base the treatment on this. Only in that case it happens again and again—I am not even saying 'may' happen for I know that this is how it is—that symptoms are overestimated or underestimated, brought together in the wrong way, so that sometimes a combination of symptoms made by homoeopaths actually is a caricature of the real thing. If you meditate on this, you meditate your way into the caricatures. If you have a genuine spiritual-scientific cause, if this determines the set of symptoms, you will not overestimate or underestimate any of the symptoms. You will have noticed that we gave the symptoms first; these are no caricatures but well-developed sets of symptoms. If you meditate you find it impossible to establish spiritual-scientific findings. And if someone says this cannot be done, I have to say: Try it, not with a set of symptoms put together arbitrarily but with a spiritual-scientifically established set of symptoms.

What is the basis of eurythmy?

In the human organism, everything is based on the fact that things which are conscious are derived from things that are unconscious. The basis of eurythmy is that when someone is born and wants to come into his own he does not lack the words for this but he lacks the ability to be fully himself in using the movements of his limbs. This element is beaten back; he must not do it and cannot do it. People do not notice it today, this beaten-back element, because it is beaten back through heredity itself. All this becomes integrated, metamorphoses, emerges bound to the air[66] and makes itself at home in speech. If we know how this has entered into speech, if we know that this is the origin of speech, we are able to go back from speech to the movements, conscious of this the other way round. And there, too, it is the case that spiritual-scientific diagnosis casts light on the set of symptoms. If you develop it and meditate on it you will in turn arrive at spiritual-scientific diagnosis.

I have to leave it at these three sessions; I hope we shall meet again. But if you come more often, this small social element will develop into the key for future activity.

It has certainly been good that we have once more been able to talk about things.

Dornach, Haus Friedwart,
im August 1920.

EINLADUNG

zu den

anthroposophischen Hochschulkursen

vom 26. September bis 16. Oktober 1920

an der

Freien Hochschule für Geisteswissenschaft
GOETHEANUM
in Dornach.

Dreiviertel Jahre vor Ausbruch des Weltkrieges wurde in Dornach, nahe an der Grenze des germanischen und romanischen Sprach- und Kulturgebietes, der Grundstein zur Freien Hochschule für Geisteswissenschaft Goetheanum gelegt. Als Arbeitsstätte für die **anthroposophisch orientierte Geisteswissenschaft**, wie sie von **Rudolf Steiner** vertreten wird, sollte dies Bauwerk in die mit Zerstörungskräften geladene abendländische Welt hineingestellt und als Quell aufbauender Kräfte in dieser Welt wirksam werden. Den verheerenden Wirkungen eines geistfremden Materialismus und einer die Welt verlierenden „Geistigkeit" sollte vom Goetheanum aus wahre Geistes*wissenschaft* entgegengestellt werden, die den Geist nicht nur — als wirklichkeitsfremdes *abstractum* — verstandesmässig erschliessen, mystisch erahnen oder verehrend anbeten will, sondern die ihn mit streng methodisch geschulter *anschauender Urteilskraft* an den einzelnen Erscheinungen der Natur und in den Lebensäusserungen der menschlichen Seele — als gegliedertes *concretum* — fasst, aus dem sittliche Stosskräfte zu sozialer Aufbauarbeit entbunden werden können.

Aus der Weltkriegskatastrophe heraus türmten sich in den folgenden Jahren Hindernisse über Hindernisse auf. Aber ihnen allen zum Trotz wurde der Dornacher Bau so weit vollendet, dass heute der innere Doppelkuppelraum im wesentlichen zu seiner endgültigen Gestalt geformt ist.

In diesem Raum sollen die Herbstkurse, zu denen hiedurch eingeladen wird, stattfinden. Sie wollen dennoch *nicht* als „Eröffnungs"veranstaltungen angesehen werden.

Denn dem Geist, der das *Gœtheanum* aus dem Boden gehoben hat, würde es widersprechen, eine „Eröffnung" als blosse Phrase vorzunehmen. Mehr als eine solche kann sie aber nicht sein, solange nicht aus der Welt, in die sich das *Gœtheanum* hineinstellt, eine Antwort kommt, die ein Verständnis dafür offenbart, dass es sich beim *Gœtheanum* um *ihre* Angelegenheit, nicht um die eines Sonderzirkels handelt.

Die Herbstkurse sollen also nicht Festveranstaltungen sein. Sie sollen in nüchterner Sachlichkeit geisteswissenschaftliche Arbeit vor die Welt stellen. Die sorgfältig ausgewählten und zusammengestellten Vorträge sollen ein erschöpfendes Bild davon geben, wie mit der geisteswissenschaftlichen Methode die Umwandlung aller Einzelwissenschaften und der Gesamtheit des wissenschaftlichen, künstlerischen, sozialen, wirtschaftlich-technischen Denkens und Schaffens in Angriff genommen wird. Sie sollen erweisen, dass Geisteswissenschaft fern von allem Dilettantismus ist, dass sie auf Untergründen baut, die in einem strengeren Sinn als wissenschaftlich zu bezeichnen sind als diejenigen der landläufigen Wissenschaften. Diesen wird ihr relativer Wert nicht abgesprochen. Doch soll gezeigt werden, wie die modernen Natur- *und* Geschichtswissenschaften durch ihre Einseitigkeit und Begrenztheit dem Menschen das allerwichtigste für sein Geistesleben nicht nur nicht geben können, sondern es ihm geradezu nehmen.

Anthroposophisch orientierte Geisteswissenschaft soll dasjenige sein, was *sie* nie werden können, sondern was sie eigentlich in seinen Anlagen zerstören. Nicht durch Kritik, sondern **durch Vorführung von positivem geisteswissenschaftlichem Wissen** soll dies erwiesen werden. Und damit soll gezeigt werden, wie aus wahrer, bis in ihre eigenen Lebenswurzeln hinein wissenschaftlicher Wissenschaft heraus die von tiefer denkenden und empfindenden Menschen seit langem angestrebte **Versöhnung von Wissenschaft, Kunst und Religion möglich ist.**

In erster Linie allerdings sollen die Herbstkurse zum *wissenschaftlichen* Gewissen der Gegenwart sprechen. Denn auf dem Felde der Wissenschaft, wo aus ungewussten Quellen die Zerstörungs- und Zersetzungskräfte kommen, die mit eindeutiger Entschiedenheit dem „Untergang des Abendlandes" entgegendrängen, muss der Geisteskampf aufgenommen und der Sieg erkämpft werden.

Zum *wissenschaftlichen* Gewissen, das sich als *Wille zu geistiger Tat* über sich selber klar wird, und zu einem aus ihm erwachsenden *neuen* künstlerischen und religiösen Gewissen will Geisteswissenschaft sprechen. Sie will dies Gewissen auch für die Einsicht wecken, dass ein *Gœtheanum,* das unfertig dasteht, und dem durch Verständnislosigkeit oder Anfeindung Hindernisse entgegengetürmt werden, zu deren Ueberwindung die einer *geistigen* Bewegung zur Verfügung stehenden Waffen nicht dienen, ein Vorwurf gegenüber der Welt ist, in der es steht.

Zum Besuche der Kurse ist jedermann eingeladen.

„Verein Gœtheanismus"
als Veranstalter,

Bund für Anthroposophische Hochschularbeit,
als Mitveranstalter.

INVITATION

to

ANTHROPOSOPHICAL COURSES OF THE

SCHOOL

26 September to 16 October 1920

at the

School of Spiritual Science

GOETHEANUM

Dornach

N ine months before the beginning of the World War, the Foundation Stone for the Independent School of Spiritual Science, Goetheanum, was laid in Dornach, close to the borders to the regions of German and Romance language and culture. As a centre for **spiritual science with anthroposophical orientation**, as represented by **Rudolf Steiner**, the building was established in the Western world which is charged with powers of destruction to be a source spring for constructive powers in this world. The devastating effects of a materialism far removed from the spirit, and a 'spirituality' losing the world were to be countered with a genuine *spiritual science* coming from the Goetheanum, where the spirit is not only studied in rational terms—as an abstract idea far removed from reality—imagined in a spirit of mysticism or the subject of reverent adoration, but grasped using powers of intuitive understanding for individual phenomena in the natural world and in the evidence of human inner life—concrete and differentiated— with the potential to give rise to moral powers for positive social endeavour.

Endless obstacles arose in the years that followed the war. But in spite of it all the building in Dornach was completed to the point where the two-domed interior space can essentially be seen in its final form.

The autumn courses to which we are inviting you are to be held in this hall. However, they are *not* to be considered 'opening' events. For it would go against the spirit which has raised the Goetheanum from the ground to have an 'opening' as mere phrase. Yet it cannot be more than that until an answer comes from the world in which the Goetheanum stands, an answer that shows understanding for the Goetheanum being *their* affair and not that of a separate group.

The autumn courses are thus not meant to be festival events. They are meant to present spiritual-scientific work done in a sober, factual way to the world. The lectures have been carefully chosen and combined to give an exhaustive picture of the way in which the spiritual-scientific method is used to transform all individual sciences and the totality of scientific, artistic, social, economic and industrial thinking and activity. They are to show that spiritual science is far removed from all amateurism, that its foundations must be considered to be scientific in a stricter sense than those of the generally accepted sciences. The value of these is not denied. But we aim to show how modern natural and historical sciences, being biased and limited, are not only unable to give humanity the things that are most important for cultural life, but do in fact deprive them of these.

Spiritual science with anthroposophical orientation is meant to be what those sciences can never be, but something which they actually destroy in its origins. We intend to demonstrate this not through criticism but by presenting **positive spiritual-scientific knowledge**. This should show that out of genuine science, scientific right down to its vital roots, it is possible to **reconcile science, art and religion**, something sought for a long time by people whose thoughts and sentience go deeper.

Primarily however the autumn courses are meant to address the conscience of our time. For the battle for the spirit must be entered into and victory gained in the field of science, where destructive, disruptive powers come from unknown sources, powers that are so clearly tending towards the 'Decline of the West'.

In spiritual science we want to address the scientific conscience which comes to see itself as the will to be active in the spirit, and a new artistic and religious conscience arising from it. We want also to awaken this conscience to the insight that the Goetheanum, incomplete as yet, with obstacles raised through lack of understanding or enmity, obstacles which the weapons available to a spiritual movement will not overcome, is a reproach to the world in which it stands.

Everyone is invited to attend the courses.

Goetheanum Association as organizer,
supported by the Alliance for anthroposophical work in the School

Programm der Anthroposophischen Hochschulkurse.

Sonntag, den 26. September, abends 5 Uhr,

Eröffnungshandlung

durch angemessene Ansprachen
(*Dr. Rudolf Steiner* über „Wissenschaft, Kunst und Religion")
und musikalisch-rezitatorisch-eurhythmische Darbietungen.

Erste Woche des Kurses:

	Montag, 27. Sept.	Dienstag, 28. Sept.	Mittwoch, 29. Sept.	Donnerst., 30. Sept.	Freitag, 1. Oktober	Samstag, 2. Oktober
9—10	Dr. Rudolf Steiner: Grenzen der Natur-Erkenntnis.					
10—11	Hermann von Baravalle: Grundprobleme der Physik im Lichte anthroposophischer Erkenntnis.			Dr. Walter Johannes Stein: „Vorstellung", „Begriff" und „Urteil" in der Lehre Rudolf Steiners.		
11—12	Dr. med. Friedrich Husemann: Fragen der heutigen Psychiatrie vom Gesichtspunkte der Anthroposophie.			Dr. Oskar Schmiedel: Licht u. Farbe im Sinne der Geisteswissenschaft.		Dr. Rudolf Steiner: Der Baugedanke von Dornach. I.
4—5	Fabrikdirektor Emil Molt: Der Industrielle in Vergangenheit und Zukunft vom Gesichtspunkt der Geisteswissenschaft. I. und II.		Rudolf Meyer, Hamburg: Geschichtsphilosophische Probleme des Christentums im Lichte anthroposophischer Forschung.			
5—6	Paul Baumann: Musik und Eurhythmische Erziehungskunst.			Emil Molt: Der Industrielle in Vergangenheit und Zukunft vom Gesichtspunkt d. Geisteswissenschaft III.	Prof. Dr. P. Boekh: Indologie und Geisteswissenschaft. I.	An den Samstag- und Sonntag-Abenden finden Eurhythmische Aufführungen statt.
6—7	Adolf Arenson: Grundzüge geisteswissenschaftlicher Methodik.		Die Kunst d. Deklamation: A. Praxis: Marie Steiner B. Theorie: Dr. Rud. Steiner	Adolf Arenson: Grundzüge geisteswissenschaftlicher Methodik.		

Zweite Woche des Kurses:

	Montag, 4. Oktober	Dienstag, 5. Oktober	Mittwoch, 6. Oktober	Donnerstag, 7. Okt.	Freitag, 8. Oktober	Samstag, 9. Oktober
9—10	Dr. Ernst Blümel: Die Hauptprobleme der modernen Mathematik in ihrer Beziehung zur Philosophie, Physik und Anthroposophie.			Dr. med. Ludwig Noll: Physiologisch-therapeutisches auf Grundlage der Geisteswissenschaft.		
10—11	Dr. Eugen Kolisko: Hypothesenfreie Chemie im Sinne der Geisteswissenschaft.			E. A. Karl Stockmeyer: Phänomenologie des Wärmewesens.		
11—12	Dr. Roman Boos: Phänomenologische Sozialwissenschaft.			Dr. Ernst Blümel: Das Element der Freiheit in den mathematischen Begriffsbestimmungen	Prof. Dr. P. Boekh: Indologie und Geisteswissenschaft. II.	Dr. Rudolf Steiner: Der Baugedanke von Dornach. II.
4—5	Rudolf Meyer, Berlin: Johann Friedrich Herbarts Lehre vom Menschen und dessen Erziehung vom Standpunkt der Anthroposophie.		Emil Leinhas: Licht- und Schattenseiten des modernen Kapitalismus.			
5—6	Dr. Rudolf Treichler: Sprachwissenschaft und Sprachunterricht.		Karl Ballmer: Künstlerisches Wollen und Anthroposophie.			An den Samstag- und Sonntag-Abenden finden Eurhythmische Aufführungen statt.
6—7	Arnold Ith: Bankwesen und Preisgestaltung in ihrer heutigen und zukünftigen Bedeutung für das Wirtschaftsleben.		Die Kunst d. Deklamation: A. Praxis: Marie Steiner B. Theorie: Dr. Rud. Steiner	Ernst Uehli: Die nordisch-germanische Mythologie als Entwicklungsgeschichte.		

Dritte Woche des Kurses:

	Montag, 11. Oktober	Dienstag, 12. Okt.	Mittwoch, 13. Okt.	Donnerstag, 14. Okt.	Freitag, 15. Oktober	Samstag, 16. Okt.
9—10	Dr. Carl Unger: Rudolf Steiners Werk.					
10—11	Dr. Hans Wohlbold: Goethes Metamorphosenlehre u. die Geisteswissenschaft.		E. Vreede, phil. doct. D. Berechtigung der Mathematik in d. Astronomie u. ihre Grenzen. I.	Dr. Karl Heyer: Anthroposophische Betrachtungen über die Geschichtswissenschaft u. aus der Geschichte.		
11—12	Dr. Caroline von Heydebrand: Pädagogische Praxis und Waldorfschule.		E. Vreede, phil. doct. D. Berechtigung der Mathematik in d. Astronomie u. ihre Grenzen. II.		Prof. Dr. P. Booth: Indologie und Geisteswissenschaft. III.	Dr. Rudolf Steiner: Der Baugedanke von Dornach. III.
4—5	Dr. J. Hugentobler: Anthroposophie und Sprachwissenschaft.		Herbert Hahn: Idee und Praxis zeitgemässer Arbeiterbildungsbestrebungen auf geisteswissenschaftlicher Grundlage.			
5—6	Ingenieur A. Strakosch: Das Signalwesen in seiner kulturgeschichtlichen Bedeutung.		Walter Kühne: Tolstois Lebensstufen.			An den Samstag- und Sonntagabenden finden Eurythmische Aufführungen statt.
6—7	Ernst Uehli: Die nordisch-germanische Mythologie als Entwicklungsgeschichte.		Die Kunst d. Rezitation: A. Praxis: Marie Steiner. B. Theorie: Dr. Rud. Steiner.	Albert Steffen: Die Krisis im Leben des Künstlers und die Geisteswissenschaft.		

Diskussion und freie Aussprache in den Zwischenstunden und Abends nach Uebereinkunft. Auf Wunsch der Teilnehmer werden Eurythmische Kurse abgehalten werden können.

Teilnehmerkarten:

Es werden ausgegeben:
1. Karten für den ganzen Kurs (ungef. 100 Stunden) zu 80 Frankes.
2. Karten für eine Woche (ungef. 33 Stunden) zu 30 Franken.
3. Karten für einzelne Vortragsreihen (nach freier Wahl) zu Preisen, die sich von 2 Franken (bis zu 6 Stunden) auf 1 Franken (über 25 Stunden) — auf die einzelne Stunde berechnet — ermässigen. (Karten für Teilvorträge werden nicht abgegeben.)

Für Teilnehmer, die nicht imstande sind, diese Beträge aufzubringen, wird in weitestgehendem Masse Ermässigung gewährt.

Vorausbestellungen sind an Dr. Roman Boos, Haus Friedwart, Dornach, zu richten.

Unterkunft:

Eine grössere Anzahl von Gruppenquartieren und Privatunterkunftsgelegenheiten zu mässigen Preisen ist bereitgestellt. Es wird jedoch notwendig sein, diese Quartiere hauptsächlich den zahlreich angemeldeten Studenten zur Verfügung zu stellen, die aus Deutschland, Oesterreich, der Tschecho-Slowakei und anderen Ländern mit darniederliegender Valuta angesagt sind. Deshalb werden alle diejenigen Teilnehmer, die sich in Basel oder in Basels Umgebung selber Privatquartiere beschaffen können, oder die imstande sind, die Kosten eines Hotel- oder Pensionsaufenthaltes zu tragen, gebeten, sich nicht in Unterkunftsfragen nach Dornach zu wenden. Studenten und andere Persönlichkeiten, die aus valutakranken Gebieten kommen wollen und auf teilweise oder völlige Entlastung von den Aufenthaltskosten angewiesen sind, wollen sich möglichst sofort in Stuttgart, Champignystr. 17, beim Arbeitsausschuss des Bundes für Anthroposophische Hochschularbeit anmelden.

Verpflegung:

In der Kantine des Goetheanum können Frühstück (ca. 50 Rp.), Mittag- und Abendessen (2 Fr.) eingenommen werden. Für unbemittelte Teilnehmer können auch hier Ermässigungen gewährt werden

Bahnverbindungen:

Basel-Hauptbahnhof SBB nach Dornach (ca. ¼ Stde.). Basel-Aeschenplatz (Birseckbahn) nach Dornach (½ Stunde) mit den fahrplanmässigen Zügen.

Finanzielle Unterstützung:

Von Freunden des Goetheanum in England, Skandinavien, Holland, Frankreich, Italien, der Schweiz u. a. Staaten sind Geldmittel gestiftet worden, mit denen deutschen, österreichischen u. a. Studenten der Besuch der Kurse ermöglicht werden kann. Es ergeht hiemit auch an weitere Kreise, denen die Bedeutung dieser Veranstaltung einleuchtet, die Bitte, durch Stiftung von Geldmitteln den Veranstaltern der Kurse die Möglichkeit zu verschaffen, in einem möglichst weitgehendem Umfang unbemittelten Personen, die teilnehmen möchten, Gastfreundschaft zu gewähren. Spenden können eingezahlt werden auf das Postcheckkonto V 5060 der Verwaltungsgesellschaft für das Goetheanum Dornach mit der, auf der Rückseite des Postcheckabschnittes anzubringenden Bemerkung „Für die Herbstkurse 1920."

Auskünfte

erteilt: Dr. Roman Boos, Haus Friedwart, Dornach, Telephon 9173.

Weitere Exemplare dieses Prospektes können kostenlos bezogen werden bei Dr. Roman Boos, Haus Friedwart, Dornach.

PROGRAMME OF THE SCHOOL'S ANTHROPOSOPHICAL COURSES

Sunday, 26 September 5 p.m.

OPENING EVENT
WITH APPROPRIATE ADDRESSES

(Dr Rudolf Steiner on 'Science, Art and Religion')
and performances in music, recitation and eurythmy

First week of the course

	Monday, 27 Sept.	Tuesday, 28 Sept.	Wednesday, 29 Sept.	Thursday, 30 Sept.	Friday, 1 Oct.	Saturday, 2 Oct.
9–10	Dr Rudolf Steiner: Limits to insight into nature					
10–11	Norman von Baravalle: Basic problems in physics in the light of anthroposophical insight			Walter Johannes Stein, Ph.D: Idea, concept and judgement in R. Steiner's teachings		
11–12	Friedrich Husemann, MD: Questions in modern psychiatry from the anthroposophical point of view			Oscar Schmiedel, Ph.D: Light and colour in terms of spiritual science		Rudolf Steiner, Ph.D: The architectural idea of Dornach
4–5	Emil Molt, managing director. The industrialist in past and future from the spiritual-scientific point of view I and II		Rudolf Meyer, Hamburg: History of philosophy problems of Christianity in terms of anthroposophical research			
5–6	Paul Baumann: Music and eurhythmic art of education			Emil Molt: The industrialist in past and future from the spiritual-scientific point of view III	Prof. Peter Beckh: Iridology and spiritual science I	
6–7	Adolf Arenson: Basic principles of spiritual-scientific methodology		The art of declamation a) practice: Marie Steiner b) theory: Dr Rud. Steiner	Adolf Arenson: Basic principles of spiritual-scientific methodology		Eurythmy performances will be given on Saturday and Sunday evenings

Second week of the course

	Monday, 4 Oct.	Tuesday, 5 Oct.	Wednesday, 6 Oct.	Thursday, 7 Oct.	Friday, 8 Oct.	Saturday, 9 Oct.
9–10	Ernst Bluemel, Ph.D: The main problems in modern mathematics as they relate to philosophy, physics and anthroposophy			Ludwig Noll, MD: Aspects of physiology and therapy based on the science of the spirit		
10–11	Eugen Kolisko, Ph.D: Chemistry free from hypotheses in spiritual-scientific terms			Karl Stockmeyer, Ph.D: Phenomenology of heat		
11–12	Roman Boos, Ph.D: Phenomenological social science			Ernst Bluemel, Ph.D: The element of freedom in mathematical definitions	Prof. P. Beckh: Iridology and spiritual science II	Dr Rudolf Steiner: The architectural idea of Dornach II
4–5	Rudolf Meyer, Berlin: Johann Friedrich Herbart's theory of man and education from the anthroposophical point of view		Emil Leinhas: The positive and negative aspects of modern capitalism			
5–6	Rudolf Treichler, MD: Linguistics and the teaching of languages		Karl Ballmer: The artist's will intent and anthroposophy			
6–7	Arnold Jth: Banking and pricing policies—present-day and future significance in economic life		The art of declamation a) practice: Marie Steiner b) theory: Dr Rud. Steiner	Ernst Uehli: Norse Germanic mythology as history of evolution		Eurythmy performances will be given on Saturday and Sunday evenings

Third week of the course

	Monday, 11 Oct.	Tuesday, 12 Oct.	Wednesday, 13 Oct.	Thursday, 14 Oct.	Friday, 15 Oct.	Saturday, 16 Oct.
9–10	Carl Unger, Ph.D					
10–11	Hans Wehlbold, Ph.D: Goethe's theory of metamorphosis and the science of the spirit		E. Vreede, Ph.D: Justification for mathematics in astronomy and their limits	Karl Heyer, Ph.D: Anthroposophical reflection on the science of history and from history		
11–12	Caroline von Heydebrand, Ph.D: Educational practice and the Waldorf School			E. Vreede, Ph.D: Justification for mathematics in astronomy and their limits II	Prof. P. Beckh: Iridology and spiritual science III	Rudolf Steiner, Ph.D: The architectural idea of Dornach III
4–5	J. Hugentobler, Ph.D: Anthroposophy and linguistics		Herbert Hahn: Idea and practice for modern workers' education on the basis of spiritual science			
5–6	Strakosch, engineer: Signals and their significance in the history of civilization		Walter Kuehne: The stages of Tolstoy's life			
6–7	Ernst Uehli: Norse Germanic mythology as history of evolution		The art of declamation a) practice: Marie Steiner b) theory: Dr Rud. Steiner	Albert Steffen: The crisis in the artist's life and the science of the spirit		Eurythmy performances will be given on Saturday and Sunday evenings

Discussion and free exchange of views in between times and in the evenings, as mutually agreed.
It will be possible to have courses in eurythmy if course members so desire.

Tickets
The following will be issued:
1) Tickets for the whole course (c. 100 sessions) at 80 francs.
2) Tickets for one week (c. 33 sessions at 30 francs.
3) Tickets for individual lecture series (open choice) at prices reduced from 2 francs (up to 6 sessions) to 1 franc (more than 25 sessions)—per session.

(Tickets are not available for part sessions)
For anyone unable to afford these prices, reductions will be made as far as possible.
Advance bookings please to Dr Roman Boos, Haus Friedwart, Dornach.

Accommodation
A fairly large number of dormitory places and private accommodation are available. It will be necessary, however, to keep these opportunities mainly for the many students coming from Germany, Austria, Czechoslovakia and other countries with poor exchange rates. We would therefore ask everyone who can organize private accommodation for themselves in Basel and environs or manage to pay for hotel accommodation not to ask us in Dornach to find accommocation. Students and others intending to come from countries with poor exchange rates and will have to depend on partial or complete support to contact the Arbeitsausschuss des Bundes fuer Anthroposophische Hochschularbeit in Stuttgart, Champignystr. 17, as soon as possible.

Meals
The Goetheanum Canteen offers breakfast at c. 50 rappen, midday and evening meal (2 francs). Reductions are possible for members who do not have the means.

Trains
Basel main station SBB to Dornach (c. ¼ hour),
Basel-Aeschenplatz (Birseckbahn) to Dornach (½ hour) as per timetable.

Financial support
Friends of the Goetheanum in England, Scandinavia, Holland, France, Italy, Switzerland and other countries have made funds available to enable people to attend the course. We would also ask others to donate money to enable the organizers of the course to offer hospitality on the broadest level possible to people without means. Donations may be paid on to the Postscheckkonto V 5080 der Verwaltungsgesellschaft fuer das Goeatheanum Dornach, adding the ref. 'Fuer die Herbstkurse 1920'.

Information
provided by Dr Roman Boos, Haus Friedwart, Dornach, telephone 9173.

Additional copies of this prospectus are available free of charge from Dr Roman Boos, Haus Friedwart, Dornach.

PROGRAMM

der vom

Klinisch-therapeutischen Institut der „Kommende Tag", Stuttgart in Aussicht genommenen medizinischen Woche.

Das Programm unserer medizinischen Woche, welche in der Zeit vom 22. bis 28. Oktober in Stuttgart, Landhausstraße 70, stattfindet, ist folgendes:

Am Sonntag, den 22. Oktober (anstatt wie zuerst vorgesehen am 21. Oktober) wird Herr Dr. Husemann um ¼11 Uhr vormittags sprechen über das Thema: »Vergangenes und Zukünftiges in der Medizin«. Nachmittags 5 Uhr wird Frau Dr. Steiner die Güte haben, uns eurythmische Kunst vorzuführen. Eine ebensolche Aufführung wird stattfinden am Mittwoch, den 25. Oktober, abends 8 Uhr. Beide Vorführungen finden Landhausstraße 70 statt.

Vom 23. bis 28. Oktober werden in der Zeit von 9—12 Uhr vormittags sprechen die Herren:

Dr. Husemann: *Lebensperioden und Krankheiten.*
Dr. Knauer: *Zur Phänomenologie der Sinne, insbesondere des Geschmackssinnes.*
Dr. Kolisko: *Einiges aus der physiologischen Chemie (mit Behandlung des periodischen Systems).*
Über das Problem der Herztätigkeit.
Dr. Noll: *Der Kieselsäure-Kohlensäure-Prozeß.*
Dr. Palmer: *Über das Problem der Entzündung und Geschwulstbildung.*
Dr. Peipers: *Prinzipielles zur Tuberkulose.*

Über spezielle Themata mit Kasuistik wird gesprochen von:

Dr. Husemann: *Versuch einer funktionellen Betrachtung der Anatomie unter Berücksichtigung der Heileurythmie.*
Dr. Knauer: *Über die Grippe.*
Dr. Noll: *Über Migräne und über Gallenstauungen und Gallensteinbildungen.*
Dr. Palmer: *Unsere seitherigen Erfahrungen über die Behandlung der Krebsgeschwulst.*
Dr. Peipers: *Kasuistisches zu Tuberkulose und Heufieber.*

Herr Dr. Steiner hat auf unsere Bitte hin seine Mitwirkung für eine Reihe von Vorträgen zugesagt. Von 5—7 Uhr nachmittags wird Gelegenheit sein, sich mit der Eurythmie im allgemeinen und mit der Heileurythmie im besonderen bekannt zu machen.

Im Hause Landhausstraße 70 ist vom Nachmittage des 21. Oktober an ein Büro eingerichtet, in dem Auskunft über alle Fragen erteilt wird; dorthin kann auch die Post nachgeschickt werden. Zur Deckung der erheblichen Unkosten soll, den Verhältnissen des Einzelnen entsprechend, ein freiwilliger Beitrag erhoben werden.

Für die beiden Eurythmieaufführungen stehen Karten (reservierte Plätze zum Preise von Mk. 50.—, 75.— und 100.—) zur Verfügung.

Für das Ärztekollegium:
Dr. Palmer.

PROGRAMME

MEDICAL WEEK PROPOSED FOR THE DER KOMMENDE TAG INSTITUTE OF CLINICAL MEDICINE IN STUTTGART

The programme of our medical week in Stuttgart, Landhausstrasse 70, 22nd–28th October will be as follows.

On Sunday, 22nd October (and not on 21st October, as originally planned), Dr Husemann will speak at 10.30 a.m. on 'Past and future elements in medicine'. At 5 p.m. Mrs Marie Steiner will be so kind as to present the art of eurythmy to us. The same performance will be given at 8 p.m. on Wednesday, 25th October. Both performances will be at Landhausstrasse 70.

From 23rd to 28th October, the morning talks will be as follows:

Dr Husemann	Life stages and diseases.
Dr Knauer	On the phenomenology of the senses, esp. the sense of taste.
Dr Kolisko	Aspects of physiological chemistry (incl. discussion of the periodic table).
Dr Noll	The silica-carbon dioxide process.
Dr Palmer	The problem of inflammation and tumour development.
Dr Peipers	Key elements of tuberculosis.

The following will speak on specific subjects, with case records.

Dr Husemann	Attempt to take a functional view of anatomy, with reference to eurythmy therapy.
Dr Knauer	Influenza
Dr Noll	Migraine, biliary stasis and gallstones.
Dr Palmer	Experience to date with the treatment of cancer.
Dr Peipers	Case studies in tuberculosis and hay fever.

Dr Steiner has acceded to our request to give a number of talks.

From 5–7 p.m., opportunity will be given to familiarize yourselves with eurythmy in general and eurythmy therapy in particular.

From the afternoon of 21st October, an office will be open at Landhausstrasse 70 to provide information on all points. You may also redirect your mail to it. To cover the considerable costs, a voluntary contribution will be requested that is is accord with individual means.

Tickets for the two eurythmy performances (reserved seats at 50, 100 and 150 Marks) are available.

For the Medical Faculty
Dr Palmer.

NOTES

Text sources: The lectures given in Dornach were taken down by Helene Finckh, a professional stenographer, the exception being the discussions in April 1924. The Stuttgart lectures were taken down by Lili Kolisko. This German edition is based on the transcripts made by the two stenographers. The texts of the Dornach lectures were compared with the original stenograms for the 2nd German edition of 1975. For the 3rd German edition in 1989, some passages were checked once more against the stenograms. It is not known who took down the discussions in April 1924; these are of a fragmentary nature. The 3rd German edition of 1989 was checked again, adding some Notes, a list of names and detailed summaries by W. Belart, MD. For the 4th German edition of 2010, the volume was checked, and a few passages were edited. Some changes were made to spelling, syntax and punctuation. The notes were reviewed and extended, an introduction was added, with additions made to the contextual and editorial details. The lecture on eurythmy therapy of 28 October 1922 was included for the first time. The title of the German volume is based on the proposed series of lectures by Dr Noll which Rudolf Steiner then took over. The title of the lecture 'Hygiene as a social issue' goes back to Rudolf Steiner, the other lecture titles were chosen by the editors of earlier editions.

Drawings in the text: Included in earlier editions, these were made by Assja Turgenieff from Rudolf Steiner's original drawings, but have not been included in this volume. Instead, reference is made to the plates showing the actual blackboard drawings at the end of the book. A facsimile of the sketch Helene Finckh made in her notebook has been included for the lecture of 7 October 1920 as the blackboard drawing made on that day has not been preserved.

The board drawings (plates): The original blackboard drawings and writing from the lectures given in Dornach (except for the lecture of 7 October 1920) were preserved by stretching black paper over the boards which was then removed and stored. They are included as plates in this volume and may also be found in vol. XXII, *Wandtafelzeichnungen zum Vortragswerk Rudolf Steiners*. The plates are referred to in the text.

1. Dr Ludwig Noll had been asked to give these lectures. Ludwig Noll (1872– 1920) was leading the branch in Kassel and the first physician with whom Rudolf Steiner collaborated. The latter thought highly of Noll's abilities and asked him to do a number of things that were important for the development of anthroposophical medicine. However, Noll was often not in a position to do them. Thus he also sent a telegram on 8 October to say that he was unable to

come and give the lectures. Rudolf Steiner was greatly dissatisfied with the situation as he would have preferred qualified medical experts to present the new points of view in medicine (see also his words at the end of the lecture given on the evening of 9 October). Concerning Ludwig Noll's nature and work, see his biography in *Anthroposopie im 20. Jahrhundert. Ein Kulturimpuls in biografischen Porträts,* Dornach 2003, Seite 565 f., and the description given by Gisbert Husemann in Peter Selg (ed.), *Anthroposophische Ärzte. Lebens- und Arbeitswege im 20. Jahrhundert,* Dornach 2000, Seite 91f.

2. The natural-scientific training of physicians in the nineteenth century in Vienna was mainly concerned with diagnosis and pathological anatomy; treatment or therapy was largely neglected. A manifesto from the faculty of medicine in Vienna in 1845 said: 'The physician has to be judged according to the sum of his knowledge and not the success of his treatment; the natural scientist in the physician must be appreciated and not the skilled practitioner.'

3. On 10 July 1897, Rudolf Steiner and Otto Erich Hartleben took on the editorship of the journal. Moriz Zitter joined them in 1898 and 1899, Chief Editor Dr Rud. Steiner, Berlin. Published by Emil Felber in Weimar, later by Siegfried Cronbach in Berlin. From 17 March to 29 September 1900 Rudolf Steiner was sole editor. At the last of these dates the journal passed into the hands of Johannes Gaulke and Franz Philips. See also Rudolf Steiner's description of this work in his autobiography.

4. Ludwig Buechner (1824–99), see essay on him in Rudolf Steiner's *Methodische Grundlagen der Anthroposophie 1884–99,* Collected Works in German No. 30.

5. 'Chemistry Free from Hypotheses' was the title of a lecture given by Dr Eugen Kolisko (1893–1939) in the course.

6. Friedrich Wilhelm Joseph Schelling (1775–1854). Rudolf Steiner would often refer to F.W.J. Schelling in his written works and in lectures. The basic details are given in *The Riddles of Philosophy,* for instance, and *The Riddle of Man.*

7. *Jahrbuecher der Medizin als Wissenschaft,* edited by A.T. Marcus and F.W.J. Schelling, Tuebingen 1805–8.

8. Literally the words are: 'To philosophize about nature is to create nature.' In F.W.J. Schelling, *Erster Entwurf eines Systems der Naturphilosophie* 1799, S. 6; in the Manfred Schroeter edition S. 13.

9. Ignaz Paul Vital Troxler (1780–1866), Swiss physician and philosopher who was highly regarded by Rudolf Steiner. Taught at Aarau, Lucerne, Basel; professor of philosophy at Berne, interested in 'theosophical and philosophical' background to medicine. Rudolf Steiner would often refer to Troxler, e.g. in *The Riddle of Man* and in the lectures given on 29 and 30 October 1916 in Bern (not translated into English).

10. Wilhelm Griesinger (1817–68). German psychiatrist and neurologist. Initiated a natural-scientific psychiatry with materialistic approach. The main work he published was on the pathology and treatment of mental diseases (Stuttgart 1845).

11. See Steiner, R., *Spiritual Science and Medicine* or *Introducing Anthroposophical Medicine.*

12. Steiner, R., *The Case for Anthroposophy,* tr. O. Barfield, Rudolf Steiner Press, London 1970.

13. In Vol. 1 of Goethe's scientific works in German.
14. Silver birch–*Betula alba* L., *Betula pendula* Roth, *B. verrucosa* Ehrh.
15. The word was not fully written out in the shorthand record which merely says 'hyper-ecz . . .' We may assume that the stenographer wrote things down purely by ear and not knowing the word did not write it down. In the given context, the 'hyper-exudation' found in earlier editions may well be correct.
16. See note 11.
17. Claudius Galenus (born AD 129 in Pergamon, died in about 216). Greek physician, writer and philosopher who greatly influenced medical theory and practice in the Middle Ages and into the seventeenth century. *Corpus Medicorum Graecorum*, compiled and translated into Latin by 'Karl Gottlob Kühn (page does not exist)' Leipzig between 1821 and 1833.
18. Steiner, R., *Knowledge of the Higher Worlds*, tr. G. Metaxa, various revisions, Rudolf Steiner Press, 1923, 1963, 2004. Alternative translation *How to Know Higher Worlds*, tr. C. Bamford, Anthroposophic Press, Hudson 1994.
19. E.g. *Occult Science. An Outline*, tr. M.B. Monges, H.B. Monges, New York & London 1939. Same title translated by G. & M. Adams, Rudolf Steiner Press, London 1962/3, rev. 1979. See also *An Outline of Esoteric Science*, tr. C.E. Creeger, Anthroposophica Press, Hudson 1997.
20. Theodor Ziehen (1862–1950), philosopher and psychologist, professor in Jena, Utrecht, Halle and Berlin, main representative of experimental psychology. Nietzsche's physician at psychiatric clinic in Jena. *Leitfaden der physiologischen Psychologie in 15 Vorlesungen* (guide to physiological psychology), 5th ed. Jena 1900. See also Steiner, R., *Von Seelenrätseln*.
21. Johann Friedrich Herbart (1776–1841), philosopher, psychologist and educationist. professor in Göttingen and Königsberg; major influence on science of education. See also Steiner, R., *The Riddles of Philosophy*, Anthroposophic Press, New York 1973.
22. Theodor Meynert (1833–92), neuropathologist and anatomist in Vienna. Meynert treated Alfred Stross, friend of the young Rudolf Steiner. Publ. *Sammlung von populaerwissenschaftlichen Vortraegen ueber den Bau und die Leistung des Gehirns*, Vienna 1892.
23. See note 12.
24. Moriz Benedikt (1835–1920). Viennese neurologist. Established criminal anthropology with Cesare Lombroso (1836–1909). Concerning the alcohol problem, see Moriz Benedikt, *Aus meinem Leben. Erinnerungen und Eroerterungen*, Vienna 1906, Chapter IX: 'Die Alkoholisten- und Abstinenzfragen' S. 404ff. Rudolf Steiner spoke about Moriz Benedikt more fully in a lecture given on 5 November 1921, published in *Cosmosophy*, Vol. 2. Published works on psychophysics of morality and law, psychology as an empirical science, biomechanical (neo-vitalist) thinking in medicine and biology, hypnotism and suggestion.
25. Full details in Steiner, R., *Spiritual Science and Medicine* (alternative translation *Introducing Anthroposophical Medicine*), end of 12th lecture, 16th and 17th lectures.
26. See also the lecture given on 28 October 1922, in this volume.

27. See also the lectures given on 28 and 29 August 1920, in *Spiritual Science as Foundation for Social Forms*, tr. M. St Goar, Collected Works in German No. 199. Also the lecture given on 22 October 1922, in *Spiritual Relations in the Human Organism*, tr. by M. Deussen, Coll. Works No. 218. Also the Questions and Answers session of 24 April 1924 in *Course for Young Doctors*, Coll. Works Vol. 316.

28. See the lecture given for physician on the same day (28 October 1922), in this volume.

29. See the lecture in this volume given for members of the medical profession on the same day (28 October 1922).

30. See the lecture of 30 December 1923 in *World History in the Light of Anthroposophy*.

31. Joseph von Hyrtl (Eisenstadt 1811–94, Perchtoldsdorf nr Vienna), famous anatomist. Hyrtl studied medicine in Vienna, was a professor in Prague from 1837, in Vienna from 1845, and a member of the Imperial Academy in that city from 1847. His *Lehrbuch der Anatomie des Menschen mit Ruecksicht auf physiologische Begruendung und praktische Anwendung* (textbook of anatomy, Vienna 1847) known well beyond Germany and translated into many languages established his reputation in the late 1840s. His gifts as a teacher and lecturer attracted students and physicians in large numbers.

32. *Astragalus exscapus*, tragacanth or hart's milk vetch.

33. Plant galls—see note 30, also *Course for Young Doctors*, lecture of 2 January 1924.

34. Both the shorthand record and the transcript say 'pocks', though 'pores' would make more sense. May be due to mishearing.

35. Dr Haakenson (1881–1933), physician in Oslo, member of the General Anthroposophical Society.

36. [any excess]—added by German editors, in accord with similar passage in the lecture of 31 December in this volume.

37. 'arsenic in its greater dilution' as per shorthand record.

38. See note 30.

39. Otto Palmer, MD (1867–1945), co-founder and head of Institute of Clinical Medicine in Stuttgart.

40. The statements made here relate to the genus and should be taken as such.

41. Dementia praecox—earlier term for schizophrenia.

42. 'I organization'—as per shorthand record.

43. 'by mouth'—as per shorthand record.

44. See *Was in der Anthroposophischen Gesellschaft vorgeht. Nachrichten fuer deren Mitglieder*.

45. Roman Boos, PhD (1889–1952), social science expert. Active representative of anthroposophy and the threefold concept as writer, speaker and editor of the monthly journal *Soziale Zukunft*. Head of social science association at the Goetheanum in Dornach.

46. Karl Marx (1818–83). Main work *Capital*, 3 volumes.
Franz Oppenheimer (1864–1944), physician, economist and sociologist, representative of Soil Reform movement. Main works *Die Siedlungsgenossenschaft* (1896) and *Theorie der reinen und politischen Oekonomie* (1910). His aim

was to break the monopoly on the soil by major land owners by establishing settlement communities.

47. See note 11.
48. First combined lower and upper school where Rudolf Steiner's ideas on education were realized. Established by Emil Molt, managing director of the Waldorf Astoria cigarette factory in Stuttgart, in 1919 for the workers' children. Conceived and guided by Rudolf Steiner. Today there are about 1000 schools around the world.
49. Steiner, R., *The Study of Man*, tr. D. Harwood, H. Fox, Rudolf Steiner Publishing Co. & Anthroposophic Press, London & New York. American edition *The Foundations of Human Experience*, tr. R.F. Lathe, N. Parsons Whittaker, H. Barnes, Anthroposophic Press, Hudson 1996.
   Steiner R., *Rhythms of Learning*, tr. R. Lathe, N. Whittaker a.o., Anthroposophic Press, Hudson 1998.
   Steiner, R., *Discussions with Teachers*, tr. H. Fox (rev.), K.E. Creeger, Anthroposophic Press, Hudson 1997. Earlier edition Rudolf Steiner Press, London 1967.
50. Steiner, R., *Towards Social Renewal*, tr. M. Barton, Rudolf Steiner Press, London 1999. Earlier translations *The Threefold Commonwealth/The Threefold Social Order/Threefold Order of the Body Social*, tr. E. Bowen-Wedgwood, Anthroposophical Publishing Co., London 1922.
51. *Soziale Zukunft*, edited by Roman Boos, Zurich 1919/1920. Rudolf Steiner's essays published in the journal have been included in Vol. 24 of his collected works.
52. The first Goetheanum, where the lecture was given. It burned down the night of New Year's Eve 1922/23.
53. Moriz Benedikt (1835–1920), see Note 24.
54. *Die Gemuetsbewegung, ihr Wesen und ihr Einfluss auf koerperliche, besonders auf krankhafte Lebenserscheinungen* (Engl. translation *The Emotions*, in 4 volumes), a medical and psychological study by Dr Carl George Lange (1834–1900), professor of pathology in Copenhagen. A copy of the German edition is in Rudolf Steiner's private library.
55. See Rudolf Steiner's autobiography.
56. See note 11.
57. Steiner, R., *The Case for Anthroposophy*, tr. O. Barfield, extracts from Vol. 21 of the works, Rudolf Steiner Press, London 1970.
58. Friedrich Husemann, MD (1887–1959), founder and head of Wiesneck Sanatorium, Buchenbach nr Freiburg i.Br., now called Friedrich-Husemann-Klinik.
59. Johann Wolfgang von Goethe, *West-Eastern Divan*, Book of the Singer, Talismans.
60. Considerably more detailed record than in the 1975 German edition, thanks to a set of more extensive notes now available.
61. Max Asch, physician and member of the German Section of the Theosophical Society from 1904. Friend of Carl Ludwig Schleich, d. March 1911 (see Steiner, R., *Karmic Relationships* Vol. 4).
62. Drawing by Dr Kolisko.

63. See Carl Ludwig Schleich, *Vom Schaltwerk der Gedanken*, Berlin 1916, p. 261. A copy of this book is in Rudolf Steiner's private library. See also *Spiritual Science and Medicine*, lecture of 23 March 1920, tr. Anon, Rudolf Steiner Press, London 1975.

64. The highly uncertain information given in fractures of percentages (½%) was changed to 'very dilute' by the editor. In another context it was also necessary to refer to the possibility of the figures being misheard (see *Education for Special Needs*, tr. M. Adams, rev.).

65. Ita Wegman, MD (1876–1943), founder and head of the Institute of Clinical Medicine in Arlesheim. See Steiner, R., Wegman, I., *Extending Practical Medicine*, tr. A.R. Meuss/*Fundamentals of Therapy*, various translations).

66. 'emerges'—notes have 'comes bound to the air', the 'out' meaning in 'emerges' was added by the editor of the German edition.

RUDOLF STEINER'S COLLECTED WORKS

The German Edition of Rudolf Steiner's Collected Works (the *Gesamtausgabe* [GA] published by Rudolf Steiner Verlag, Dornach, Switzerland) presently runs to 354 titles, organized either by type of work (written or spoken), chronology, audience (public or other), or subject (education, art, etc.). For ease of comparison, the Collected Works in English [CW] follows the German organization exactly. A complete listing of the CWs follows with literal translations of the German titles. Other than in the case of the books published in his lifetime, titles were rarely given by Rudolf Steiner himself, and were often provided by the editors of the German editions. The titles in English are not necessarily the same as the German; and, indeed, over the past seventy-five years have frequently been different, with the same book sometimes appearing under different titles.

For ease of identification and to avoid confusion, we suggest that readers looking for a title should do so by CW number. Because the work of creating the Collected Works of Rudolf Steiner is an ongoing process, with new titles being published every year, we have not indicated in this listing which books are presently available. To find out what titles in the Collected Works are currently in print, please check our website at www.rudolfsteinerpress.com (or www.steinerbooks.org for US readers).

Written Work

CW 1	Goethe: Natural-Scientific Writings, Introduction, with Footnotes and Explanations in the text by Rudolf Steiner
CW 2	Outlines of an Epistemology of the Goethean World View, with Special Consideration of Schiller
CW 3	Truth and Science
CW 4	The Philosophy of Freedom
CW 4a	Documents to 'The Philosophy of Freedom'
CW 5	Friedrich Nietzsche, A Fighter against His Own Time
CW 6	Goethe's Worldview
CW 6a	Now in CW 30
CW 7	Mysticism at the Dawn of Modern Spiritual Life and Its Relationship with Modern Worldviews
CW 8	Christianity as Mystical Fact and the Mysteries of Antiquity
CW 9	Theosophy: An Introduction into Supersensible World Knowledge and Human Purpose
CW 10	How Does One Attain Knowledge of Higher Worlds?
CW 11	From the Akasha-Chronicle

CW 12	Levels of Higher Knowledge
CW 13	Occult Science in Outline
CW 14	Four Mystery Dramas
CW 15	The Spiritual Guidance of the Individual and Humanity
CW 16	A Way to Human Self-Knowledge: Eight Meditations
CW 17	The Threshold of the Spiritual World. Aphoristic Comments
CW 18	The Riddles of Philosophy in Their History, Presented as an Outline
CW 19	Contained in CW 24
CW 20	The Riddles of the Human Being: Articulated and Unarticulated in the Thinking, Views and Opinions of a Series of German and Austrian Personalities
CW 21	The Riddles of the Soul
CW 22	Goethe's Spiritual Nature And Its Revelation In 'Faust' and through the 'Fairy Tale of the Snake and the Lily'
CW 23	The Central Points of the Social Question in the Necessities of Life in the Present and the Future
CW 24	Essays Concerning the Threefold Division of the Social Organism and the Period 1915–1921
CW 25	Cosmology, Religion and Philosophy
CW 26	Anthroposophical Leading Thoughts
CW 27	Fundamentals for Expansion of the Art of Healing according to Spiritual-Scientific Insights
CW 28	The Course of My Life
CW 29	Collected Essays on Dramaturgy, 1889–1900
CW 30	Methodical Foundations of Anthroposophy: Collected Essays on Philosophy, Natural Science, Aesthetics and Psychology, 1884–1901
CW 31	Collected Essays on Culture and Current Events, 1887–1901
CW 32	Collected Essays on Literature, 1884–1902
CW 33	Biographies and Biographical Sketches, 1894–1905
CW 34	Lucifer-Gnosis: Foundational Essays on Anthroposophy and Reports from the Periodicals 'Lucifer' and 'Lucifer-Gnosis,' 1903–1908
CW 35	Philosophy and Anthroposophy: Collected Essays, 1904–1923
CW 36	The Goetheanum-Idea in the Middle of the Cultural Crisis of the Present: Collected Essays from the Periodical 'Das Goetheanum,' 1921–1925
CW 37	Now in CWs 260a and 251
CW 38	Letters, Vol. 1: 1881–1890
CW 39	Letters, Vol. 2: 1890–1925
CW 40	Truth-Wrought Words
CW 40a	Sayings, Poems and Mantras; Supplementary Volume
CW 42	Now in CWs 264–266
CW 43	Stage Adaptations
CW 44	On the Four Mystery Dramas. Sketches, Fragments and Para-lipomena on the Four Mystery Dramas
CW 45	Anthroposophy: A Fragment from the Year 1910

Public Lectures

Lectures to the Members of the Anthroposophical Society

CW 217a	Youth's Cognitive Task
CW 218	Spiritual Connections in the Forming of the Human Organism
CW 219	The Relationship of the World of the Stars to the Human Being, and of the Human Being to the World of the Stars. The Spiritual Communion of Humanity
CW 220	Living Knowledge of Nature. Intellectual Fall and Spiritual Redemption
CW 221	Earth-Knowing and Heaven-Insight
CW 222	The Imparting of Impulses to World-Historical Events through Spiritual Powers
CW 223	The Cycle of the Year as Breathing Process of the Earth and the Four Great Festival-Seasons. Anthroposophy and the Human Heart (Gemüt)
CW 224	The Human Soul and its Connection with Divine-Spiritual Individualities. The Internalization of the Festivals of the Year
CW 225	Three Perspectives of Anthroposophy. Cultural Phenomena observed from a Spiritual-Scientific Perspective
CW 226	Human Being, Human Destiny, and World Development
CW 227	Initiation-Knowledge
CW 228	Science of Initiation and Knowledge of the Stars. The Human Being in the Past, the Present, and the Future from the Viewpoint of the Development of Consciousness
CW 229	The Experiencing of the Course of the Year in Four Cosmic Imaginations
CW 230	The Human Being as Harmony of the Creative, Building, and Formative World-Word
CW 231	The Supersensible Human Being, Understood Anthroposophically
CW 232	The Forming of the Mysteries
CW 233	World History Illuminated by Anthroposophy and as the Foundation for Knowledge of the Human Spirit
CW 233a	Mystery Sites of the Middle Ages: Rosicrucianism and the Modern Initiation-Principle. The Festival of Easter as Part of the History of the Mysteries of Humanity
CW 234	Anthroposophy. A Summary after 21 Years
CW 235	Esoteric Observations of Karmic Relationships in 6 Volumes, Vol. 1
CW 236	Esoteric Observations of Karmic Relationships in 6 Volumes, Vol. 2
CW 237	Esoteric Observations of Karmic Relationships in 6 Volumes, Vol. 3: The Karmic Relationships of the Anthroposophical Movement
CW 238	Esoteric Observations of Karmic Relationships in 6 Volumes, Vol. 4: The Spiritual Life of the Present in Relationship to the Anthroposophical Movement
CW 239	Esoteric Observations of Karmic Relationships in 6 Volumes, Vol. 5

CW 240   Esoteric Observations of Karmic Relationships in 6 Volumes, Vol. 6
CW 243   The Consciousness of the Initiate
CW 245   Instructions for an Esoteric Schooling
CW 250   The Building-Up of the Anthroposophical Society. From the Beginning to the Outbreak of the First World War
CW 251   The History of the Goetheanum Building-Association
CW 252   Life in the Anthroposophical Society from the First World War to the Burning of the First Goetheanum
CW 253   The Problems of Living Together in the Anthroposophical Society. On the Dornach Crisis of 1915. With Highlights on Swedenborg's Clairvoyance, the Views of Freudian Psychoanalysts, and the Concept of Love in Relation to Mysticism
CW 254   The Occult Movement in the 19th Century and Its Relationship to World Culture. Significant Points from the Exoteric Cultural Life around the Middle of the 19th Century
CW 255   Rudolf Steiner during the First World War
CW 255a   Anthroposophy and the Reformation of Society. On the History of the Threefold Movement
CW 255b   Anthroposophy and Its Opponents, 1919–1921
CW 256   How Can the Anthroposophical Movement Be Financed?
CW 256a   Futurum, Inc. / International Laboratories, Inc.
CW 256b   The Coming Day, Inc.
CW 257   Anthroposophical Community-Building
CW 258   The History of and Conditions for the Anthroposophical Movement in Relationship to the Anthroposophical Society. A Stimulus to Self-Contemplation
CW 259   The Year of Destiny 1923 in the History of the Anthroposophical Society. From the Burning of the Goetheanum to the Christmas Conference
CW 260   The Christmas Conference for the Founding of the General Anthroposophical Society
CW 260a   The Constitution of the General Anthroposophical Society and the School for Spiritual Science. The Rebuilding of the Goetheanum
CW 261   Our Dead. Addresses, Words of Remembrance, and Meditative Verses, 1906–1924
CW 262   Rudolf Steiner and Marie Steiner-von Sivers: Correspondence and Documents, 1901–1925
CW 263/1 Rudolf Steiner and Edith Maryon: Correspondence: Letters, Verses, Sketches, 1912–1924
CW 264   On the History and the Contents of the First Section of the Esoteric School from 1904 to 1914. Letters, Newsletters, Documents, Lectures
CW 265   On the History and from the Contents of the Ritual-Knowledge Section of the Esoteric School from 1904 to 1914. Documents, and Lectures from the Years 1906 to 1914, as Well as on New Approaches to Ritual-Knowledge Work in the Years 1921–1924

CW 342   Lectures and Courses on Christian Religious Work, Vol. 1: Anthroposophical Foundations for a Renewed Christian Religious Working

CW 343   Lectures and Courses on Christian Religious Work, Vol. 2: Spiritual Knowledge—Religious Feeling—Cultic Doing

CW 344   Lectures and Courses on Christian Religious Work, Vol. 3: Lectures at the Founding of the Christian Community

CW 345   Lectures and Courses on Christian Religious Work, Vol. 4: Concerning the Nature of the Working Word

CW 346   Lectures and Courses on Christian Religious Work, Vol. 5: The Apocalypse and the Work of the Priest

CW 347   The Knowledge of the Nature of the Human Being According to Body, Soul and Spirit. On Earlier Conditions of the Earth

CW 348   On Health and Illness. Foundations of a Spiritual-Scientific Doctrine of the Senses

CW 349   On the Life of the Human Being and of the Earth. On the Nature of Christianity

CW 350   Rhythms in the Cosmos and in the Human Being. How Does One Come To See the Spiritual World?

CW 351   The Human Being and the World. The Influence of the Spirit in Nature. On the Nature of Bees

CW 352   Nature and the Human Being Observed Spiritual-Scientifically

CW 353   The History of Humanity and the World-Views of the Folk Cultures

CW 354   The Creation of the World and the Human Being. Life on Earth and the Influence of the Stars

SIGNIFICANT EVENTS IN THE LIFE OF
RUDOLF STEINER

1829: June 23: birth of Johann Steiner (1829–1910)—Rudolf Steiner's father—in Geras, Lower Austria.

1834: May 8: birth of Franciska Blie (1834–1918)—Rudolf Steiner's mother—in Horn, Lower Austria. 'My father and mother were both children of the glorious Lower Austrian forest district north of the Danube.'

1860: May 16: marriage of Johann Steiner and Franciska Blie.

1861: February 25: birth of *Rudolf Joseph Lorenz Steiner* in Kraljevec, Croatia, near the border with Hungary, where Johann Steiner works as a telegrapher for the South Austria Railroad. Rudolf Steiner is baptized two days later, February 27, the date usually given as his birthday.

1862: Summer: the family moves to Mödling, Lower Austria.

1863: The family moves to Pottschach, Lower Austria, near the Styrian border, where Johann Steiner becomes stationmaster. 'The view stretched to the mountains ... majestic peaks in the distance and the sweet charm of nature in the immediate surroundings.'

1864: November 15: birth of Rudolf Steiner's sister, Leopoldine (d. November 1, 1927). She will become a seamstress and live with her parents for the rest of her life.

1866: July 28: birth of Rudolf Steiner's deaf-mute brother, Gustav (d. May 1, 1941).

1867: Rudolf Steiner enters the village school. Following a disagreement between his father and the schoolmaster, whose wife falsely accused the boy of causing a commotion, Rudolf Steiner is taken out of school and taught at home.

1868: A critical experience. Unknown to the family, an aunt dies in a distant town. Sitting in the station waiting room, Rudolf Steiner sees her 'form,' which speaks to him, asking for help. 'Beginning with this experience, a new soul life began in the boy, one in which not only the outer trees and mountains spoke to him, but also the worlds that lay behind them. From this moment on, the boy began to live with the spirits of nature ...'

1869: The family moves to the peaceful, rural village of Neudorfl, near Wiener-Neustadt in present-day Austria. Rudolf Steiner attends the village school. Because of the 'unorthodoxy' of his writing and spelling, he has to do 'extra lessons.'

1870: Through a book lent to him by his tutor, he discovers geometry: 'To grasp something purely in the spirit brought me inner happiness. I know that I first learned happiness through geometry.' The same tutor allows him to draw, while other students still struggle with their reading and writing. 'An artistic element' thus enters his education.

1871: Though his parents are not religious, Rudolf Steiner becomes a 'church child,' a favorite of the priest, who was 'an exceptional character.' 'Up to the age of ten or eleven, among those I came to know, he was far and away the most significant.' Among other things, he introduces Steiner to Copernican, heliocentric cosmology. As an altar boy, Rudolf Steiner serves at Masses, funerals, and Corpus Christi processions. At year's end, after an incident in which he escapes a thrashing, his father forbids him to go to church.

1872: Rudolf Steiner transfers to grammar school in Wiener-Neustadt, a five-mile walk from home, which must be done in all weathers.

1873–75: Through his teachers and on his own, Rudolf Steiner has many wonderful experiences with science and mathematics. Outside school, he teaches himself analytic geometry, trigonometry, differential equations, and calculus.

1876: Rudolf Steiner begins tutoring other students. He learns bookbinding from his father. He also teaches himself stenography.

1877: Rudolf Steiner discovers Kant's *Critique of Pure Reason*, which he reads and rereads. He also discovers and reads von Rotteck's *World History*.

1878: He studies extensively in contemporary psychology and philosophy.

1879: Rudolf Steiner graduates from high school with honors. His father is transferred to Inzersdorf, near Vienna. He uses his first visit to Vienna 'to purchase a great number of philosophy books'—Kant, Fichte, Schelling, and Hegel, as well as numerous histories of philosophy. His aim: to find a path from the 'I' to nature.

October 1879–1883: Rudolf Steiner attends the Technical College in Vienna—to study mathematics, chemistry, physics, mineralogy, botany, zoology, biology, geology, and mechanics—with a scholarship. He also attends lectures in history and literature, while avidly reading philosophy on his own. His two favorite professors are Karl Julius Schröer (German language and literature) and Edmund Reitlinger (physics). He also audits lectures by Robert Zimmerman on aesthetics and Franz Brentano on philosophy. During this year he begins his friendship with Moritz Zitter (1861–1921), who will help support him financially when he is in Berlin.

1880: Rudolf Steiner attends lectures on Schiller and Goethe by Karl Julius Schröer, who becomes his mentor. Also 'through a remarkable combination of circumstances,' he meets Felix Koguzki, a 'herb gatherer' and healer, who could 'see deeply into the secrets of nature.' Rudolf Steiner will meet and study with this 'emissary of the Master' throughout his time in Vienna.

1881: January: '... I didn't sleep a wink. I was busy with philosophical problems until about 12:30 a.m. Then, finally, I threw myself down on my couch. All my striving during the previous year had been to research whether the following statement by Schelling was true or not: *Within everyone dwells a secret, marvelous capacity to draw back from the stream of time—out of the self clothed in all that comes to us from outside—into our innermost being and there, in the immutable form of the Eternal, to look into ourselves.* I believe, and I am still quite certain of it, that I discovered this capacity in myself; I had long had an inkling of it. Now the whole of idealist philosophy stood before me in modified form. What's a sleepless night compared to that!'

Rudolf Steiner begins communicating with leading thinkers of the day, who send him books in return, which he reads eagerly.

July: 'I am not one of those who dives into the day like an animal in human form. I pursue a quite specific goal, an idealistic aim—knowledge of the truth! This cannot be done offhandedly. It requires the greatest striving in the world, free of all egotism, and equally of all resignation.'

August: Steiner puts down on paper for the first time thoughts for a 'Philosophy of Freedom.' 'The striving for the absolute: this human yearning is freedom.' He also seeks to outline a 'peasant philosophy,' describing what the worldview of a 'peasant'—one who lives close to the earth and the old ways—really is.

1881–1882: Felix Koguzki, the herb gatherer, reveals himself to be the envoy of another, higher initiatory personality, who instructs Rudolf Steiner to penetrate Fichte's philosophy and to master modern scientific thinking as a preparation for right entry into the spirit. This 'Master' also teaches him the double (evolutionary and involutionary) nature of time.

1882: Through the offices of Karl Julius Schröer, Rudolf Steiner is asked by Joseph Kurschner to edit Goethe's scientific works for the *Deutschen National-Literatur* edition. He writes 'A Possible Critique of Atomistic Concepts' and sends it to Friedrich Theodore Vischer.

1883: Rudolf Steiner completes his college studies and begins work on the Goethe project.

1884: First volume of Goethe's *Scientific Writings* (CW 1) appears (March). He lectures on Goethe and Lessing, and Goethe's approach to science. In July, he enters the household of Ladislaus and Pauline Specht as tutor to the four Specht boys. He will live there until 1890. At this time, he meets Josef Breuer (1842–1925), the coauthor with Sigmund Freud of *Studies in Hysteria*, who is the Specht family doctor.

1885: While continuing to edit Goethe's writings, Rudolf Steiner reads deeply in contemporary philosophy (Edouard von Hartmann, Johannes Volkelt, and Richard Wahle, among others).

1886: May: Rudolf Steiner sends Kurschner the manuscript of *Outlines of Goethe's Theory of Knowledge* (CW 2), which appears in October, and which he sends out widely. He also meets the poet Marie Eugenie Delle Grazie and writes 'Nature and Our Ideals' for her. He attends her salon, where he meets many priests, theologians, and philosophers, who will become his friends. Meanwhile, the director of the Goethe Archive in Weimar requests his collaboration with the *Sophien* edition of Goethe's works, particularly the writings on color.

1887: At the beginning of the year, Rudolf Steiner is very sick. As the year progresses and his health improves, he becomes increasingly 'a man of letters,' lecturing, writing essays, and taking part in Austrian cultural life. In August–September, the second volume of Goethe's *Scientific Writings* appears.

1888: January–July: Rudolf Steiner assumes editorship of the 'German Weekly' (*Deutsche Wochenschrift*). He begins lecturing more intensively, giving, for example, a lecture titled 'Goethe as Father of a New Aesthetics.' He meets and becomes soul friends with Friedrich Eckstein (1861–1939), a vegetarian, philosopher of symbolism, alchemist, and musician, who will introduce him to various spiritual currents (including Theosophy) and with whom he will meditate and interpret esoteric and alchemical texts.

1889: Rudolf Steiner first reads Nietzsche (*Beyond Good and Evil*). He encounters Theosophy again and learns of Madame Blavatsky in the Theosophical circle around Marie Lang (1858–1934). Here he also meets well-known figures of Austrian life, as well as esoteric figures like the occultist Franz Hartman and Karl Leinigen-Billigen (translator of C.G. Harrison's *The Transcendental Universe*). During this period, Steiner first reads A.P. Sinnett's *Esoteric Buddhism* and Mabel Collins's *Light on the Path*. He also begins traveling, visiting Budapest, Weimar, and Berlin (where he meets philosopher Edouard von Hartmann).

1890: Rudolf Steiner finishes volume 3 of Goethe's scientific writings. He begins his doctoral dissertation, which will become *Truth and Science* (CW 3). He also meets the poet and feminist Rosa Mayreder (1858–1938), with whom he can exchange his most intimate thoughts. In September, Rudolf Steiner moves to Weimar to work in the Goethe-Schiller Archive.

1891: Volume 3 of the Kurschner edition of Goethe appears. Meanwhile, Rudolf Steiner edits Goethe's studies in mineralogy and scientific writings for the *Sophien* edition. He meets Ludwig Laistner of the Cotta Publishing Company, who asks for a book on the basic question of metaphysics. From this will result, ultimately, *The Philosophy of Freedom* (CW 4), which will be published not by Cotta but by Emil Felber. In October, Rudolf Steiner takes the oral exam for a doctorate in philosophy, mathematics, and mechanics at Rostock University, receiving his doctorate on the twenty-sixth. In November, he gives his first lecture on Goethe's 'Fairy Tale' in Vienna.

1892: Rudolf Steiner continues work at the Goethe-Schiller Archive and on his *Philosophy of Freedom*. *Truth and Science*, his doctoral dissertation, is published. Steiner undertakes to write introductions to books on Schopenhauer and Jean Paul for Cotta. At year's end, he finds lodging with Anna Eunike, née Schulz (1853–1911), a widow with four daughters and a son. He also develops a friendship with Otto Erich Hartleben (1864–1905) with whom he shares literary interests.

1893: Rudolf Steiner begins his habit of producing many reviews and articles. In March, he gives a lecture titled 'Hypnotism, with Reference to Spiritism.' In September, volume 4 of the Kurschner edition is completed. In November, *The Philosophy of Freedom* appears. This year, too, he meets John Henry Mackay (1864–1933), the anarchist, and Max Stirner, a scholar and biographer.

1894: Rudolf Steiner meets Elisabeth Förster Nietzsche, the philosopher's sister, and begins to read Nietzsche in earnest, beginning with the as yet unpublished *Antichrist*. He also meets Ernst Haeckel (1834–1919). In the fall, he begins to write *Nietzsche, A Fighter against His Time* (CW 5).

1895: May, *Nietzsche, A Fighter against His Time* appears.

1896: January 22: Rudolf Steiner sees Friedrich Nietzsche for the first and only time. Moves between the Nietzsche and the Goethe-Schiller Archives, where he completes his work before year's end. He falls out with Elisabeth Förster Nietzsche, thus ending his association with the Nietzsche Archive.

1897: Rudolf Steiner finishes the manuscript of *Goethe's Worldview* (CW 6). He moves to Berlin with Anna Eunike and begins editorship of the *Magazin für Literatur*. From now on, Steiner will write countless reviews, literary and philosophical articles, and so on. He begins lecturing at the 'Free Literary Society.' In September, he attends the Zionist Congress in Basel. He sides with Dreyfus in the Dreyfus affair.

1898: Rudolf Steiner is very active as an editor in the political, artistic, and theatrical life of Berlin. He becomes friendly with John Henry Mackay and poet Ludwig Jacobowski (1868–1900). He joins Jacobowski's circle of writers, artists, and scientists—'The Coming Ones' (*Die Kommenden*)— and contributes lectures to the group until 1903. He also lectures at the 'League for College Pedagogy.' He writes an article for Goethe's ses- quicentennial, 'Goethe's Secret Revelation,' on the 'Fairy Tale of the Green Snake and the Beautiful Lily.'

1898–99: 'This was a trying time for my soul as I looked at Christianity. . . . I was able to progress only by contemplating, by means of spiritual perception, the evolution of Christianity. . . . Conscious knowledge of real Chris- tianity began to dawn in me around the turn of the century. This seed continued to develop. My soul trial occurred shortly before the beginning of the twentieth century. It was decisive for my soul's development that I stood spiritually before the Mystery of Golgotha in a deep and solemn celebration of knowledge.'

1899: Rudolf Steiner begins teaching and giving lectures and lecture cycles at the Workers' College, founded by Wilhelm Liebknecht (1826–1900). He will continue to do so until 1904. Writes: *Literature and Spiritual Life in the Nineteenth Century; Individualism in Philosophy; Haeckel and His Opponents; Poetry in the Present;* and begins what will become (fifteen years later) *The Riddles of Philosophy* (CW 18). He also meets many artists and writers, including Käthe Kollwitz, Stefan Zweig, and Rainer Maria Rilke. On October 31, he marries Anna Eunike.

1900: 'I thought that the turn of the century must bring humanity a new light. It seemed to me that the separation of human thinking and willing from the spirit had peaked. A turn or reversal of direction in human evolution seemed to me a necessity.' Rudolf Steiner finishes *World and Life Views in the Nineteenth Century* (the second part of what will become *The Riddles of Philosophy*) and dedicates it to Ernst Haeckel. It is published in March. He continues lecturing at *Die Kommenden*, whose leadership he assumes after the death of Jacobowski. Also, he gives the Gutenberg Jubilee lecture before 7,000 typesetters and printers. In September, Rudolf Steiner is invited by Count and Countess Brockdorff to lecture in the Theosophical Library. His first lecture is on Nietzsche. His second lecture is titled 'Goethe's Secret Revelation.' October 6, he begins a lecture cycle on the mystics that will become *Mystics after Modernism* (CW 7). November-December: 'Marie von Sivers appears in the audience....' Also in November, Steiner gives his first lecture at the Giordano Bruno Bund (where he will continue to lecture until May, 1905). He speaks on Bruno and modern Rome, focusing on the importance of the philosophy of Thomas Aquinas as monism.

1901:   In continual financial straits, Rudolf Steiner's early friends Moritz Zitter and Rosa Mayreder help support him. In October, he begins the lecture cycle *Christianity as Mystical Fact* (CW 8) at the Theosophical Library. In November, he gives his first 'Theosophical lecture' on Goethe's 'Fairy Tale' in Hamburg at the invitation of Wilhelm Hubbe-Schleiden. He also attends a gathering to celebrate the founding of the Theosophical Society at Count and Countess Brockdorff's. He gives a lecture cycle, 'From Buddha to Christ,' for the circle of the *Kommenden*. November 17, Marie von Sivers asks Rudolf Steiner if Theosophy needs a Western-Christian spiritual movement (to complement Theosophy's Eastern emphasis). 'The question was posed. Now, following spiritual laws, I could begin to give an answer....' In December, Rudolf Steiner writes his first article for a Theosophical publication. At year's end, the Brockdorffs and possibly Wilhelm Hubbe-Schleiden ask Rudolf Steiner to join the Theosophical Society and undertake the leadership of the German section. Rudolf Steiner agrees, on the condition that Marie von Sivers (then in Italy) work with him.

1902:   Beginning in January, Rudolf Steiner attends the opening of the Workers' School in Spandau with Rosa Luxemburg (1870–1919). January 17, Rudolf Steiner joins the Theosophical Society. In April, he is asked to become general secretary of the German Section of the Theosophical Society, and works on preparations for its founding. In July, he visits London for a Theosophical congress. He meets Bertram Keightly, G.R.S. Mead, A.P. Sinnett, and Annie Besant, among others. In September, *Christianity as Mystical Fact* appears. In October, Rudolf Steiner gives his first public lecture on Theosophy ('Monism and Theosophy') to about three hundred people at the Giordano Bruno Bund. On October 19–21, the German Section of the Theosophical Society has its first meeting; Rudolf Steiner is the general secretary, and Annie Besant attends. Steiner lectures on practical karma studies. On October 23, Annie Besant inducts Rudolf Steiner into the Esoteric School of the Theosophical Society. On October 25, Steiner begins a weekly series of lectures: 'The Field of Theosophy.' During this year, Rudolf Steiner also first meets Ita Wegman (1876–1943), who will become his close collaborator in his final years.

1903:   Rudolf Steiner holds about 300 lectures and seminars. In May, the first issue of the periodical *Luzifer* appears. In June, Rudolf Steiner visits

London for the first meeting of the Federation of the European Sections of the Theosophical Society, where he meets Colonel Olcott. He begins to write *Theosophy* (CW 9).

1904: Rudolf Steiner continues lecturing at the Workers' College and elsewhere (about 90 lectures), while lecturing intensively all over Germany among Theosophists (about 140 lectures). In February, he meets Carl Unger (1878–1929), who will become a member of the board of the Anthroposophical Society (1913). In March, he meets Michael Bauer (1871–1929), a Christian mystic, who will also be on the board. In May, *Theosophy* appears, with the dedication: 'To the spirit of Giordano Bruno.' Rudolf Steiner and Marie von Sivers visit London for meetings with Annie Besant. June: Rudolf Steiner and Marie von Sivers attend the meeting of the Federation of European Sections of the Theosophical Society in Amsterdam. In July, Steiner begins the articles in *Luzifer-Gnosis* that will become *How to Know Higher Worlds* (CW 10) and *Cosmic Memory* (CW 11). In September, Annie Besant visits Germany. In December, Steiner lectures on Freemasonry. He mentions the High Grade Masonry derived from John Yarker and represented by Theodore Reuss and Karl Kellner as a blank slate 'into which a good image could be placed.'

1905: This year, Steiner ends his non-Theosophical lecturing activity. Supported by Marie von Sivers, his Theosophical lecturing—both in public and in the Theosophical Society—increases significantly: 'The German Theosophical Movement is of exceptional importance.' Steiner recommends reading, among others, Fichte, Jacob Boehme, and Angelus Silesius. He begins to introduce Christian themes into Theosophy. He also begins to work with doctors (Felix Peipers and Ludwig Noll). In July, he is in London for the Federation of European Sections, where he attends a lecture by Annie Besant: 'I have seldom seen Mrs. Besant speak in so inward and heartfelt a manner....' 'Through Mrs. Besant I have found the way to H.P. Blavatsky.' September to October, he gives a course of thirty-one lectures for a small group of esoteric students. In October, the annual meeting of the German Section of the Theosophical Society, which still remains very small, takes place. Rudolf Steiner reports membership has risen from 121 to 377 members. In November, seeking to establish esoteric 'continuity,' Rudolf Steiner and Marie von Sivers participate in a 'Memphis-Misraim' Masonic ceremony. They pay forty-five marks for membership. 'Yesterday, you saw how little remains of former esoteric institutions.' 'We are dealing only with a "framework"... for the present, nothing lies behind it. The occult powers have completely withdrawn.'

1906: Expansion of Theosophical work. Rudolf Steiner gives about 245 lectures, only 44 of which take place in Berlin. Cycles are given in Paris, Leipzig, Stuttgart, and Munich. Esoteric work also intensifies. Rudolf Steiner begins writing *An Outline of Esoteric Science* (CW 13). In January, Rudolf Steiner receives permission (a patent) from the Great Orient of the Scottish A & A Thirty-Three Degree Rite of the Order of the Ancient

Freemasons of the Memphis-Misraim Rite to direct a chapter under the name 'Mystica Aeterna.' This will become the 'Cognitive-Ritual Section' (also called 'Misraim Service') of the Esoteric School. (See: *Freemasonry and Ritual Work: The Misraim Service*, CW 265). During this time, Steiner also meets Albert Schweitzer. In May, he is in Paris, where he visits Edouard Schuré. Many Russians attend his lectures (including Konstantin Balmont, Dimitri Mereszkovski, Zinaida Hippius, and Maximilian Woloshin). He attends the General Meeting of the European Federation of the Theosophical Society, at which Col. Olcott is present for the last time. He spends the year's end in Venice and Rome, where he writes and works on his translation of H.P. Blavatsky's *Key to Theosophy*.

1907: Further expansion of the German Theosophical Movement according to the Rosicrucian directive to 'introduce spirit into the world'—in education, in social questions, in art, and in science. In February, Col. Olcott dies in Adyar. Before he dies, Olcott indicates that 'the Masters' wish Annie Besant to succeed him: much politicking ensues. Rudolf Steiner supports Besant's candidacy. April-May: preparations for the Congress of the Federation of European Sections of the Theosophical Society—the great, watershed Whitsun 'Munich Congress,' attended by Annie Besant and others. Steiner decides to separate Eastern and Western (Christian-Rosicrucian) esoteric schools. He takes his esoteric school out of the Theosophical Society (Besant and Rudolf Steiner are 'in harmony' on this). Steiner makes his first lecture tours to Austria and Hungary. That summer, he is in Italy. In September, he visits Edouard Schuré, who will write the introduction to the French edition of *Christianity as Mystical Fact* in Barr, Alsace. Rudolf Steiner writes the autobiographical statement known as the 'Barr Document.' In *Luzifer-Gnosis*, 'The Education of the Child' appears.

1908: The movement grows (membership: 1,150). Lecturing expands. Steiner makes his first extended lecture tour to Holland and Scandinavia, as well as visits to Naples and Sicily. Themes: St. John's Gospel, the Apocalypse, Egypt, science, philosophy, and logic. *Luzifer-Gnosis* ceases publication. In Berlin, Marie von Sivers (with Johanna Mücke (1864–1949) forms the *Philosophisch-Theosophisch* (after 1915 *Philosophisch-Anthroposophisch*) *Verlag* to publish Steiner's work. Steiner gives lecture cycles titled *The Gospel of St. John* (CW 103) and *The Apocalypse* (104).

1909: *An Outline of Esoteric Science* appears. Lecturing and travel continues. Rudolf Steiner's spiritual research expands to include the polarity of Lucifer and Ahriman; the work of great individualities in history; the Maitreya Buddha and the Bodhisattvas; spiritual economy (CW 109); the work of the spiritual hierarchies in heaven and on earth (CW 110). He also deepens and intensifies his research into the Gospels, giving lectures on the Gospel of St. Luke (CW 114) with the first mention of two Jesus children. Meets and becomes friends with Christian Morgenstern (1871–1914). In April, he lays the foundation stone for the Malsch model—the building that will lead to the first Goetheanum. In May, the International Congress of the Federation of European Sections of the

Theosophical Society takes place in Budapest. Rudolf Steiner receives the Subba Row medal for *How to Know Higher Worlds*. During this time, Charles W. Leadbeater discovers Jiddu Krishnamurti (1895–1986) and proclaims him the future 'world teacher,' the bearer of the Maitreya Buddha and the 'reappearing Christ.' In October, Steiner delivers seminal lectures on 'anthroposophy,' which he will try, unsuccessfully, to rework over the next years into the unfinished work, *Anthroposophy (A Fragment)* (CW 45).

1910: New themes: *The Reappearance of Christ in the Etheric* (CW 118); *The Fifth Gospel; The Mission of Folk Souls* (CW 121); *Occult History* (CW 126); the evolving development of etheric cognitive capacities. Rudolf Steiner continues his Gospel research with *The Gospel of St. Matthew* (CW 123). In January, his father dies. In April, he takes a month-long trip to Italy, including Rome, Monte Cassino, and Sicily. He also visits Scandinavia again. July–August, he writes the first mystery drama, *The Portal of Initiation* (CW 14). In November, he gives 'psychosophy' lectures. In December, he submits 'On the Psychological Foundations and Episte-mological Framework of Theosophy' to the International Philosophical Congress in Bologna.

1911: The crisis in the Theosophical Society deepens. In January, 'The Order of the Rising Sun,' which will soon become 'The Order of the Star in the East,' is founded for the coming world teacher, Krishnamurti. At the same time, Marie von Sivers, Rudolf Steiner's coworker, falls ill. Fewer lectures are given, but important new ground is broken. In Prague, in March, Steiner meets Franz Kafka (1883–1924) and Hugo Bergmann (1883-1975). In April, he delivers his paper to the Philosophical Congress. He writes the second mystery drama, *The Soul's Probation* (CW 14). Also, while Marie von Sivers is convalescing, Rudolf Steiner begins work on *Calendar 1912/1913*, which will contain the 'Calendar of the Soul' meditations. On March 19, Anna (Eunike) Steiner dies. In September, Rudolf Steiner visits Einsiedeln, birthplace of Paracelsus. In December, Friedrich Rittelmeyer, future founder of the Christian Community, meets Rudolf Steiner. The *Johannes-Bauverein*, the 'building committee,' which would lead to the first Goetheanum (first planned for Munich), is also founded, and a preliminary committee for the founding of an indepen-dent association is created that, in the following year, will become the Anthroposophical Society. Important lecture cycles include *Occult Phy-siology* (CW 128); *Wonders of the World* (CW 129); *From Jesus to Christ* (CW 131). Other themes: esoteric Christianity; Christian Rosenkreutz; the spiritual guidance of humanity; the sense world and the world of the spirit.

1912: Despite the ongoing, now increasing crisis in the Theosophical Society, much is accomplished: *Calendar 1912/1913* is published; eurythmy is created; both the third mystery drama, *The Guardian of the Threshold* (CW 14) and *A Way of Self-Knowledge* (CW 16) are written. New (or renewed) themes included life between death and rebirth and karma and reincarnation. Other lecture cycles: *Spiritual Beings in the Heavenly Bodies and in the Kingdoms of Nature* (CW 136); *The Human Being in the Light of Occultism, Theosophy, and Philosophy* (CW 137); *The Gospel of St. Mark* (CW 139); and *The Bhagavad Gita and the Epistles of Paul* (CW 142). On May 8, Rudolf Steiner celebrates White Lotus Day, H.P. Blavatsky's death day, which he had faithfully observed for the past decade, for the last time. In August, Rudolf Steiner suggests the 'independent association' be called the 'Anthroposophical Society.' In September, the first eurythmy course takes place. In October, Rudolf Steiner declines recognition of a Theosophical Society lodge dedicated to the Star of the East and decides to expel all Theosophical Society members belonging to the order. Also, with Marie von Sivers, he first visits Dornach, near Basel, Switzerland, and they stand on the hill where the Goetheanum will be built. In November, a Theosophical Society lodge is opened by direct mandate from Adyar (Annie Besant). In December, a meeting of the German section occurs at which it is decided that belonging to the Order of the Star of the East is incompatible with membership in the Theosophical Society. December 28: informal founding of the Anthroposophical Society in Berlin.

1913:   Expulsion of the German section from the Theosophical Society. February 2–3: Foundation meeting of the Anthroposophical Society. Board members include: Marie von Sivers, Michael Bauer, and Carl Unger. September 20: Laying of the foundation stone for the *Johannes Bau* (Goetheanum) in Dornach. Building begins immediately. The third mystery drama, *The Soul's Awakening* (CW 14), is completed. Also: *The Threshold of the Spiritual World* (CW 147). Lecture cycles include: *The Bhagavad Gita and the Epistles of Paul* and *The Esoteric Meaning of the Bhagavad Gita* (CW 146), which the Russian philosopher Nikolai Berdyaev attends; *The Mysteries of the East and of Christianity* (CW 144); *The Effects of Esoteric Development* (CW 145); and *The Fifth Gospel* (CW 148). In May, Rudolf Steiner is in London and Paris, where anthroposophical work continues.

1914:   Building continues on the *Johannes Bau* (Goetheanum) in Dornach, with artists and coworkers from seventeen nations. The general assembly of the Anthroposophical Society takes place. In May, Rudolf Steiner visits Paris, as well as Chartres Cathedral. June 28: assassination in Sarajevo ('Now the catastrophe has happened!'). August 1: War is declared. Rudolf Steiner returns to Germany from Dornach—he will travel back and forth. He writes the last chapter of *The Riddles of Philosophy*. Lecture cycles include: *Human and Cosmic Thought* (CW 151); *Inner Being of Humanity between Death and a New Birth* (CW 153); *Occult Reading and Occult Hearing* (CW 156). December 24: marriage of Rudolf Steiner and Marie von Sivers.

1915:   Building continues. Life after death becomes a major theme, also art. Writes: *Thoughts during a Time of War* (CW 24). Lectures include: *The Secret of Death* (CW 159); *The Uniting of Humanity through the Christ Impulse* (CW 165).

1916:   Rudolf Steiner begins work with Edith Maryon (1872–1924) on the sculpture 'The Representative of Humanity' ('The Group'—Christ, Lucifer, and Ahriman). He also works with the alchemist Alexander von Bernus on the quarterly *Das Reich*. He writes *The Riddle of Humanity* (CW 20). Lectures include: *Necessity and Freedom in World History and Human Action* (CW 166); *Past and Present in the Human Spirit* (CW 167); *The Karma of Vocation* (CW 172); *The Karma of Untruthfulness* (CW 173).

1917:   Russian Revolution. The U.S. enters the war. Building continues. Rudolf Steiner delineates the idea of the 'threefold nature of the human being' (in a public lecture March 15) and the 'threefold nature of the social organism' (hammered out in May-June with the help of Otto von Lerchenfeld and Ludwig Polzer-Hoditz in the form of two documents titled *Memoranda*, which were distributed in high places). August–September: Rudolf Steiner writes *The Riddles of the Soul* (CW 20). Also: commentary on 'The Chemical Wedding of Christian Rosenkreutz' for Alexander Bernus (*Das Reich*). Lectures include: *The Karma of Materialism* (CW 176); *The Spiritual Background of the Outer World: The Fall of the Spirits of Darkness* (CW 177).

1918:   March 18: peace treaty of Brest-Litovsk—'Now everything will truly enter chaos! What is needed is cultural renewal.' June: Rudolf Steiner visits Karlstein (Grail) Castle outside Prague. Lecture cycle: *From Symptom to Reality in Modern History* (CW 185). In mid-November, Emil Molt, of the Waldorf-Astoria Cigarette Company, has the idea of founding a school for his workers' children.

1919:   Focus on the threefold social organism: tireless travel, countless lectures, meetings, and publications. At the same time, a new public stage of Anthroposophy emerges as cultural renewal begins. The coming years will see initiatives in pedagogy, medicine, pharmacology, and agriculture. January 27: threefold meeting: ' We must first of all, with the money we have, found free schools that can bring people what they need.' February: first public eurythmy performance in Zurich. Also: 'Appeal to the German People' (CW 24), circulated March 6 as a newspaper insert. In April, *Towards Social Renewal* (CW 23) appears— 'perhaps the most widely read of all books on politics appearing since the war.' Rudolf Steiner is asked to undertake the 'direction and leadership' of the school founded by the Waldorf-Astoria Company. Rudolf Steiner begins to talk about the 'renewal' of education. May 30: a building is selected and purchased for the future Waldorf School. August–September, Rudolf Steiner gives a lecture course for Waldorf teachers, *The Foundations of Human Experience (Study of Man)* (CW 293). September 7: Opening of the first Waldorf School. December (into January): first science course, the *Light Course* (CW 320).

1920:   The Waldorf School flourishes. New threefold initiatives. Founding of limited companies *Der Kommende Tag* and *Futurum A.G.* to infuse spiritual values into the economic realm. Rudolf Steiner also focuses on the sciences. Lectures: *Introducing Anthroposophical Medicine* (CW 312); *The Warmth Course* (CW 321); *The Boundaries of Natural Science* (CW 322); *The Redemption of Thinking* (CW 74). February: Johannes Werner

Klein—later a cofounder of the Christian Community—asks Rudolf Steiner about the possibility of a 'religious renewal,' a 'Johannine church.' In March, Rudolf Steiner gives the first course for doctors and medical students. In April, a divinity student asks Rudolf Steiner a second time about the possibility of religious renewal. September 27–October 16: anthroposophical 'university course.' December: lectures titled *The Search for the New Isis* (CW 202).

1921:   Rudolf Steiner continues his intensive work on cultural renewal, including the uphill battle for the threefold social order. 'University' arts, scientific, theological, and medical courses include: *The Astronomy Course* (CW 323); *Observation, Mathematics, and Scientific Experiment* (CW 324); the *Second Medical Course* (CW 313); *Color*. In June and September–October, Rudolf Steiner also gives the first two 'priests' courses' (CW 342 and 343). The 'youth movement' gains momentum. Magazines are founded: *Die Drei* (January), and—under the editorship of Albert Steffen (1884–1963)—the weekly, *Das Goetheanum* (August). In February–March, Rudolf Steiner takes his first trip outside Germany since the war (Holland). On April 7, Steiner receives a letter regarding 'religious renewal,' and May 22–23, he agrees to address the question in a practical way. In June, the Klinical-Therapeutic Institute opens in Arlesheim under the direction of Dr. Ita Wegman. In August, the Chemical-Pharmaceutical Laboratory opens in Arlesheim (Oskar Schmiedel and Ita Wegman are directors). The Clinical Therapeutic Institute is inaugurated in Stuttgart (Dr. Ludwig Noll is director); also the Research Laboratory in Dornach (Ehrenfried Pfeiffer and Gunther Wachsmuth are directors). In November–December, Rudolf Steiner visits Norway.

1922:   The first half of the year involves very active public lecturing (thousands attend); in the second half, Rudolf Steiner begins to withdraw and turn toward the Society—'The Society is asleep.' It is 'too weak' to do what is asked of it. The businesses—*Der Kommende Tag* and *Futurum A.G.*—fail. In January, with the help of an agent, Steiner undertakes a twelve-city German lecture tour, accompanied by eurythmy performances. In two weeks he speaks to more than 2,000 people. In April, he gives a 'university course' in The Hague. He also visits England. In June, he is in Vienna for the East–West Congress. In August–September, he is back in England for the Oxford Conference on Education. Returning to Dornach, he gives the lectures *Philosophy, Cosmology, and Religion* (CW 215), and gives the third priests' course (CW 344). On September 16, The Christian Community is founded. In October–November, Steiner is in Holland and England. He also speaks to the youth: *The Youth Course* (CW 217). In December, Steiner gives lectures titled *The Origins of Natural Science* (CW 326), and *Humanity and the World of Stars: The Spiritual Communion of Humanity* (CW 219). December 31: Fire at the Goetheanum, which is destroyed.

1923:   Despite the fire, Rudolf Steiner continues his work unabated. A very hard year. Internal dispersion, dissension, and apathy abound. There is conflict—between old and new visions—within the Society. A wake-up call is needed, and Rudolf Steiner responds with renewed lecturing vitality. His focus: the spiritual context of human life; initiation science; the course of the year; and community building. As a foundation for an artistic school, he creates a series of pastel sketches. Lecture cycles: *The Anthroposophical Movement; Initiation Science* (CW 227) (in England at the Penmaenmawr Summer School); *The Four Seasons and the Archangels* (CW 229); *Harmony of the Creative Word* (CW 230); *The Supersensible Human* (CW 231), given in Holland for the founding of the Dutch society. On November 10, in response to the failed Hitler-Ludendorf putsch in Munich, Steiner closes his Berlin residence and moves the *Philosophisch-Anthroposophisch Verlag* (Press) to Dornach. On December 9, Steiner begins the serialization of his *Autobiography: The Course of My Life* (CW 28) in *Das Goetheanum*. It will continue to appear weekly, without a break, until his death. Late December–early January: Rudolf Steiner re-founds the Anthroposophical Society (about 12,000 members internationally) and takes over its leadership. The new board members are: Marie Steiner, Ita Wegman, Albert Steffen, Elizabeth Vreede, and Guenther Wachsmuth. (See *The Christmas Meeting for the Founding of the General Anthroposophical Society*, CW 260). Accompanying lectures: *Mystery Knowledge and Mystery Centers* (CW 232); *World History in the Light of Anthroposophy* (CW 233). December 25: the Foundation Stone is laid (in the hearts of members) in the form of the 'Foundation Stone Meditation.'

1924: January 1: having founded the Anthroposophical Society and taken over its leadership, Rudolf Steiner has the task of 'reforming' it. The process begins with a weekly newssheet ('What's Happening in the Anthroposophical Society') in which Rudolf Steiner's 'Letters to Members' and 'Anthroposophical Leading Thoughts' appear (CW 26). The next step is the creation of a new esoteric class, the 'first class' of the 'University of Spiritual Science' (which was to have been followed, had Rudolf Steiner lived longer, by two more advanced classes). Then comes a new language for Anthroposophy—practical, phenomenological, and direct; and Rudolf Steiner creates the model for the second Goetheanum. He begins the series of extensive 'karma' lectures (CW 235–40); and finally, responding to needs, he creates two new initiatives: biodynamic agriculture and curative education. After the middle of the year, rumors begin to circulate regarding Steiner's health. Lectures: January–February, *Anthroposophy* (CW 234); February: *Tone Eurythmy* (CW 278); June: *The Agriculture Course* (CW 327); June–July: *Speech Eurythmy* (CW 279); *Curative Education* (CW 317); August: (England, 'Second International Summer School'), *Initiation Consciousness: True and False Paths in Spiritual Investigation* (CW 243); September: *Pastoral Medicine* (CW 318). On September 26, for the first time, Rudolf Steiner cancels a lecture. On September 28, he gives his last lecture. On September 29, he withdraws to his studio in the carpenter's shop; now he is definitively ill. Cared for by Ita Wegman, he continues working, however, and writing the weekly installments of his *Autobiography* and *Letters to the Members/Leading Thoughts* (CW 26).

1925: Rudolf Steiner, while continuing to work, continues to weaken. He finishes *Extending Practical Medicine* (CW 27) with Ita Wegman.
On March 30, around ten in the morning, Rudolf Steiner dies.

INDEX

PLATES

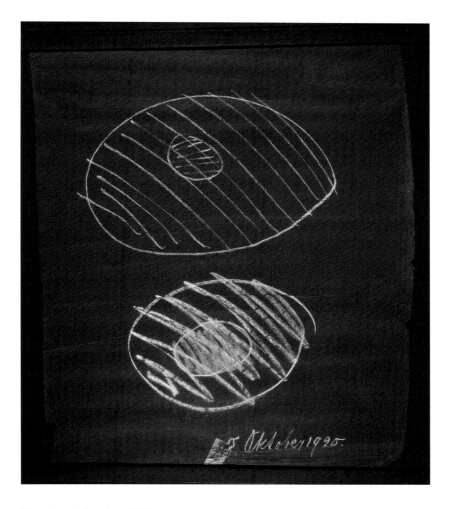

Plate 1   8 October 1920

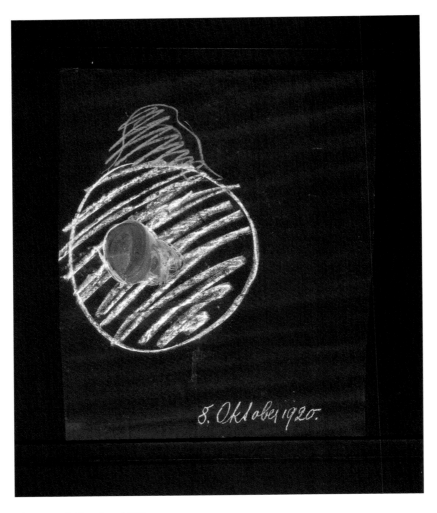

Plate 2   8 October 1920

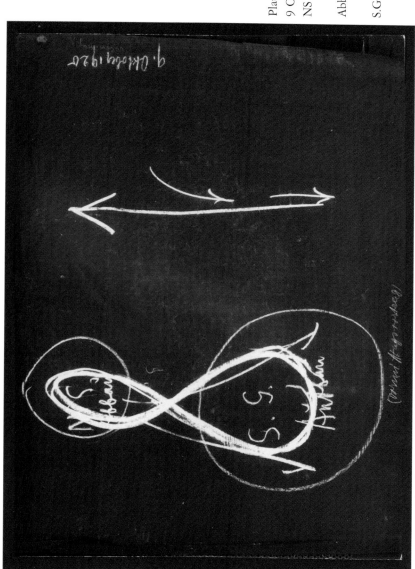

Plate 3
9 October 1920
NS = neurosensory
system
Abbau = destruction
catabolism
S.G. = system of
metabolism
and limbs

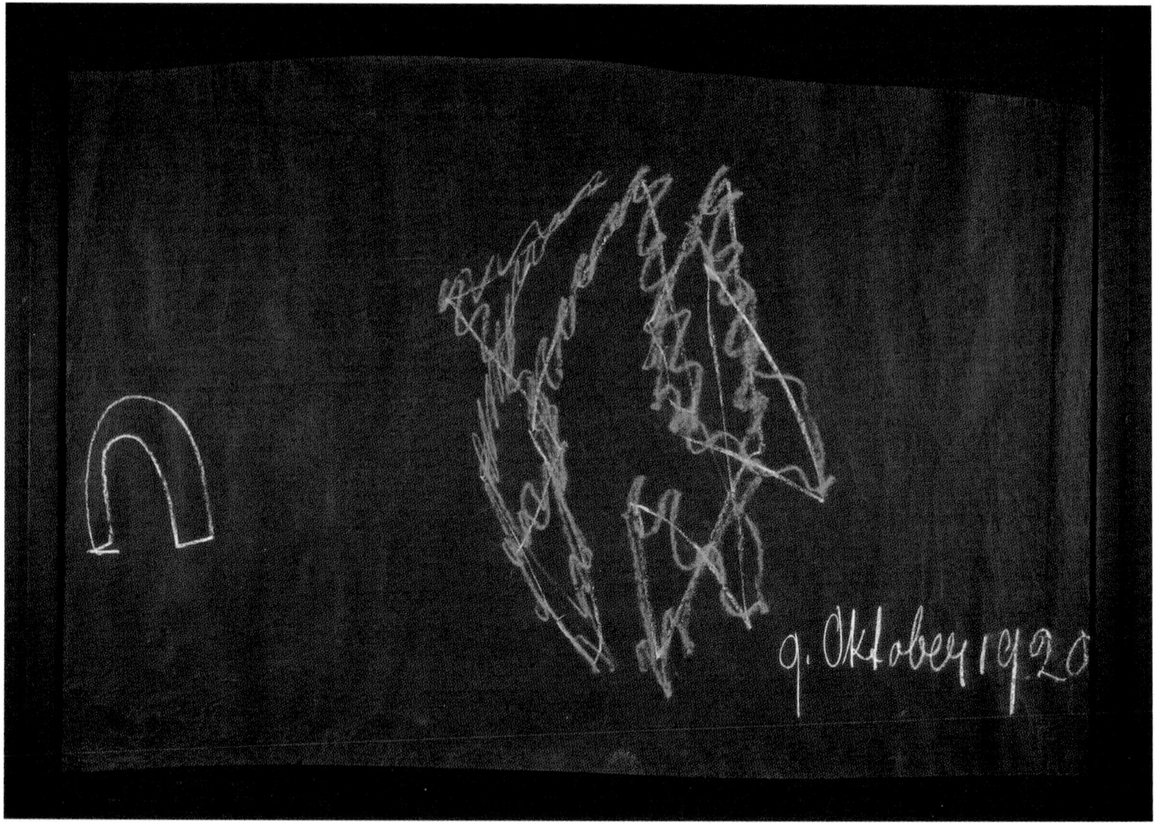

Plate 4

9 October 1920

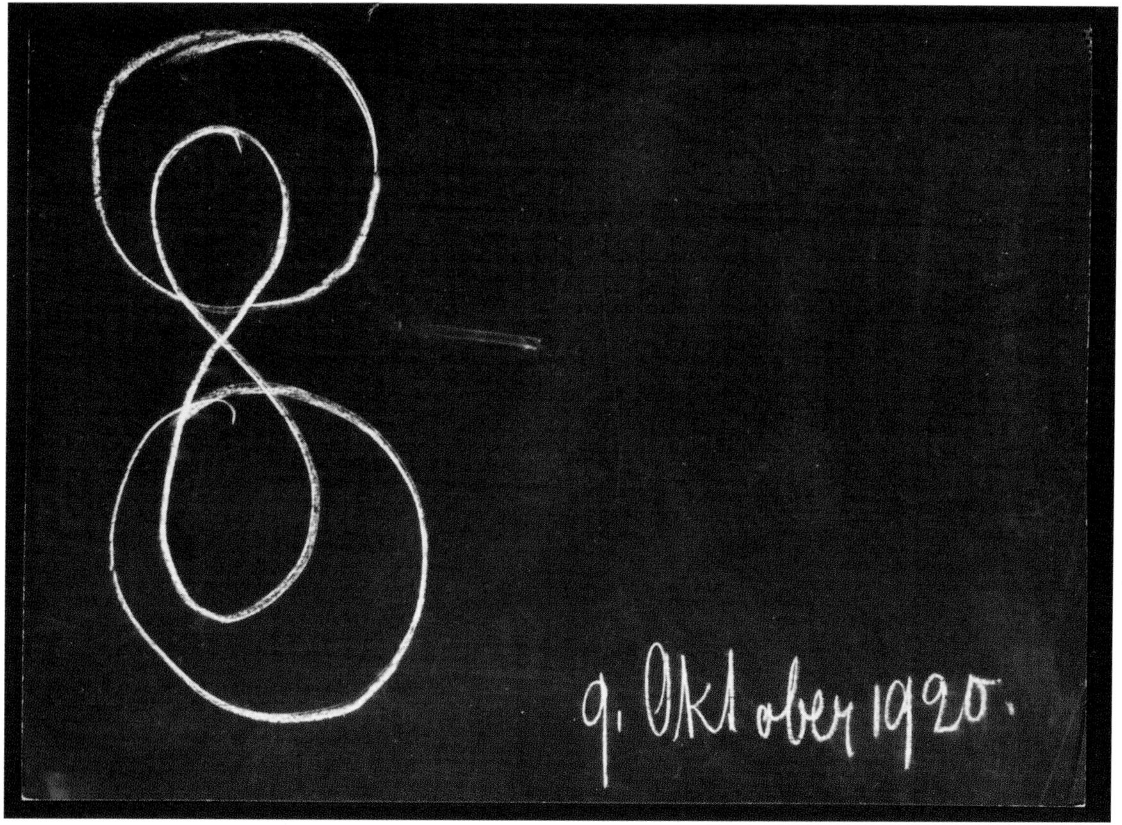

9. Oktober 1920.

Plate 5
9 October 1920

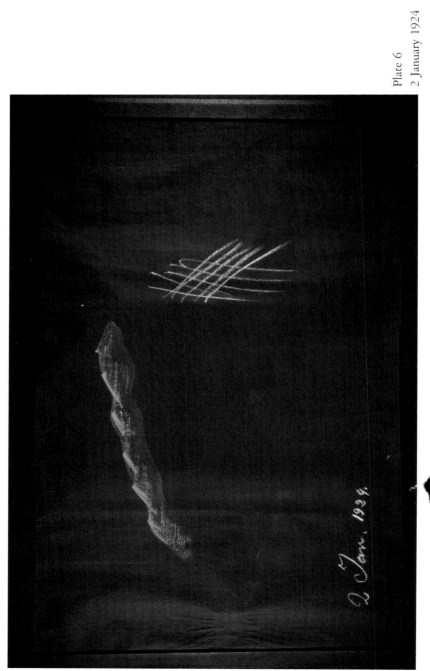

Plate 6
2 January 1924

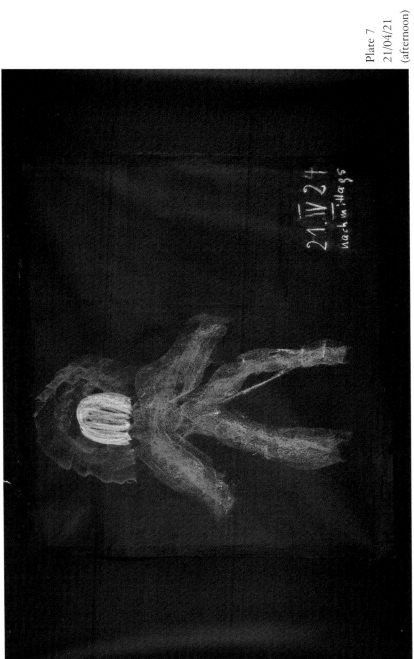

Plate 7
21/04/21
(afternoon)

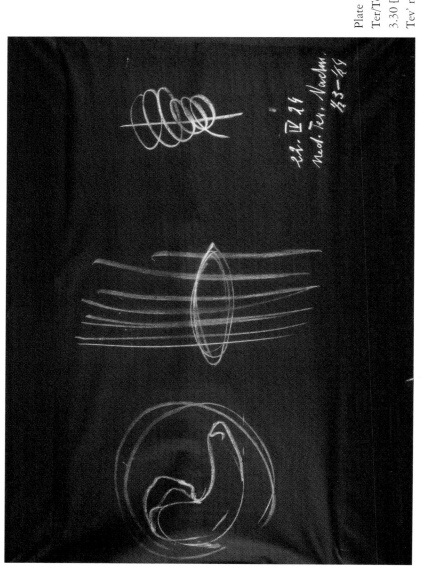

Plate 8   22/04/24 med.
Ter/Tev afternoon 2.30–
3.30 [Can't say what 'Ter/
Tev' means. Translator]

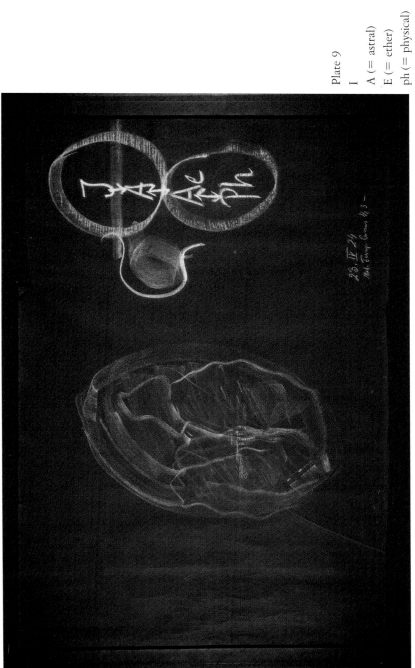

Plate 9

I

A (= astral)

E (= ether)

ph (= physical)